T0259515

Pulmonary Diseases

Editor

DANIEL M. GOODENBERGER

MEDICAL CLINICS
OF NORTH AMERICA

www.medical.theclinics.com

Consulting Editor
JACK ENDE

November 2022 • Volume 106 • Number 6

ELSEVIER

1600 John F. Kennedy Boulevard • Suite 1800 • Philadelphia, Pennsylvania, 19103-2899

http://www.theclinics.com

MEDICAL CLINICS OF NORTH AMERICA Volume 106, Number 6
November 2022 ISSN 0025-7125, ISBN-13: 978-0-323-93863-1

Editor: Taylor Hayes
Developmental Editor: Arlene Campos

Photocopying

Single photocopies of single articles may be made for personal use as allowed by national copyright laws. Permission of the Publisher and payment of a fee is required for all other photocopying, including multiple or systematic copying, copying for advertising or promotional purposes, resale, and all forms of document delivery. Special rates are available for educational institutions that wish to make photocopies for non-profit educational classroom use. For information on how to seek permission visit www.elsevier.com/permissions or call: (+44) 1865 843830 (UK)/(+1) 215 239 3804 (USA).

Derivative Works

Subscribers may reproduce tables of contents or prepare lists of articles including abstracts for internal circulation within their institutions. Permission of the Publisher is required for resale or distribution outside the institution. Permission of the Publisher is required for all other derivative works, including compilations and translations (please consult www.elsevier.com/permissions).

Electronic Storage or Usage

Permission of the Publisher is required to store or use electronically any material contained in this periodical, including any article or part of an article (please consult www.elsevier.com/permissions). Except as outlined above, no part of this publication may be reproduced, stored in a retrieval system or transmitted in any form or by any means, electronic, mechanical, photocopying, recording or otherwise, without prior written permission of the Publisher.

Notice

No responsibility is assumed by the Publisher for any injury and/or damage to persons or property as a matter of products liability, negligence or otherwise, or from any use or operation of any methods, products, instructions or ideas contained in the material herein. Because of rapid advances in the medical sciences, in particular, independent verification of diagnoses and drug dosages should be made.

Although all advertising material is expected to conform to ethical (medical) standards, inclusion in this publication does not constitute a guarantee or endorsement of the quality or value of such product or of the claims made of it by its manufacturer.

Medical Clinics of North America (ISSN 0025-7125) is published bimonthly by Elsevier Inc., 360 Park Avenue South, New York, NY 10010-1710. Months of publication are January, March, May, July, September, and November. Business and editorial offices: 1600 John F. Kennedy Boulevard, Suite 1800, Philadelphia, PA 19103-2899. Periodicals postage paid at New York, NY, and additional mailing offices. Subscription prices are USD $316.00 per year (US individuals), $956.00 per year (US institutions), $100.00 per year (US Students), $396.00 per year (Canadian individuals), $1,004.00 per year (Canadian institutions), $200.00 per year for (foreign students), $100.00 per year for (Canadian students), $439.00 per year (foreign individuals), and $1,004.00 per year (foreign institutions). To receive student/resident rate, orders must be accompanied by name of affiliated institution, date of term, and the signature of program/residency coordinator on institution letterhead. Orders will be billed at individual rate until proof of status is received. Foreign air speed delivery is included in all Clinics' subscription prices. All prices are subject to change without notice. **POSTMASTER:** Send address changes to *Medical Clinics of North America*, Elsevier Health Sciences Division, Subscription Customer Service, 3251 Riverport Lane, Maryland Heights, MO 63043. **Customer Service: Telephone: 1-800-654-2452** (U.S. and Canada); **1-314-447-8871** (outside U.S. and Canada). **Fax: 314-447-8029. E-mail: journalscustomerserviceusa@ elsevier.com** (for print support); **journalsonlinesupport-usa@elsevier.com** (for online support).

Reprints. For copies of 100 or more of articles in this publication, please contact the Commercial Reprints Department, Elsevier Inc., 360 Park Avenue South, New York, NY 10010-1710. Tel.: 212-633-3874; Fax: 212-633-3820; E-mail: reprints@elsevier.com.

Medical Clinics of North America is also published in Spanish by McGraw-Hill Interamericana Editores S. A., P.O. Box 5-237, 06500 Mexico, D.F., Mexico.

Medical Clinics of North America is covered in *MEDLINE/PubMed (Index Medicus), Current Contents, ASCA, Excerpta Medica, Science Citation Index, and ISI/BIOMED.*

PROGRAM OBJECTIVE
The goal of the *Medical Clinics of North America* is to keep practicing physicians up to date with current clinical practice by providing timely articles reviewing the state of the art in patient care.

TARGET AUDIENCE
All practicing physicians and other healthcare professionals.

LEARNING OBJECTIVES
Upon completion of this activity, participants will be able to:
1. Review the treatment, therapies, and management therapies, traditional and novel, for pulmonary diseases.
2. Explain how the recommended screening and evaluation tools, assessments, and diagnostic studies can be utilized to determine and identify patients who can benefit from them.
3. Discuss the impact of racial, gender, and economic disparities and biases on pulmonary disease patients and populations.

ACCREDITATION
The Elsevier Office of Continuing Medical Education (EOCME) is accredited by the Accreditation Council for Continuing Medical Education (ACCME) to provide continuing medical education for physicians.

The EOCME designates this journal-based CME activity for a maximum of 14 *AMA PRA Category 1 Credit*(s)™. Physicians should claim only the credit commensurate with the extent of their participation in the activity.

All other healthcare professionals requesting continuing education credit for this enduring material will be issued a certificate of participation.

DISCLOSURE OF CONFLICTS OF INTEREST
The EOCME assesses conflict of interest with its instructors, faculty, planners, and other individuals who are in a position to control the content of CME activities. All relevant conflicts of interest that are identified are thoroughly vetted by EOCME for fair balance, scientific objectivity, and patient care recommendations. EOCME is committed to providing its learners with CME activities that promote improvements or quality in healthcare and not a specific proprietary business or a commercial interest.

The planning committee, staff, authors, and editors listed below have identified no financial relationships or relationships to products or devices they or their spouse/life partner have with commercial interest related to the content of this CME activity:
Thaddeus Bartter, MD, FCCP; Marcel A. Behr, MD, MSc, FRCPC; Whitney Buckel, PharmD; Humberto K. Choi, MD, FCCP; John M. Coleman, MD; Gerard J. Criner, MD, FACP, FACCP; Alejandra Ellison-Barnes, MD, MPH; Christopher H. Fanta, MD; Adam W. Gaffney, MD, MPH; Panagis Galiatsatos, MD, MHS; Daniel M. Goodenberger, MD; Munish Goyal, MD; Max Hockstein, MD; Raksha Jain, MD, MSc; Anita Joshi, BDS, MPH; Manish Joshi, MD, FCCP; Hasmeena Kathuria, MD; Megan A. Koster, MD, PharmD; Bilal H. Lashari, MD, MScPH; Lindsay M. Leither, DO; Madalina Macrea, MD, PhD, MPH; Dick Menzies, MD; Kristina Montemayor, MD, MHS; Edgar Ortiz-Brizuela, MSc; Merlin Packiam; Rory Spiegel, MD; Doreen Thomas-Payne, MSN, BSN, RN, PMHNP-BC; Jessica Waters, MD

The planning committee, staff, authors, and editors listed below have identified financial relationships or relationships to products or devices they or their spouse/life partner have with commercial interest related to the content of this CME activity:
Samuel M. Brown, MD, MS: Research support: Faron, Janssen, Sedana Medical

Peter J. Mazzone, MD, MPH, FCCP: Researcher: Adele, Delfi, Exact Sciences, Necleix

UNAPPROVED/OFF-LABEL USE DISCLOSURE
The EOCME requires CME faculty to disclose to the participants;
1. When products or procedures being discussed are off-label, unlabelled, experimental, and/or investigational (not US Food and Drug Administration [FDA] approved); and
2. Any limitations on the information presented, such as data that are preliminary or that represent ongoing research, interim analyses, and/or unsupported opinions. Faculty may discuss information about pharmaceutical agents that is outside of FDA-approved labelling. This information is intended solely for CME and is not intended to promote off-label use of these medications. If you have any questions, contact the medical affairs department of the manufacturer for the most recent prescribing information.

TO ENROLL

To enroll in the *Medical Clinics of North America* Continuing Medical Education program, call customer service at 1-800-654-2452 or sign up online at http//www.theclinics.com/home/cme. The CME program is available to subscribers for an additional annual fee of USD 324.00.

METHOD OF PARTICIPATION

In order to claim credit, participants must complete the following;

1. Complete enrolment as indicated above.
2. Read the activity.
3. Complete the CME Test and Evaluation. Participants must achieve a score of 70% on the test. All CME Tests and Evaluations must be completed online.

CME INQUIRIES/SPECIAL NEEDS

For all CME inquiries or special needs, please contact elsevierCME@elsevier.com.

MEDICAL CLINICS OF NORTH AMERICA

Contributors

CONSULTING EDITOR

JACK ENDE, MD, MACP
The Schaeffer Professor of Medicine, Perelman School of Medicine, University of Pennsylvania, Philadelphia, Pennsylvania, USA

EDITOR

DANIEL M. GOODENBERGER, MD, MACP, FRCP (London)
Professor of Medicine, Washington University, St Louis, Missouri, USA

AUTHORS

THADDEUS BARTTER, MD, FCCP
Professor of Medicine, Pulmonary and Critical Care Division, University of Arkansas for Medical Sciences, Central Arkansas Veterans Healthcare System, Little Rock, Arkansas, USA

MARCEL A. BEHR, MD, MSc, FRCPC
Departments of Epidemiology, Biostatistics & Occupational Health, Department of Medicine, McGill University, McGill International TB Centre, Research Institute of the McGill University Health Centre, Montreal, Quebec, Canada

SAMUEL M. BROWN, MD, MS
Department of Internal Medicine, University of Utah School of Medicine, Salt Lake City, Utah, USA

WHITNEY BUCKEL, PHARMD
Pharmacy Services, Intermountain Healthcare, Taylorsville, Utah, USA

HUMBERTO K. CHOI, MD, FCCP
Assistant Professor of Medicine of Lerner College of Medicine of Case Western Reserve University, Respiratory Institute, Cleveland Clinic, Cleveland, Ohio, USA

JOHN M. COLEMAN III, MD
Associate Professor, Division of Pulmonary and Critical Care Medicine, Department of Neurology, Northwestern University Feinberg School of Medicine, Chicago, Illinois, USA

GERARD J. CRINER, MD, FACP, FACCP
Professor and Chair, Department of Thoracic Medicine and Surgery, Lewis Katz School of Medicine at Temple University, Temple Lung Center, Temple University Hospital, Philadelphia, Pennsylvania, USA

ALEJANDRA ELLISON-BARNES, MD, MPH
The Tobacco Treatment and Cancer Screening Clinic, The Johns Hopkins Health System, Division of General Internal Medicine, Johns Hopkins School of Medicine, Baltimore, Maryland, USA

CHRISTOPHER H. FANTA, MD
Director of Partners Asthma Centre, Member, Pulmonary and Critical Care Medicine Division, Brigham and Women's Hospital, Professor of Medicine, Harvard Medical School, Boston, Massachusetts, USA

ADAM W. GAFFNEY, MD, MPH
Assistant Professor, Harvard Medical School, Cambridge Health Alliance, Cambridge, Massachusetts, USA

PANAGIS GALIATSATOS, MD, MHS
The Tobacco Treatment and Cancer Screening Clinic, The Johns Hopkins Health System, Division of Pulmonary and Critical Care Medicine, Johns Hopkins School of Medicine, Baltimore, Maryland, USA

MUNISH GOYAL, MD
Professor of Emergency Medicine, Georgetown University School of Medicine, Department of Emergency Medicine, MedStar Washington Hospital Center, Washington, DC, USA

MAX HOCKSTEIN, MD
Assistant Professor of Emergency Medicine, Georgetown University School of Medicine, Departments of Emergency Medicine, and Critical Care Medicine, MedStar Washington Hospital Center, Washington, DC, USA

RAKSHA JAIN, MD, MSC
Department of Medicine, Associate Professor of Medicine, University of Texas Southwestern, Dallas, Texas, USA

ANITA JOSHI, BDS, MPH
Department of Epidemiology, Fay W. Boozman College of Public Health, University of Arkansas for Medical Sciences, Little Rock, Arkansas, USA

MANISH JOSHI, MD, FCCP
Professor of Medicine, Pulmonary and Critical Care Division, University of Arkansas for Medical Sciences, Central Arkansas Veterans Healthcare System, Little Rock, Arkansas, USA

HASMEENA KATHURIA, MD
Associate Professor, The Pulmonary Center, Boston University School of Medicine, Boston, Massachusetts, USA

MEGAN A. KOSTER, MD, PharmD
Division of Pulmonary and Critical Care, Department of Medicine, Mount Auburn Hospital, Harvard Medical School, Cambridge, Massachusetts, USA

BILAL H. LASHARI, MD, MScPH
Fellow in Pulmonary and Critical Care Medicine, Department of Thoracic Medicine and Surgery, Temple Lung Center, Temple University Hospital, Philadelphia, Pennsylvania, USA

LINDSAY M. LEITHER, DO
Department of Internal Medicine, University of Utah School of Medicine, Salt Lake City, Utah, USA

MADALINA MACREA, MD, PhD, MPH
Associate Professor, Division of Pulmonary and Sleep Medicine, Salem VA Medical Center, Salem, Virginia, USA; Department of Medicine, University of Virginia, Charlottesville, Virginia, USA

PETER J. MAZZONE, MD, MPH, FCCP
Section Head, Thoracic Oncology, Respiratory Institute, Cleveland Clinic, Cleveland, Ohio, USA

DICK MENZIES, MD, MSc
Departments of Epidemiology, Biostatistics & Occupational Health, McGill University, Department of Medicine, McGill International TB Centre, Research Institute of the McGill University Health Centre, Montreal, Quebec, Canada

KRISTINA MONTEMAYOR, MD, MHS
Department of Medicine, Assistant Professor, Johns Hopkins University, Baltimore, Maryland, USA

EDGAR ORTIZ-BRIZUELA, MD, MSc
Departments of Epidemiology, Biostatistics & Occupational Health, McGill University, McGill International TB Centre, Research Institute of the McGill University Health Centre, Montreal, Quebec, Canada; Department of Medicine, Insituto Nacional de Ciencias Médicas y Nutrición Salvador Zubirán, Tlalpan, Mexico City, Mexico

RORY SPIEGEL, MD
Assistant Professor of Emergency Medicine, Georgetown University School of Medicine, Departments of Emergency Medicine, and Critical Care Medicine, MedStar Washington Hospital Center, Washington, DC, USA

JESSICA WATERS, MD
Critical Care Medicine Fellow Physician, Department of Emergency Medicine, MedStar Washington Hospital Center, Washington, DC, USA

Contents

> After infection with Mycobacterium tuberculosis, a minority of individuals will progress to tuberculosis disease (TB). The risk is higher among persons with well-established risk factors and within the first year after infection. Testing and treating individuals at high risk of progression maximizes the benefits of TB preventive therapy; avoiding testing of low-risk persons will limit potential harms. Several treatment options are available; rifamycin-based regimens offer the best efficacy-safety balance. In this review, we present an overview of the diagnosis and treatment of TB infection, and summarize common clinical scenarios.

> In late 2019, SARS-CoV-2 caused the greatest global health crisis in a century, impacting all aspects of society. As the COVID-19 pandemic evolved throughout 2020 and 2021, multiple variants emerged, contributing to multiple surges in cases of COVID-19 worldwide. In 2021, highly effective vaccines became available, although the pandemic continues into 2022. There has been tremendous expansion of basic, translational, and clinical knowledge about SARS-CoV-2 and COVID-19 since the pandemic's onset. Treatment options have been rapidly explored, attempting to repurpose preexisting medications in tandem with development and evaluation of novel agents. Care of the seriously ill patient is examined.

> Despite the heterogeneity of data on the role of noninvasive ventilation (NIV) in severe stable chronic obstructive pulmonary disease with chronic hypercapnia, the current evidence supports the use of NIV in select populations and phenotypes. The Center for Medicare and Medicaid Services reimbursement criteria are complex, and the practice of navigating the most efficient method to initiate NIV therapy continues to be challenging. These patients optimally require referral to a medical center that has physicians with specific training in pulmonary and sleep medicine, who can navigate the specific needs for the use of NIV.

disorders. As the understanding of the pathogenesis has evolved, it led to targeting mechanical aspects of the disease to improve patient symptoms and quality of life. Modern management of COPD offers a variety of mechanical and surgical treatments for patients with advanced disease who do not achieve benefit from medical therapy alone. These treatments include therapies aimed at lung volume reduction, through surgical or bronchoscopic techniques. While these techniques are established and have proven benefit, others are still under development. Herein we discuss these techniques, aimed at improving clinician recognition of patients that may benefit from these interventions.

Lung health reflects the inequities of our society. Asthma and chronic obstructive pulmonary disease are 2 lung conditions commonly treated in general clinical practice; each imposes a disproportionate burden on disadvantaged patients. Numerous factors mediate disparities in lung health, including air pollution, allergen exposures, tobacco, and respiratory infections. Members of racial/ethnic minorities and those of low socioeconomic status also have inferior access to high-quality medical care, compounding disparities in disease burden. Physicians can work against disparities in their practice, but wide-ranging policy reforms to achieve better air quality, housing, workplace safety, and healthcare for all are needed to achieve equity in lung health.

Lung cancer screening with low-dose computed tomography (LDCT) reduces lung cancer deaths by early detection. The United States Preventive Services Task Force recommends lung cancer screening with LDCT in adults of age 50 years to 80 years who have at least a 20 pack-year smoking history and are currently smoking or have quit within the past 15 years. The implementation of a lung-cancer-screening program is complex. High-quality screening requires the involvement of a multidisciplinary team. The aim of a screening program is to find balance between mortality reduction and avoiding potential harms related to false-positive findings, overdiagnosis, invasive procedures, and radiation exposure. Components and processes of a high-quality lung-cancer-screening program include the identification of eligible individuals, shared decision-making, performing and reporting LDCT results, management of screen-detected lung nodules and non-nodule findings, smoking cessation, ensuring adherence, data collection, and quality improvement.

This summary highlights updated definitions, terminology, and classification systems proposed in the diagnosis of hypersensitivity pneumonitis. Clinical presentation, epidemiology, and pathophysiology are reviewed from the most recent data. Radiographic and histopathologic diagnostic criteria are presented in a manner relevant to the practice of general medicine internists, including new guideline recommendations. The role of adjunctive tests, such as serum IgG testing, bronchoalveolar lavage lymphocyte analysis, and pulmonary function testing is discussed in the context of supporting diagnostic confidence for hypersensitivity pneumonitis diagnosis. Finally, new diagnostic algorithms are synthesized and applied to the general internal medicine setting.

There is a strong evidence base for the use of existing pharmacotherapies to support tobacco cessation, alone or in combination, ideally with concurrent behavioral interventions. Future pharmacotherapies under development may assist in the most refractory cases. Incorporating current and future therapies into a longitudinal chronic care model for tobacco dependence will help a diverse range of patients achieve independence from nicotine addiction.

Electronic cigarettes (e-cigarettes) are battery-powered devices that use heat to aerosolize a liquid containing a variety of substances (usually nicotine and/or cannabinoids, flavorings, and glycerol or propylene glycol base) that is then inhaled. E-cigarettes are rapidly evolving over time, so the true health effects of e-cigarettes are difficult to study and remain largely unknown. We review the effects of e-cigarettes on nicotine addiction and on pulmonary disease including the effects of dual use and switching from combustible cigarettes to e-cigarettes. Studies show that e-cigarette use can increase the risk to nicotine dependence and combustible tobacco use. Studies show an association between e-cigarette use and pulmonary disease. Some studies suggest reduced harm from e-cigarette use compared with smoking, but this requires further study. Most adults who use e-cigarettes also smoke cigarettes; epidemiologic studies suggest that the combination of e-cigarettes and cigarettes is more harmful than using either product alone.

Human beings have used marijuana products for centuries. Relatively recent data showing extensive cannabinoid receptors, particularly in the brain, help to explain the impacts of cannabinoids on symptoms/diseases, such as pain and seizures, with major nervous system components. Marijuana can cause bronchitis, but a moderate body of literature suggests that distal airway/parenchymal lung disease does not occur; marijuana does not cause chronic obstructive pulmonary disease and probably does not cause lung cancer, distinctly different from tobacco. Potentials for cognitive impairment and for damage to the developing brain are contextually important as its beneficial uses are explored.

Even well-intentioned policies have great potential to cause harm. This statement is vividly illustrated by the influential, yet controversial, Surviving Sepsis Campaign guidelines and subsequent CMS benchmarks. Despite low-quality evidence, tendentious industry ties, and rebuke from the Infectious Disease Society of America (IDSA), these benchmarks continue to eschew therapy driven by clinician expertise and individual patient needs in favor of mandating an arbitrary, one-size-fits-all approach that suspends clinical judgment and promotes indiscriminate use of treatments that have the potential to cause great harm.

Foreword

Specialists Without Borders

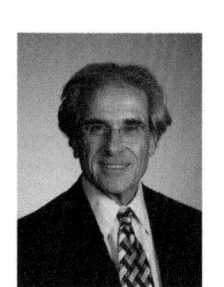

Jack Ende, MD, MACP
Consulting Editor

It was 30 years ago that the iconic medical sociologist, Barbara Starfield, in her ground-breaking book, *Primary Care: Concept Evaluation and Policy*,[1] laid out the tenets of primary care. These have come to be known as the 4 C's: First Contact, Comprehensiveness, Coordination, and Continuity, and serve as aspirational goals of general internal medicine, family medicine, and primary care overall. This is what we stand for. This is what we hope to provide. As a general internist myself, I have strived to represent and provide the 4 C's.

This issue of *Medical Clinics of North America*, "Pulmonary Diseases," however, gives me pause. Not because I doubt the critical role of the 4 C's in defining primary care but, rather, that primary care is not the only branch of medicine concerned with these values. This issue has reminded me that these values can be expressed in subspecialty medicine just as in primary care.

Perhaps first contact is most directly associated with primary care, but what of the other C's? Look at the topics covered in this issue. They highlight the importance of long-term care; the critical association of race and gender in medical care disparities; screening and prevention; and substance abuse. In choosing the topics and authors as he did, our Guest Editor, Daniel Goodenberger, has demonstrated a comprehensive and patient-focused perspective in the subspecialty of pulmonary medicine and demonstrated as well the central role of socioeconomic determinants of health in this field. My view of primary care as the branch of medicine that "owns" the 4 C's may have been clouded by hubris. I now appreciate that specialization need not be synonymous with constricted focus, just as primary care is not synonymous with lack of depth.

I hope you find the issue of *Medical Clinics of North America* as eye-opening as I did. Along with gaining up-to-date knowledge of the important pulmonary problems that our patients deal with, it just may expand your view of what a subspecialty can be and should be, and convince you that all physicians, primary care providers, and

Med Clin N Am 106 (2022) xvii–xviii
https://doi.org/10.1016/j.mcna.2022.08.009
0025-7125/22/© 2022 Published by Elsevier Inc.

subspecialists alike should be striving for the same outcomes and representing the same values.

Jack Ende, MD, MACP
Perelman School of Medicine of the
University of Pennsylvania
5033 West Gates Pavilion
3400 Spruce Street
Philadelphia, PA 19104, USA

E-mail address:
jack.ende@uphs.upenn.edu

REFERENCE

1. Starfield B. Primary Care: Concept, Evaluation, and Policy. New York: Oxford University Press, Inc; 1992.

Preface

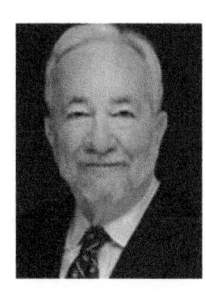

Daniel M. Goodenberger, MD, MACP, FRCP (London)
Editor

When Dr Ende approached me about editing an issue of the *Medical Clinics of North America* on pulmonary diseases, I was skeptical. The last issue dealing with respiratory problems had come out in May 2019, fewer than three years earlier. My initial inclination was to say that it was too soon, and there were not enough "new things" worth bringing to the attention of the internal medicine community.

However, it's hard to say no to Jack, so I did a little due diligence. I read through the issues of the major respiratory journals of the preceding several years, looking for ideas for topics, and I spoke with a number of my very fine colleagues in the pulmonary division at Washington University for their thoughts. Both my review and their recommendations allowed identification of a group of highly qualified subject matter experts on topics that have little overlap with the preceding issue. The organizing principle was to bring forward information that would represent an update on respiratory diseases that are important in adults, are very likely to manifest themselves in an internist's office, and about which there is important new information on diagnosis, therapy, and/or decision on referral. We were also mindful regarding the increasing importance of changes in the medicolegal and social environment around substance use, and on health care disparities.

One of the pleasures of undertaking an editorial role is the opportunity to be educated by experts, and that certainly happened here. I am confident that you will have a similarly enjoyable experience. I am grateful to the authors, who have given freely of their time and expertise to produce this issue, and the editorial staff at Elsevier for their skill and patience.

Daniel M. Goodenberger, MD, MACP, FRCP (London)
Washington University
St. Louis, MO, USA

E-mail address:
dgoodenb@wustl.edu

Med Clin N Am 106 (2022) xix
https://doi.org/10.1016/j.mcna.2022.07.003
medical.theclinics.com

Testing and Treating *Mycobacterium tuberculosis* Infection

Edgar Ortiz-Brizuela, MD, MSc[a,b,c], Dick Menzies, MD, MSc[a,b,d], Marcel A. Behr, MD, MSc, FRCPC[a,b,d],*

KEYWORDS

- Tuberculosis • *Mycobacterium tuberculosis* • Diagnosis • Treatment

KEY POINTS

- Tuberculosis (TB) preventive therapy (TPT) offers benefits for individuals and populations by reducing the risk of progression to TB disease, which also acts to reduce transmission.
- Testing and treating those at high or very high risk of progression to TB provides the greatest opportunity for TB prevention.
- A decision to test for TB infection must entail a likely benefit for the individual and a commitment to treat by the physician.
- Newer, TPT regimens containing rifamycin offer the same efficacy as those based on isoniazid but with a better safety profile and shorter duration.

INTRODUCTION

Globally, the incidence of tuberculosis (TB) is estimated at 9.9 million per year, of whom nearly 1.5 million succumb to disease.[1] A subset of these individuals will never be detected, and consequently, not treated. Those fortunate to be diagnosed are often identified months after they are contagious. Therefore, by the time these people receive treatment of TB, which rapidly reduces their contagiousness, many have already seeded new infections. If individuals with TB infection (TBI) are identified before they progress to disease, TB preventive therapy (TPT) can be expected to reduce individual morbidity and mortality, and the number of new infections they

Funded by: CANADALETR.
[a] Department of Epidemiology, Biostatistics & Occupational Health, McGill University, 1020 Pine Avenue, West Montreal, H3A 1A2, Canada; [b] McGill International TB Centre, Research Institute of the McGill University Health Centre, 5252 boul.de Maisonneuve, West Montreal, Quebec, H4A 3S5, Canada; [c] Department of Medicine, Insituto Nacional de Ciencias Médicas y Nutrición Salvador Zubirán. Vasco de Quiroga 15, Belisario Domínguez Secc 16, Tlalpan, Mexico City, 14000, Mexico; [d] Department of Medicine, McGill University, 1001 Decarie Boulevard, Montreal, Quebec, H4A 3J1, Canada
* Corresponding author. 1001 boul. Décarie, E05.1808, Montréal, Quebec H4A 3J1, Canada.
E-mail address: marcel.behr@mcgill.ca

generate should in theory be diminished. The number of people globally infected with *Mycobacterium tuberculosis* is not directly measured, and that there are different estimates depending on the models and the assumptions used therein.[2,3] Empiric data for the effect of TPT on global TB burden is lacking but mathematical modeling suggests that a concerted effort to identify individuals with TBI and provide TPT could contribute substantially to the World Health Organization (WHO) TB elimination goals.[4]

To understand how TPT could provide individual and potentially public health benefits, we first review the natural history of infection. Following the inhalation of *M. tuberculosis*, a subset of individuals develops TBI of whom a minority progresses to TB. There are at least 4 lines of evidence for a median incubation period of less than 1 year in those who progress: (1) longitudinal studies published in the preantibiotic era reported that most cases developed 3 to 9 months after exposure[5]; (2) follow-up of individuals with a new tuberculin conversion from the British Medical Research Council's trial of Bacillus Calmette–Guérin (BCG) showed 60% of cases occurred within the first year[6]; (3) molecular epidemiology studies have shown that the geometric mean serial interval between case pairs that have a matching bacterial genotype was 29.5 weeks[7]; and (4) in a low-incidence country with discrete TB outbreaks, most of genomically defined secondary cases occur within 1 year.[8,9] Given the delays in diagnosing contagious source cases, by the time contacts are identified and investigated, some of them have already progressed to disease. The goal of TPT is to identify those who have been infected, have not progressed, but are at risk of future progression, and offer antibiotic therapy to interrupt the natural history (**Fig. 1**).

To perform a benefit/risk evaluation for which individuals are most likely to benefit from TPT, 2 parameters must be known: what is the potential benefit from the intervention and what is the potential harm? Regarding the latter, the risk of harm has been established in well-controlled trials, and this has been shown to be lower with newer, shorter rifamycin-containing regimens than older isoniazid-based regimens. Regarding the potential benefit, one needs to know the efficacy of the treatment and the absolute risk of progression. The efficacy has been established in randomized controlled trials. Therefore, the critical parameter to prioritize TPT is the absolute risk of TB in specific patient populations.[10]

In this review, we focus on a health-care provider's perspective, asking who is at risk of progressing to TB and how can we optimally offer TPT to those who will most likely benefit. This will not be a review of basic science concepts surrounding latent infection and what it means (this is addressed elsewhere).[11] Although we acknowledge that there is a spectrum from *M tuberculosis* infection to disease, including subclinical and clinical disease, for pragmatic reasons, this review is focused on the individuals without symptoms and without positive microbiologic cultures.[12,13] Because different terminologies have been applied by national and international agencies, and by clinical and fundamental researchers, we use TBI for infection and TB for disease and avoid terms used elsewhere, such as latent TB infection, active disease, and reactivation disease. Given the need to detect individuals with *M tuberculosis* infection to intervene, we start with an overview of diagnosis, including tests that are available, before discussing specific risk groups, along with the evidence-base for offering TPT in these scenarios.

Who Should Be Tested for Tuberculosis Infection?

Although testing for TBI may be required by regulations in certain settings (eg, health-care workers, immigration requirements), in this review, we focus on testing for clinical indications. A decision to test for TBI implies a decision to treat if the result is positive, or not treat if the result is negative. Since the benefits of TPT are greatest for persons

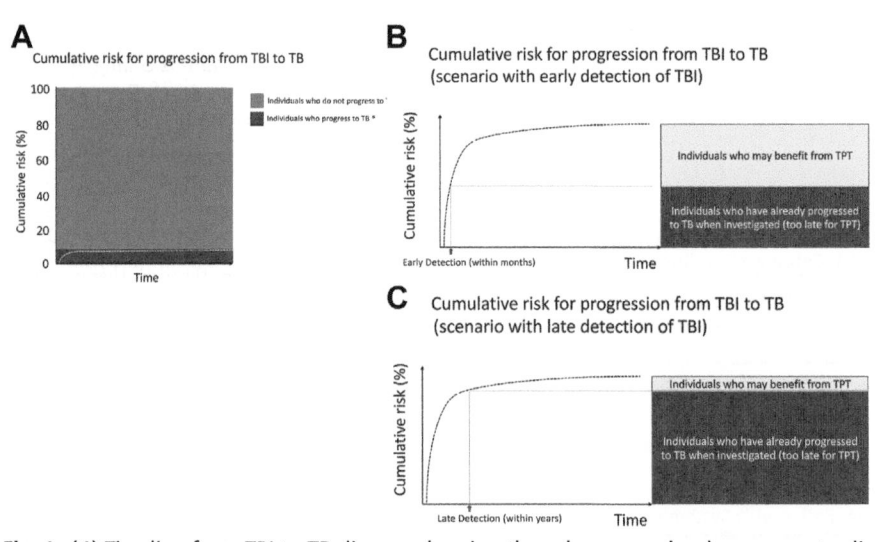

Fig. 1. (*A*) Timeline from TBI to TB disease, showing the subgroups who do progress to disease (*red*) and those who do not progress to disease (*green*). The asterisk indicates that the cumulative risk is greater in some groups (eg, children aged younger than 5 years) than other groups (eg, people aged older than 15 years). (*B, C*) Timeline of the subset who progress to show the time-dependent opportunity for TPT. Those who have already progressed to disease are presented in red. Those who have yet to progress are presented in yellow. In panel (*B*), infection is detected early (within several months of exposure, such as household contacts). In panel (*C*), infection is detected years after exposure and there is no new cause of immune suppression (eg, preemployment screening of healthy foreign-born health-care workers). These concepts are based largely on data from household contacts, presented in Sloot *and colleagues,*[86] Trauer *and colleagues,*[87] and Behr *and colleagues,* 2018.[4]

who are at increased risk of TB disease, it is essential to identify these risk groups based on their clinical, epidemiologic, and demographic features, which are summarized in **Tables 1–4**. As shown in these tables, the risk of disease for each condition varies widely across studies and populations. However, it is evident that there is a very low risk of TB among healthy individuals with no apparent risk factors and a very high risk in individuals having recent contact with patients diagnosed with TB disease. Given the enormous gradient of risk summarized in **Table 1**, priority for diagnosis of TBI, and subsequent treatment should be given to persons at high and very high risk. In contrast, testing the lowest risk group will provide minimal individual benefit, and the harms of TPT may exceed the benefits. The decision to test persons considered at moderate risk, such as persons with diabetes, malnutrition, or history of alcohol or cigarette consumption, should be individualized, based on the expected balance of benefits and harms from TPT.

What Are the Benefits of Testing for Tuberculosis Infection?

WHO has recommended testing for TBI (tests detailed below) before offering TPT for all high-risk groups, except child contacts aged younger than 5 years. However, access to TBI diagnostic tests is limited in many settings, so they have recommended that TBI testing should not be a barrier to initiation of TPT. This means that, in high-risk individuals, TPT should be offered, even without TBI testing. Recognizing this pragmatic limitation, there are 3 lines of evidence that support TBI testing of all groups,

Table 1
Absolute risks for progression to tuberculosis using information from multiple studies in very high-risk and low-risk populations

Risk Category Condition	Campbell et al,[10] 2020 Systematic Review (Annual Risk)	Gupta et al,[88] 2020 IPD-MA (5-y risk)	Martinez et al,[89] 2020 IPD-MA (2-y risk)
Very high risk			
Contacts—Younger than 5 y	2.9%–14.6%	27.7%	19.0%
5–14 y		13.4%	8.8%–9.0%
Adults (15+ y)	0.8%–3.7%	4.8%	10.6% (aged 15–17 y)
Low risk			
Danish general population	0.06%		
Navy recruits	0.10%		

Campbell et al[10]: Systematic review and aggregate data meta-analysis, 122 studies and 33,811 persons. Gupta et al[88]: Systematic review and individual patient meta-analysis, 18 cohorts and 80,468 persons. This study also estimated risk of disease among immune-compromised but did not stratify because of immune suppression. Martinez et al[89]: Systematic review and Individual patient meta-analysis, 46 cohorts and 137,647 children. Low risk: Studies in Danish population ([90]) and Navy recruits ([91]) not included in Campbell et al.

Abbreviation: IPD-MA, individual patient data meta-analysis.

Table 2
Absolute and relative risks for progression to tuberculosis associated with specific medical conditions or habits

Risk Category Condition	Relative Risks ([b])	Absolute Annual risks ([c])
Very high risk		
HIV infection	50–170	1.7%–2.7%
Silicosis	30	3.7%
High risk		
Renal failure (dialysis or predialysis)	10–25	0.3%–1.2%
Solid organ transplant	20–74	0.1%–0.7%
Biologics (TNF alpha)	1.5–46	0.5%
Glucocorticoids	4.9–7.7	a
Cancer—hematologic	26	a
Dolid organ	7.0	0.1%–0.4%
Fibronodular changes on Chest X-ray	6–19	0.2%–0.6%
Moderate risk		
Diabetes mellitus	2.0–3.6	0.1%–0.2%
Heavy alcohol use	3.0–4.0	0.1%–0.2%
Underweight (<90% Ideal body weight)	2.0–3.0	a
Cigarette smoking (current)	1.8–3.5	0.1%
Granuloma on chest X-ray	2.0	0.1%

[a] Indicates no study found that reported absolute risks for a given condition.
[b] Relative risks largely taken from Ref.[92]
[c] Absolute risks from Refs.[10,52,88,89]

Table 3
Relative risk of tuberculosis with a positive versus negative tuberculous infection test in persons with various risk factors

Risk Factor	Test and Cutoff	N Cohorts	Relative Risk	Pooled Estimates of TB 95% Confidence interval
Contacts—all ages	IGRA positive (vs negative)	7	8.4	5.2, 13.5
	TST: 5+mm vs 0–4 mm	4	12.5	6.9, 22.5
	TST: 10+mm vs 0–9 mm	5	6.9	3.3, 14.4
Contacts: Children (aged < 18 y)	TST: 5+mm vs 0–4 mm	2	20.1	2.9, 141.0
	TST: 10+mm vs 0–9 mm	3	21.2	6.4, 70.0
PLHIV	IGRA positive (vs negative)	7	11.0	4.6, 26.2
	TST: 10+mm vs 0–9 mm	7	11.1	6.2, 19.9
Dialysis	TST: 10+mm vs 0–9 mm	3	2.6	1.4, 4.8
Solid organ transplant	IGRA positive (vs negative)	6	2.5	1.0, 6.0
	TST: 5+mm vs 0–4 mm	7	0.6	0.1, 3.0
	TST: 10+mm vs 0–9 mm	3	2.4	0.9, 6.4

(Pooled estimates from systematic review and meta-analysis by Campbell et al.[10] Estimates based on single studies, not shown.)
Abbreviations: PLHIV, people living with HIV; TB, tuberculosis; TST tuberculin skin test.

if feasible, before offering TPT. First, studies that have estimated the relative risk of developing disease in persons with positive compared with negative TBI tests (summarized in **Table 2**) show that the relative risks significantly exceed 1.0 for almost all conditions and, for people living with human immunodeficiency virus (HIV) infection (PLHIV), the relative risk is greater than 10. Second, more than a dozen randomized trials have compared the protection provided by TPT in persons with positive and negative tests. These have been summarized in 2 systematic reviews,[14,15] which concluded that TPT provided significant benefits only in persons with positive TBI tests, and nonsignificant benefits in those without. Subsequent large-scale randomized trials have confirmed this, with a few exceptions.[16,17] Third, even in countries with TB incidence greater than 100/10,000, most individuals tested will be negative, given that systematic reviews estimated pooled prevalence of 30% to 50% of positive tests among adults.[18,19] Treatment of all, without testing, will expose many persons to unnecessary harms, and add burden and costs to health services for the initial management and follow-up of those placed on TPT. Together, these studies strongly support offering TBI testing to all high risk and very high-risk individuals and offering TPT only to those with positive tests.

What Tests Are in Use for the Diagnosis of Tuberculosis Infection?

Tuberculin skin testing

The tuberculin skin test (TST) was first introduced in 1908 by Charles Mantoux; he administered intradermally a mixture of products from killed *M tuberculosis*. During the next 100 years, not much changed, although refinements of production resulted in a more standardized purified protein derivative (PPD) from *M tuberculosis*. Current tuberculin manufacturers standardized their PPD against the PPD lot produced by Florence Seibert in 1970 (named PPDS). We will refer to all such tuberculin materials as PPDS. The advantages of testing with PPDS are several. The safety of the material is very well established. Allergic reactions, which are mainly localized rashes, occur in

Table 4
Summary of tuberculosis preventive therapy recommendations according to the high-risk population

Population at Risk	Testing Algorithm	TPT Regimen by Order of Preference
Contacts of patients with respiratory drug-susceptible TB	After ruling out TB (based on a clinical ± radiological evaluation), perform either TST or IGRA. Individuals with a TST induration ≥5 mm or a positive IGRA are diagnosed with TBI and TPT must be considered If initial results are negative but tests were performed within 8 wk of exposure, consider a second TST after 8 wk of contact (otherwise, the result is considered a true negative and observation is warranted)	First lines of therapy: 3HP or 4R Preferred alternatives: 9H or 6H Other alternatives: 3HR
Patients living with HIV	After ruling out TB (based on a clinical ± radiological evaluation), perform either TST or IGRA. Individuals with a TST induration ≥5 mm or a positive IGRA are diagnosed with TBI and TPT must be considered. Consider repeating TBI test(s) after 6–12 mo of ARV therapy	First lines of therapy: 3HP (consider interactions) Preferred alternatives: 4R (consider interactions) Other alternatives: 9H, 6H, 3HR
Anti-TNF alpha therapy	Perform TST (cutoff ≥5 mm) or IGRAs after ruling out TB (consider alternative strategies to increase sensitivity such as sequential or simultaneous testing with both, the TST and IGRAs)	No particular regimen recommended (consider rifamycin-based shorter regimens)
Solid transplant candidates Stem cell transplant candidates	Perform either the TST (cutoff ≥5 mm) or IGRA (if possible, on the waiting list) after ruling out TB. If the initial TST is negative, consider repeating test 2 wk after	No regimen recommended (consider rifamycin-based shorter regimens on the waiting list). For candidates for liver transplantation, consider administering therapy after transplant
End-stage renal disease (dialysis patients)	Perform either the TST (cutoff ≥5 mm) or IGRA after ruling out TB	No particular regimen recommended (consider rifamycin-based shorter regimens). Administer anti-TB drugs postdialysis
Silicosis	Perform either the TST (cutoff ≥10 mm) or IGRA after ruling out TB. Periodic chest-X-rays are advised	No particular regimen recommended (consider rifamycin-based shorter regimens)

Abbreviations: 3HP, 3 mo once weekly directly observed isoniazid and rifapentine; 4R, 4 mo daily self-administered Rifampin; 6–9H, daily self-administered monotherapy with isoniazid 6 to 9 mo; 3HR, 3 mo daily self-administered isoniazid and rifampin; IGRA, interferon-gamma release assay; TB, tuberculosis; TBI, tuberculosis infection; TPT, tuberculosis preventive therapy; TST tuberculin skin testing.

less than 1%, and anaphylaxis is very rare, occurring approximately 1 per million doses administered. The other major advantage is that there are decades of longitudinal data on the occurrence of TB in individuals with negative and positive tests. However, there are also certain limitations. PPDS contains a broad mix of mycobacterial antigens, many of which are also found in nontuberculous mycobacteria and in the vaccine strain, *Mycobacterium bovis* BCG. This compromises the specificity of tuberculin testing, particularly in BCG-vaccinated populations. The other major problem of PPDS, which is an issue of all currently available tests for TB infection, is its low predictive ability. As seen in **Table 1**, even in the very high-risk population, less than 30% among those with a positive test will develop TB. Whether this low-predictive value is because of a chronically contained infection or a cleared infection with residual immunity is unknown. Given that most individuals with a positive TST who are subject to natural or iatrogenic immunosuppression do not progress to TB, it has been argued that a sizable proportion of those with a positive TST are no longer infected.[5]

New more specific tuberculins
In April 2022, 3 new tuberculins were approved by WHO for the diagnosis of TBI.[20] The 3 tests are C-Tb (developed by Statens Serum Institut, Denmark, and produced by Serum Institute of India, India), C-TST (formerly known as ESAT6-CFP10 test, developed and produced by Anhui Zhifei Longcom, China), and Diaskintest (developed and produced by Generium, Russian Federation). All 3 of these tuberculins contain ESAT-6 and CFP10 proteins, specific to *M tuberculosis*; hence, they have similar sensitivity to PPDS but better specificity, especially among persons who have received BCG vaccination. The 3 new tuberculins have a safety profile comparable to PPDS, although safety data is based on thousands instead of millions of test doses (for the PPDS). Although these are very promising results, none of the 3 new tests have been approved by the Food and Drug Administration, Health Canada, the European Medicines Agency, or other similar regulatory authority.

Interferon gamma release assays
The past 20 years have seen the introduction and rapid expansion of the use of interferon gamma (IFN-γ) release assays (IGRAs). These tests incubate blood samples in the presence of the *M tuberculosis*-specific antigens ESAT6 and CFP10 and measure the production of IFN-γ by lymphocytes that have been previously sensitized to these antigens. This IFN-γ is then quantified by enzyme-linked immunosorbent assay (ELISA; QuantiFERON–TB [Qiagen, Hilden, Germany], Qiagen; Wantai TB IGRA [Beijing Wantai Biological Pharmacy Enterprise, Beijing, China]) or by enumerating IFN-γ producing cells by enzyme-linked immune absorbent spot (ELISpot; T-SPOT.TB [Oxford Immunotec, Abingdon, United Kingdom], Oxford Immunotec). When the IGRA tests were developed, their validation was principally done in patients newly diagnosed with TB as the reference standard. These studies reported that sensitivity of ELISA-based IGRAs was similar to that of TST[21,22], whereas the sensitivity of the T-SPOT.TB was somewhat higher, particularly in immunocompromised hosts. Specificity of IGRA was estimated in populations considered at a very low risk of prior *M tuberculosis* exposure. These studies indicated that IGRA tests were more specific than TST, particularly in populations that had received BCG vaccination after infancy or more than once.[21,22] Despite their superior specificity, the ability of IGRAs to predict future risk of TB (positive predictive value) in longitudinal studies is low, and not much different from that of TST.[23] This observation that the TST and IGRAs have limited ability to predicting future TB, despite different platforms and antigens, provides further support for the possibility that these tests cannot distinguish who is currently infected

from who was previously infected. For this reason, tests for TBI will be of greatest value when used selectively, namely in those who are known to be at high risk of disease if the test result is positive.

What Are the Recommended Regimes for Tuberculosis Preventive Therapy?

TPT involves offering antibiotic therapy to patients with indirect evidence of TBI (positive TST or IGRA) but no clinical or microbiologic evidence of disease. Treatment of TBI was first introduced in the 1960s; a series of large-scale placebo-controlled trials evaluated 6 to 12 months of monotherapy with isoniazid (INH) in several populations. These demonstrated consistent benefit in reduction of TB risk with INH. In 1970, this evidence was used as the basis for recommendations by the American Thoracic Society to treat TBI in individuals with a wide variety of risk factors.

Daily, self-administered monotherapy with isoniazid for 6 or 9 months

From the 1960s until recently, monotherapy of INH has been the preferred regimen in most countries. In placebo-controlled trials, efficacy has been estimated to be as high as 93% with 12 months,[24,25] 90% with 9 months INH (9H),[26] and 70% with 6 months INH (6H).[25] The trade-off between duration and efficacy led some authorities to recommend 9H of therapy,[27,28] whereas others opted for 6H as completion was better.[29] However, regardless of recommended duration, completion rates are poor,[30] substantially reducing the effectiveness of INH treatment. In addition, the risk of severe hepatotoxicity, which can be fatal, reduced acceptance by patients and providers, further limiting the potential public health benefits of this treatment. Because of these problems, INH is now considered a second-line regimen in the United States[31] and Canada.[32]

Rifamycin-based regimens

A large number of trials have compared the completion, safety, and efficacy of INH regimens with shorter regimens containing rifapentine or rifampin. These 2 drugs have excellent sterilizing ability against *M tuberculosis*, which means that treatment of TBI can be shortened. The 3 most commonly used rifamycin-containing regimens for TBI treatment are 3 months of INH plus rifapentine, 4 months of rifampin, and 3 months of INH plus rifampin. These are described in detail below. Several network meta-analyses of TPT trials have concluded that these regimens were consistently associated with better completion, having a similar or better efficacy than monotherapy with INH for 6H to 9H, and reduced hepatotoxicity,[33–35] although only for 2 of the 3 regimens (see later discussion). In a network meta-analysis of trials in PLHIV, regimens with these 2 rifamycins were also associated with significantly lower overall mortality.[33]

The greatest disadvantage of the rifamycin-based regimens is the potential for drug–drug interactions. Both rifapentine and rifampin increase the hepatic metabolism of many other drugs currently in use. Resultant clinical effects occur within 1 to 2 weeks (and resolve again 1–2 weeks after completion of these regimens). As examples, the rifamycins have a major impact of *increasing* metabolism of hormonal contraceptives, many antiretroviral (ARV) medications, transplant rejection drugs, antidiabetic, and antihypertensive medications. For treatment of HIV infection, alternative regimens are available whose efficacy is not diminished by rifamycins, such as regimens based on efavirenz or dolutegravir (with increased doses of dolutegravir). For some drugs (eg, phenytoin), serum levels can be measured, and doses adjusted, whereas for hypertension, diabetes, or hypothyroidism, the end effect can be measured. However, for some medications such as direct-acting oral anticoagulants or transplant rejection medications, the degree of interaction is difficult to predict or measure; in patients on these drugs, the rifamycin regimens are best avoided. Several websites that we find helpful to identify potential drug–drug interactions are available.[36–38]

Three months once weekly directly observed isoniazid and rifapentine

Rifapentine is similar in structure to rifampin but has a longer half-life (13–14 vs 2–3 hours) and an active metabolite (25-desacetyl rifapentine) that has a comparably long half-life.[39] Based on these considerations, rifapentine can be given once weekly. Trials have combined rifapentine and isoniazid given once weekly, despite the much shorter half-life of isoniazid (1–4 hours). When given together for 3 months, the TPT regimen is abbreviated as 3HP. In PLHIV,[40,41] HIV uninfected adults,[42] and children,[43] 3 months once weekly directly isoniazid and rifapentine (3HP) has consistently demonstrated superior completion rates compared with 6H or 9H INH. These trials also reported lower rates of hepatotoxicity, with similar efficacy to protect against TB progression. As a result, this regimen is now recommended as first-line therapy in the United States[31] and Canada[32] and is increasingly used globally. However, other adverse events can be serious enough to result in discontinuation of the regimen in 3% to 5% of subjects. Because this is given once a week, all doses of this regimen have been directly observed in randomized trials. One randomized trial compared self-administered 3HP to directly observed 3HP.[44] In this trial completion in the self-administered arm was significantly worse than the directly observed arm. Given this evidence, we suggest that every dose of this regimen should be directly observed; exceptions can be made on a case-by-case basis. The requirement for observed dosing may render this regimen impractical in many settings, and possibly less acceptable to certain providers and patients.

Four months daily self-administered rifampin

Several clinical trials and observational studies have demonstrated superior safety and completion rates with 4 months of rifampin (4R) compared with 6H or 9H INH.[45–48] Hepatotoxicity and other adverse events leading to drug discontinuation are significantly lower with 4R than with 9H INH, making 4R the only regimen with significantly fewer discontinuations for adverse events, compared with the 9H INH standard. In randomized trials, the efficacy is similar to that of 9H INH, suggesting that the efficacy of 4R is expected around 90%. As a result, this regimen is recommended as first-line therapy for TB infection in the United States[31] and Canada.[32]

Three months daily self-administered isoniazid and rifampin

The major source of evidence for this regimen has been observational studies, although randomized trials have been performed among people living with HIV. A systematic review and meta-analysis of these trials concluded that the efficacy of 3 months daily self-administered isoniazid and rifampin (3HR) was similar to that of 6H of INH but the toxicity was also similar, particularly hepatotoxicity.[49] This regimen therefore combines the hepatotoxicity risks of daily isoniazid, plus the drug–drug interactions of rifampin, without conferring an advantage in efficacy or completion. Hence, this regimen is not recommended in Canada[32] and is conditionally recommended as an alternative in the United States.[31] We suggest this regimen should be reserved for settings where rifampin is available only in fixed dose combination tablets with INH, and rifapentine is not yet available.

Other regimens: suspected drug-resistant tuberculosis infection, or first-line regimens cannot be used

Contacts of persons with TB due to drug-resistant organisms (DR-TB) often develop drug-resistant disease. Therefore, it is recommended that therapy for contacts of patients with DR-TB receive TPT that is based on the drug susceptibility test of the isolate from the presumed source. INH monoresistance or polydrug resistance (INH resistance without rifampin resistance) is the most common form of drug-resistance. Contacts of persons with INH monoresistance or polyresistance should be given 4R. Contacts of persons with TB due to rifampin monoresistant *M tuberculosis* (ie, with organisms that are sensitive to INH) should be given INH because this has well-established efficacy. Contacts of patients with multidrug resistant TB—MDR TB—(ie, resistant to INH and rifampin) should be given 6H levofloxacin or moxifloxacin. A systematic review of observational studies suggested that this was an effective regimen.[50] A large-scale randomized trial testing this regimen in contacts of MDR TB patients has completed enrollment and follow-up, so better evidence for this therapy should be forthcoming within a year.[51] In patients who are allergic to or intolerant of rifamycins, 9H is usually given. However, in patients with preexisting liver disease (eg, preliver transplant), or older age, where INH is not a good option, we suggest 6H levofloxacin or moxifloxacin can be given, although we acknowledge there is limited evidence to support this.

Common Scenarios in Clinical Practice

Tuberculosis contacts

Individuals with a recent exposure to a patient with respiratory TB (ie, pulmonary, laryngeal, or pleural) during its infectious period are at high risk for progression to TB, the risk being higher in adolescents than in adults, and higher still in children.[10,52,53] There are different definitions of what a "contact" is in the literature[54,55]; however, anyone with whom a source case had prolonged and close interaction (eg, household members, close friends, close work contacts) is at risk of TBI/TB.[55] A systematic review reported that 3.1% of contacts are found to have TB (also called coprevalent TB) and that the incidence of new cases is highest in the first year (0.5%–1.5% depending on the setting) before declining thereafter.[19] For this reason, TB contacts should be evaluated as soon as possible to rule out TB and to assess the need for TPT (practitioners should prioritize the evaluation of those with a higher risk, based on the patient's characteristics and the intensity of exposure).[52,55,56] The initial evaluation should include questions about TB symptoms (eg, cough, fever), comorbidities that may increase the risk of TB (eg, HIV infection, if unknown, an HIV diagnostic test may be offered), and the characteristics of the exposure (ie, setting, duration, intensity).[57] Based on the initial assessment, further studies may be required (eg, chest X-ray, microbiological examinations). In HIV-negative contacts, the absence of TB symptoms and of chest X-ray abnormalities may rule out TB.[54]

A conversion from a negative to a positive TST or IGRA test (suggestive of a recently acquired TBI) is expected to occur between 3 and 8 weeks after contact.[58] Therefore, a repeat testing may be required. A limitation of this approach is the possibility of false-positive conversions as a consequence of the intraperson variability of all TBI tests.[59] Because there is no consensus on the clinical significance of a conversion when using IGRAs, the TST may be preferred for contact investigation.[52] The recommended cutoff for positivity for the initial TST is 5 mm[52,55]; if the result is negative (<5 mm) but the test was performed within 8 weeks of exposure, a second TST is indicated 8 weeks after the contact (otherwise, the result is considered a true negative and observation is warranted).[52] If the first TST has a diameter of 5 mm or greater, or the second of 10 mm or greater, the patient should be evaluated for TPT.[52] As a side note, even if the TST conversion could be due to a booster effect, a recent exposure to a patient with TB increases pretest probability of infection. Therefore, a conversion in this context is considered a true positive.[52]

After confirming the diagnosis of a TBI (and properly ruling out TB),[57] contacts should be evaluated for TPT. The decision to treat must be shared with the patient and, if TPT is not accepted, close monitoring of warning signs and symptoms may be appropriate and should be offered on a case-by-case basis.[56] The eighth edition of the Canadian Tuberculosis Standards and the National Tuberculosis Controllers Association/Centers for Disease Control and Prevention (CDC) guidelines consider as first lines of treatment—for contacts of patients with drug susceptible TB—either 3HP or 4R.[56,60] Factors such as drug-availability, pill burden, costs, and the potential of adverse events (see earlier discussion) may aid in the decision between both regimens.[56] If these regimens are not an option (eg, contraindications, poor tolerability) the preferred alternatives by both organizations are 9H and 6H, whereas regimens such as 3HR are considered as last options by the Canadian Tuberculosis Standards for reasons described before.[56] Given that children aged younger than 5 years who are contacts of a bacteriologically confirmed case have a higher risk of TB and a higher proportion of severe forms of TB, the WHO recommends providing them TPT even if TBI testing is unavailable—but after ruling out TB.[54] However, TPT may also be justifiable for those aged older than 5 years in the absence of TBI tests based on an individual risk/benefit assessment.[54]

People living with human immunodeficiency virus

PLHIV are at a particularly high risk of progression to TB, which may depend, among other factors, on the degree of immunosuppression and on the use of ARV therapy.[61] Although ARV treatment alone is effective for the prevention of TB, several studies have found additional and independent benefits for TB prevention with the administration of TPT.[17,62,63] Therefore, all PLHIV, with a low probability of concurrent TB, should be considered for TPT, regardless of their immune or ARV status.[54] TB must be ruled out before the administration of TPT. This is especially relevant for PLHIV because they have a higher risk of subclinical disease and, consequently, of receiving inappropriate anti-TB therapy.[60,64] There are several clinical rules that may help identify patients with a low risk of TB. The WHO currently recommends the use of a 4-symptom screening rule (ie, of current cough, fever, weight loss, or night sweats).[54] However, its sensitivity is relatively poor, especially in patients under ARV treatment (51.0% vs 89.4% in patients naïve to ARV).[65] The diagnostic accuracy of this clinical rule is improved with the addition of a chest radiography (sensitivity of 84.6%).[65]

According to the WHO, TPT is recommended for PLHIV even if TBI diagnostic tests are not available.[54] However, previous studies have shown that the benefit of TPT is greater among patients with a laboratory confirmation of TBI (see earlier discussion). Therefore, TBI diagnostic testing (either TST or IGRAs) aids to identify patients with a higher probability of benefit with TPT.[52] Nevertheless, it is important to consider that the sensitivity of the TBI diagnostic tests is diminished in PLHIV (TST and IGRAs sensitivities ~60% to 70%).[66,67] One explanation for a false-negative result with an initial test (ie, TST <5 mm or a negative IGRA) is a severe degree of immunosuppression. Therefore, a strategy to increase sensitivity is performing a second test 6 to 12 months after initiation of ARV therapy (this is mainly recommended for patients with advanced immunosuppression and at a higher risk of adverse TB outcomes).[52] A second strategy that may increase the sensitivity of the algorithm is performing both TBI tests (ie, TST and IGRAs) after a negative initial test.[55]

Rifamycin-based regimens are as effective and safer than isoniazid-based regimens in PLHIV.[33] The National Tuberculosis Controllers Association/CDC guidelines consider 3HP as first-line in adults and children aged older than 2 years, even in PLHIV.[60] This recommendation is based on clinical trials comparing 3HP with 6H to

9H that showed noninferiority in the prevention of TB but higher tolerability with 3HP.[40,42] However, the evidence for the use of 4R in this group of patients is limited.[56,60] Despite the clear benefits of rifamycin-based regimens, a limitation (introduced above) to their wide use among PLHIV is the possibility of drug–drug interactions with ARVs, which should be thoroughly evaluated before their administration (a specialist consultation may be advised). Finally, in settings where the risk of TB transmission is very high (TB incidence ≥500 per 100,000), a treatment option recommended by WHO is isoniazid for at least 36 months for adults and adolescents living with HIV; however, the decision to use this regimen should be based on national local recommendations.[54]

Selected Other Populations at Risk

Evidence of TPT benefits in other high-risk groups is limited. Based on their benefit-risk profile, the WHO recommends a systematic evaluation for TPT for patients who will start immune therapy with inhibitors of tumor necrosis factor (TNF)-alpha (eg, infliximab, adalimumab, etanercept), those on renal replacement therapy, candidates or recipients of solid organ or hematopoietic cell transplants, and patients with silicosis.[54] We briefly describe each of these settings.

Antitumor necrosis factor-alpha therapy

One major adverse effect of the anti-TNF agents, a group of drugs used to inflammatory diseases (eg, rheumatoid arthritis, inflammatory bowel disease), is an increased risk of infectious diseases, including TB (Odds Ratio [OR] of 1.94).[68] Therefore, before their administration, patients should be evaluated for TBI and treated accordingly. The American College of Rheumatology recommends performing either the TST or IGRA for all patients with rheumatoid arthritis who will start anti-TNF therapy and, if the result is positive (TST ≥5 mm),[52,55] performing a chest X-ray to rule out TB.[69] Candidates for anti-TNF therapy are often immunocompromised; therefore, the possibility of false-negative results with the TBI tests should be considered (alternative strategies to increase sensitivity are sequential or simultaneous testing with both, the TST and IGRAs).[69,70] TPT should be offered to those patients with confirmed TBI after ruling out TB. There is no evidence about an ideal regimen for this group of patients. Nonetheless, given the severity of the underlying conditions and the urgency of starting immunosuppressive therapies, the WHO favors the use of short TPT regimens in this group of patients such as 1HP or 3HP.[54] The American College of Rheumatology recommends completing at least 1 month of TPT before initiating biologic therapy.[69]

Solid organ and stem cell transplant

Solid organ transplant recipients and stem cell transplant recipients have an increased risk of TB (eg, 15 times the risk in the general population with lung transplant and 6–10 times the risk in the general population for stem cell transplants).[71] Hence, every transplant candidate (or recipient, if not evaluated before) should be assessed for TBI using either the TST (cutoff ≥5 mm) and/or an IGRA.[52] If the TST is used for screening and the result is negative, a second test after 7 to 10 days may be appropriate to increase its sensitivity (booster-effect).[72] A crucial consideration in these patients is the ideal timing, relative to the transplantation date, for TPT administration. In most cases, it is recommended that patients complete TPT before transplantation.[71] However, an exception to this recommendation are candidates for liver transplant, in whom TPT administration may trigger fulminant hepatitis and, therefore, posttransplant TPT is advised.[71] If TPT was initiated while the patient was on the waiting list and the transplantation was performed before completion of TPT, the former should be completed in the posttransplant period.[71] There is no regimen of choice in this context, nevertheless, a barrier to the use of rifamycin-based regimens is the risk of drug–drug interactions with immunosuppressants.[56] This limitation favors the administration of TPT in the pretransplant period whenever possible.[71]

End-stage renal disease (dialysis patients)

Patients with end-stage renal disease and renal replacement therapy have a risk of TB 3 to 25 times higher than the general population.[73] Given the congregation of patients in hemodialysis units, unrecognized patients with TB represent an important risk to other patients and health-care workers in the same units, causing occasional outbreaks in these centers.[74] Therefore, screening for TBI using IGRAs and/or the TST (cutoff point of positivity is $\geq$5 mm)[52] and offering TPT—if results are positive and after ruling out TB—is recommended.[54] The TPT regimen of choice for this group is also undefined. However, it is important to note that patients with renal replacement present a higher risk of adverse events with TPT, requiring close monitoring after its initiation.[56] Drugs such as isoniazid, rifapentine, and rifampicin do not require dose adjustment; however, their administration should be preferably postdialysis.[56,75]

Silicosis

Silicosis is caused by chronic inhalation of free silica particles because of occupational exposures such as mining, masonry, glass or ceramic manufacturing, among others.[76] Exposure to silica dust, with or without silicosis, increases the risk of TB (Risk Ratio [RR] of 4.0 among individuals with silicosis vs 1.9 among people without silicosis but with silica exposure).[77,78] Screening for TB must include a clinical evaluation, imaging studies, and IGRA or TST (cutoff for positivity $\geq$10 mm).[52,79] It is important to note that, in this group of patients, it is often difficult to discriminate TB from the chronic respiratory symptoms and radiographic findings due to silicosis.[80] Strategies to help identify TB before the administration of TPT are periodic chest X-rays, as well a thorough microbiological evaluation.[80] Regarding therapy, an RCT performed in Hong Kong showed a reduction in the risk of developing TB in patients with silicosis who received TPT 6H, 3HR, 3R (5-year risk of TB of 27% in the placebo group vs 13% in patients with TPT).[81] However, a recent cluster-randomized trial comparing 9H versus standard of care in South African gold miners found no benefit in preventing TB (Rate ratio in the intervention clusters, 1.00; 95% confidence interval [CI], 0.75 to 1.34; $P=0.98$)).[82] The discrepancy between these trials may be a consequence of differences in TB burden and the reinfection risk in the latter study.[77] There is no evidence in favor of one of the TPT regimens for this specific group of patients; factors such as patient baseline characteristics and preference, risk of reinfection, and treatment availability should dictate the treatment of choice.

FUTURE PERSPECTIVES

TPT has been practiced for more than a half-century and is, therefore, based on decades of data on tests and drugs. Despite the tremendous amount of information available, there remain some areas of uncertainty for which newer tools might provide improved and better approaches in the future. The 2 drivers of TPT utility are the ability to predict TB and the benefit/risk ratio of the intervention. For the former, current tests provide indirect evidence for TBI as a one-time dichotomous outcome. Yet, evidence have emerged that a sustained quantitative IGRA response is associated with an increased risk of subsequent TB relative to a transient response, and that higher IGRA values are also associated with a higher risk.[83,84] Furthermore, among those classified as having a "positive" test, additional biomarker-based assays may ultimately be able to identify those with the highest risk, who will benefit from TPT, or those with the lowest risk, for which it is not beneficial.[85] How these observations can be operationalized remains a challenge but such challenges have been overcome in other fields of preventive medicine, for instance cholesterol reduction. The other driver of the TPT uptake is the complexity of the intervention. In other infectious diseases, preventive treatment can be as short as a single dose of an antihelminthic drug. It follows that the risk strata in **Table 1** that benefit from the intervention would be expanded if shorter, nontoxic regimens become available. Ideally, tests that can detect who is infected today, and is at risk of developing TB, would be combined with shorter, nontoxic regimens, and then TPT could optimally be offered to all those who will derive benefit but only those individuals.

DISCLOSURE

The authors have nothing to disclose.

REFERENCES

1. World Health O. Global tuberculosis report 2021. Geneva: World Health Organization; 2021.
2. Houben RM, Dodd PJ. The Global Burden of Latent Tuberculosis Infection: A Re-estimation Using Mathematical Modelling. Plos Med 2016;13(10):e1002152. https://doi.org/10.1371/journal.pmed.1002152.
3. Emery JC, Richards AS, Dale KD, et al. Self-clearance of Mycobacterium tuberculosis infection: implications for lifetime risk and population at-risk of tuberculosis disease. Proc Biol Sci 2021;288(1943):20201635. https://doi.org/10.1098/rspb.2020.1635.
4. Dye C, Glaziou P, Floyd K, et al. Prospects for tuberculosis elimination. Annu Rev Public Health 2013;34:271–86. https://doi.org/10.1146/annurev-publhealth-031912-114431.
5. Behr MA, Edelstein PH, Ramakrishnan L. Revisiting the timetable of tuberculosis. Bmj 2018;362:k2738. https://doi.org/10.1136/bmj.k2738.
6. Sutherland I, Svandová E, Radhakrishna S. The development of clinical tuberculosis following infection with tubercle bacilli. 1. A theoretical model for the development of clinical tuberculosis following infection, linking from data on the risk of tuberculous infection and the incidence of clinical tuberculosis in the Netherlands. Tubercle 1982;63(4):255–68. https://doi.org/10.1016/s0041-3879(82)80013-5.
7. ten Asbroek AH, Borgdorff MW, Nagelkerke NJ, et al. Estimation of serial interval and incubation period of tuberculosis using DNA fingerprinting. Int J Tuberc Lung Dis 1999;3(5):414–20.
8. Hatherell HA, Didelot X, Pollock SL, et al. Declaring a tuberculosis outbreak over with genomic epidemiology. Microb Genom 2016;2(5):e000060. https://doi.org/10.1099/mgen.0.000060.
9. Lee RS, Radomski N, Proulx JF, et al. Reemergence and amplification of tuberculosis in the Canadian arctic. J Infect Dis 2015;211(12):1905–14. https://doi.org/10.1093/infdis/jiv011.
10. Campbell JR, Winters N, Menzies D. Absolute risk of tuberculosis among untreated populations with a positive tuberculin skin test or interferon-gamma release assay result: systematic review and meta-analysis. BMJ (Clinical research ed) 2020;368:m549.

11. Behr MA, Kaufmann E, Duffin J, et al. Latent Tuberculosis: Two Centuries of Confusion. Am J Respir Crit Care Med 2021;204(2):142–8.
12. Esmail H, Macpherson L, Coussens AK, et al. Mind the gap - Managing tuberculosis across the disease spectrum. Ebiomedicine 2022;17:103928.
13. Wong EB. It Is Time to Focus on Asymptomatic Tuberculosis. Clin Infect Dis 2021; 72(12):e1044–6.
14. Akolo C, Adetifa I, Shepperd S, et al. Treatment of latent tuberculosis infection in HIV infected persons. Cochrane Database Syst Rev 2010;(1):CD000171.
15. Smieja MJ, Marchetti CA, Cook DJ, et al. Isoniazid for preventing tuberculosis in non-HIV infected persons. Cochrane Database Syst Rev 2000;2:CD001363. https://doi.org/10.1002/14651858.CD001363.
16. Rangaka MX, Wilkinson RJ, Boulle A, et al. Isoniazid plus antiretroviral therapy to prevent tuberculosis: a randomised double-blind, placebo-controlled trial. Lancet 2014;384(9944):682–90.
17. Group TAS, Danel C, Moh R, et al. A Trial of Early Antiretrovirals and Isoniazid Preventive Therapy in Africa. N Engl J Med 2015;373(9):808–22.
18. Morrison J, Pai M, Hopewell P. Tuberculosis and latent tuberculosis infection in close contacts of people with pulmonary tuberculosis in low-income andmiddle -income countries:a systematic review and meta-analysis. Lancel Infect Dis 2008;8(359):368. Not in File.
19. Fox GJ, Barry SE, Britton WJ, et al. Contact investigation for tuberculosis: a systematic review and meta-analysis. Eur Respir J 2013;41(1):140–56.
20. Rapid communication: TB antigen-based skin tests for the diagnosis of TB infection. Geneva: World Health Organization; 2022 (WHO/UCN/TB/2022.1). Licence: CC BY-NC-SA 3.0 IGO.
21. Menzies D, Pai M, Comstock G. Meta-analysis: New Tests for the Diagnosis of Latent Tuberculosis Infection: Areas of Uncertainty and Recommendations for Research. Ann Intern Med 2007;146(5):340–54. https://doi.org/10.7326/0003-4819-146-5-200703060-00006.
22. Pai M, Zwerling A, Menzies D. Systematic review: T-cell-based assays for the diagnosis of latent tuberculosis infection: an update. Ann Intern Med 2008; 149(3):177–84.
23. Rangaka M, Wilkinson KA, Glynn J, et al. Predictive value of interferon-gamma release assays for incident active tuberculosis: a systematic review and meta-analysis. Lancet Infect Dis 2012;12(1):45–55.
24. Sh F. Controlled chemoprophylaxis trials in tuberculosis. Adv Tuberc Res 1969; 17:28–106. In File.
25. IUATCo Prophylaxis. Efficacy of various durations of isoniazid preventive therapy for tuberculosis: five years of follow-up in the IUAT trial. Bull World Health Organ 1982;60(4):555–64.
26. Comstock G. How much isoniazid is needed for prevention of tuberculosis in immunocompetent adults? Int J Tuberc Lung Dis 1999;3(10):847–50.
27. Society AT. Targeted tuberculin testing and treatment of latent tuberculosis infection. MMWR Recomm Rep 2000;49(RR-6):1–51. Not in File.
28. Menzies D, editor. Canadian Tuberculosis Standards. Canadian lung association. Ottawa: Public Health Agency of Canada; 2013.
29. World Health Organization. Guidelines on the Management of Latent Tuberculosis Infection. Geneva: World Health Organization; 2015.
30. Hirsch-Moverman Y, Daftary A, Franks J, et al. Adherence to treatment for latent tuberculosis infection:systematic review of students in theUS and Canada. Int J Tuberc Lung Dis 2008;12(11):1235–54. Not in File.

31. Sterling T, Njie G, Zenner D, et al. Guidelines for the Treatment of Latent Tuberculosis Infection: Recommendations from the National Tuberculosis Controllers Association and CDC. MMWR 2020;69(No.RR-1):1–11. https://doi.org/10.15585/mmwr.rr6901a1external icon.

32. De M, editor. Canadian tuberculosis standards. 8th edition. Canadian Thoracic Society; 2022.

33. Yanes-Lane M, Ortiz-Brizuela E, Campbell J, et al. Tuberculosis preventive therapy for people living with HIV: A systematic review and network meta-analysis. PLoS Med 2021;18(9):e1003738.

34. Pease C, Hutton B, Yazdi F, et al. Efficacy and completion rates of rifapentine and isoniazid (3HP) compared to other treatment regimens for latent tuberculosis infection: a systematic review with network meta-analyses. BMC Infect Dis 2017;17(1):265.

35. Zenner D, Beer N, Harris R, et al. Treatment of Latent Tuberculosis Infection: An Updated Network Meta-analysis. Ann Intern Med 2017;167(4):248–55.

36. Medscape drug interaction checker. Available at: https://reference.medscape.com/drug-interactionchecker. Accessed June 1, 2022.

37. University of Liverpool HIV Drug Interactions checker. Available at: https://www.hiv-druginteractions.org/checker. Accessed June 1 2022.

38. HIV/HCV drug therapy guide from toronto interactions checker. Available at: https://hivclinic.ca/wp-content/plugins/php/app.php. Accessed June 1 2022.

39. Zurlinden TJ, Eppers GJ, Reisfeld B. Physiologically Based Pharmacokinetic Model of Rifapentine and 25-Desacetyl Rifapentine Disposition in Humans. Antimicrob Agents Chemother 2016;60(8):4860–8.

40. Martinson N, Barnes G, Moulton L, et al. New regimens to prevent tuberculosis in adults with HIV infection. N Engl J Med 2011;365(1):11–20. In File.

41. Sterling T, Villarino M, Borisov A, et al. Three months of rifapentine and isoniazid for latent tuberculosis infection. N Engl J Med 2011;(23):365. In File.

42. Sterling TR, Scott NA, Miro JM, et al. Three months of weekly rifapentine and isoniazid for treatment of Mycobacterium tuberculosis infection in HIV-coinfected persons. AIDS 2016;30(10):1607–15.

43. Villarino M, Scott N, Weis S, et al. Treatment for Preventing Tuberculosis in Children and Adolescents. JAMA Pediatr 2015;169(3):247.

44. Belknap R, Holland D, Feng P, et al. Self-administered Versus Directly Observed Once-Weekly Isoniazid and Rifapentine Treatment of Latent Tuberculosis Infection: A Randomized Trial. Ann Intern Med 2017;167(10):689–97.

45. KR P, F S, R MdO, et al. Improved adherence and less toxicity with rifampin vs isoniazid for treatment of latent tuberculosis: a retrospective study. Arch Intern Med 2006;166(17):1863–70. Not in File.

46. D M, MJ D, B R, et al. Treatment completion and costs of a randomized trial of rifampin for 4 months versus isoniazid for 9 months. Am J Respir Crit Care Med 2004;170(4):445–9. Not in File.

47. Menzies D, Long R, Trajman A, et al. Adverse Events with 4 Months of Rifampin Therapy or 9 Months of Isoniazid Therapy for Latent Tuberculosis Infection. Ann Intern Med 2008;(10):149.

48. Menzies D, Adjobimey M, Ruslami R, et al. Four Months of Rifampin or Nine Months of Isoniazid for Latent Tuberculosis in Adults. N Engl J Med 2018;(5):379.

49. Ena J, Valls V. Short-Course Therapy with Rifampin plus Isoniazid, Compared with Standard Therapy with Isoniazid, for Latent Tuberculosis Infection: A Meta-analysis. Clin Infect Dis 2005;40(5).

50. Marks S, Mase S, Morris S. Systematic Review, Meta-Analysis, and Cost-Effectiveness of Treatment of Latent Tuberculosis to Reduce Progression to Multidrug-Resistant Tuberculosis. Clin Infect Dis 2017;64(2):1670–7.

51. Fox GJ, Nguyen CB, Nguyen TA, et al. Levofloxacin versus placebo for the treatment of latent tuberculosis among contacts of patients with multidrug-resistant tuberculosis (the VQUIN MDR trial): a protocol for a randomised controlled trial. BMJ Open 2020;10(1):e033945.

52. Campbell JR, Pease C, Daley P, et al. Chapter 4: Diagnosis of tuberculosis infection. Can J Respir Crit Care Sleep Med 2022;6(sup1):49–65.

53. Sutherland I. Recent studies in the epidemiology of tuberculosis, based on the risk of being infected with tubercle bacilli. Adv Tuberc Res 1976;19:1–63.

54. World Health O. WHO consolidated guidelines on tuberculosis: module 1: prevention: tuberculosis preventive treatment. Geneva: World Health Organization; 2020.

55. Cole B, Nilsen DM, Will L, et al. Essential Components of a Public Health Tuberculosis Prevention, Control, and Elimination Program: Recommendations of the Advisory Council for the Elimination of Tuberculosis and the National Tuberculosis Controllers Association. MMWR Recomm Rep 2020;69(7):1–27.

56. Alvarez GG, Pease C, Menzies D. Chapter 6: Tuberculosis preventive treatment in adults. Can J Respir Crit Care Sleep Med 2022;6(sup1):77–86.

57. Guidelines for the investigation of contacts of persons with infectious tuberculosis. Recommendations from the National Tuberculosis Controllers Association and CDC. MMWR Recomm Rep 2005;54(Rr-15):1–47.

58. Menzies D. Interpretation of repeated tuberculin tests. Boosting, conversion, and reversion. Am J Respir Crit Care Med 1999;159(1):15–21.

59. Pai M, O'Brien R. Serial testing for tuberculosis: can we make sense of T cell assay conversions and reversions? Plos Med 2007;4(6):e208.

60. Sterling TR, Njie G, Zenner D, et al. Guidelines for the Treatment of Latent Tuberculosis Infection: Recommendations from the National Tuberculosis Controllers Association and CDC, 2020. MMWR Recomm Rep 2020;69(1):1–11.

61. Suthar AB, Lawn SD, del Amo J, et al. Antiretroviral therapy for prevention of tuberculosis in adults with HIV: a systematic review and meta-analysis. Plos Med 2012;9(7):e1001270.

62. Ross JM, Badje A, Rangaka MX, et al. Isoniazid preventive therapy plus antiretroviral therapy for the prevention of tuberculosis: a systematic review and meta-analysis of individual participant data. Lancet HIV 2021;8(1):e8–15.

63. Hakim J, Musiime V, Szubert AJ, et al. Enhanced Prophylaxis plus Antiretroviral Therapy for Advanced HIV Infection in Africa. N Engl J Med 2017;377(3):233–45.

64. Chaisson LH, Naufal F, Delgado-Barroso P, et al. A systematic review of the number needed to screen for active TB among people living with HIV. Int J Tuberc Lung Dis 2021;25(6):427–35.

65. Hamada Y, Lujan J, Schenkel K, et al. Sensitivity and specificity of WHO's recommended four-symptom screening rule for tuberculosis in people living with HIV: a systematic review and meta-analysis. Lancet HIV 2018;5(9):e515–23.

66. Santin M, Munoz L, Rigau D. Interferon-gamma release assays for the diagnosis of tuberculosis and tuberculosis infection in HIV-infected adults: a systematic review and meta-analysis. PLoS One 2012;7(3):e32482.

67. Huo ZY, Peng L. Accuracy of the interferon-gamma release assay for the diagnosis of active tuberculosis among HIV-seropositive individuals: a systematic review and meta-analysis. BMC Infect Dis 2016;16:350.

68. Zhang Z, Fan W, Yang G, et al. Risk of tuberculosis in patients treated with TNF-alpha antagonists: a systematic review and meta-analysis of randomised controlled trials. BMJ Open 2017;7(3):e012567.

69. Singh JA, Saag KG, Bridges SL Jr, et al. 2015 American College of Rheumatology Guideline for the Treatment of Rheumatoid Arthritis. Arthritis Rheumatol 2016; 68(1):1–26.

70. O'Young CKY, Ho KM, So H, et al. Recommendations on Management of Latent Tuberculosis Infection in Patients Initiating Anti-tumor Necrosis Factor Biologics. J Clin Rheumatol Immunol 2021;21(02):51–7.

71. Hasan T, Au E, Chen S, et al. Screening and prevention for latent tuberculosis in immunosuppressed patients at risk for tuberculosis: a systematic review of clinical practice guidelines. BMJ Open 2018;8(9):e022445.

72. Aguado JM, Torre-Cisneros J, Fortun J, et al. Tuberculosis in solid-organ transplant recipients: consensus statement of the group for the study of infection in transplant recipients (GESITRA) of the Spanish Society of Infectious Diseases and Clinical Microbiology. Clin Infect Dis 2009;48(9):1276–84.

73. Romanowski K, Clark EG, Levin A, et al. Tuberculosis and chronic kidney disease: an emerging global syndemic. Kidney Int 2016;90(1):34–40.

74. Centers for Disease C Prevention. Tuberculosis transmission in a renal dialysis center–Nevada, 2003. MMWR Morb Mortal Wkly Rep 2004;53(37):873–5.

75. Nahid P, Dorman SE, Alipanah N, et al. Official American Thoracic Society/Centers for Disease Control and Prevention/Infectious Diseases Society of America Clinical Practice Guidelines: Treatment of Drug-Susceptible Tuberculosis. Clin Infect Dis 2016;63(7):e147–95.

76. Lanzafame M, Vento S. Mini-review: Silico-tuberculosis. J Clin Tuberc Other Mycobact Dis 2021;23:100218.

77. Leung CC, Yu IT, Chen W. Silicosis Lancet 2012;379(9830):2008–18.

78. Ehrlich R, Akugizibwe P, Siegfried N, et al. The association between silica exposure, silicosis and tuberculosis: a systematic review and meta-analysis. BMC Public Health 2021;21(1):953.

79. Churchyard GJ, Fielding K, Roux S, et al. Twelve-monthly versus six-monthly radiological screening for active case-finding of tuberculosis: a randomised controlled trial. Thorax 2011;66(2):134–9.

80. Rees D, Murray J. Silica, silicosis and tuberculosis. Int J Tuberc Lung Dis 2007; 11(5):474–84.

81. A double-blind placebo-controlled clinical trial of three antituberculosis chemoprophylaxis regimens in patients with silicosis in Hong Kong. Hong Kong Chest Service/Tuberculosis Research Centre, Madras/British Medical Research Council. Am Rev Respir Dis 1992;145(1):36–41.

82. Churchyard GJ, Fielding KL, Lewis JJ, et al. A trial of mass isoniazid preventive therapy for tuberculosis control. N Engl J Med 2014;370(4):301–10.

83. Andrews JR, Hatherill M, Mahomed H, et al. The dynamics of QuantiFERON-TB gold in-tube conversion and reversion in a cohort of South African adolescents. Am J Respir Crit Care Med 2015;191(5):584–91.

84. Ledesma JR, Ma J, Zheng P, et al. Interferon-gamma release assay levels and risk of progression to active tuberculosis: a systematic review and dose-response meta-regression analysis. BMC Infect Dis 2021;21(1):467.

85. Broderick C, Cliff JM, Lee JS, et al. Host transcriptional response to TB preventive therapy differentiates two sub-groups of IGRA-positive individuals. Tuberculosis (Edinb) 2021;127:102033.

86. Sloot R, Schim van der Loeff MF, Kouw PM, et al. Risk of tuberculosis after recent exposure. A 10-year follow-up study of contacts in Amsterdam. Am J Respir Crit Care Med 2014;190(9):1044–52.
87. Trauer JM, Moyo N, Tay EL, et al. Risk of Active Tuberculosis in the Five Years Following Infection . . . 15%? Chest 2016;149(2):516–25.
88. Gupta RK, Calderwood CJ, Yavlinsky A, et al. Discovery and validation of a personalized risk predictor for incident tuberculosis in low transmission settings. Nat Med 2020;26(12):1941–9.
89. Martinez L, Cords O, Horsburgh CR, et al. The risk of tuberculosis in children after close exposure: a systematic review and individual-participant meta-analysis. Lancet 2020;395(10228):973–84.
90. Horwitz O, Knudsen J. A follow-up study of tuberculosis incidence and general mortality in various occupational-social groups of the Danish population. Bull World Health Organ 1961;24:793–805.
91. Comstock GW, Edwards LB, Livesay VT. Tuberculosis morbidity in the U.S. Navy: its distribution and decline. Am Rev Respir Dis 1974;110(5):572–80.
92. Pai M, Kunimoto D, Jamieson F, et al. Chapter 4: Diagnosis of Latent Tuberculosis Infection. Can J Respir Crit Care Sleep Med 2013;1–32.

Care of the Seriously Ill Patient with SARS-CoV-2

Lindsay M. Leither, DO[a,b,*], Whitney Buckel, PharmD[c], Samuel M. Brown, MD, MS[a,b]

KEYWORDS

- COVID-19 • Treatment • Critical care

KEY POINTS

- High-quality supportive ICU care is paramount, including established therapies for acute respiratory distress syndrome.
- Therapeutic interventions for COVID-19 include virologic and immunologic therapies.
- COVID-19 can be complicated by thromboembolic events and multisystem inflammatory syndrome.

INTRODUCTION

Common COVID-19 symptoms include fever, dyspnea, cough, and fatigue. Dyspnea is more often reported by those who develop severe infection and correlates with worse prognosis.[1,2] COVID-19 disease results in a dynamic balance between antiviral immune defense and excessive inflammation, often conceptualized into a biphasic disease: an initial "viral phase" followed by either recovery or a "hyperinflammatory phase" driven by host-mediated organ damage resulting in severe illness, sometimes referred to as "cytokine storm."[3] Histopathologic evidence has demonstrated end-organ damage even in the absence of viral particles, supporting the notion that excessive host response contributes to mortality.[4] In general, virus-targeted therapies tend to be most effective early in disease and host-focused or inflammatory focused therapies tend to be most effective later in the course of illness. In addition to the "biphasic model," distinction has emerged over the past year regarding patient serologic status and viral load in relation to therapeutic efficacy. Notably, a subset of patients are unable to limit viral replication, and this inability to control the virus may contribute to the development of respiratory failure. Thus, although antivirals are most effective early in

[a] Division of Pulmonary & Critical Care Medicine, Department of Medicine, Intermountain Medical Center, 5121 South Cottonwood Street, Salt Lake City, UT 84107, USA; [b] Division of Pulmonary & Critical Care Medicine, Department of Internal Medicine, University of Utah School of Medicine, Salt Lake City, UT, USA; [c] Pharmacy Services, Intermountain Healthcare, 4393 S Riverboat Road, Taylorsville, UT 84123, USA
* Corresponding author. Division Pulmonary, Intermountain Medical Center, 5121 South Cottonwood Street, Murray, UT 84107.
E-mail address: Lindsay.Leither@imail.org

Med Clin N Am 106 (2022) 949–960
https://doi.org/10.1016/j.mcna.2022.08.002
0025-7125/22/© 2022 Elsevier Inc. All rights reserved.

the disease, subgroups of patients with severe or critical disease may benefit from antiviral therapy (**Fig. 1**).[5–9]

Morta among critically ill patients receiving invasive mechanical ventilation have varied significantly throughout the pandemic. Contemporary meta-analysis suggests that mortality in this population is around 45%, although notable heterogeneity exists among published cohorts.[10,11] Several studies have detected an association between increased mortality and case load or patient volumes, suggesting an impact of limited resources on outcomes.[12,13]

SUPPORTIVE CARE

The mainstay of treatment for all critically ill patients is high-quality supportive intensive care unit (ICU) care. In the most severe cases of COVID-19, patients develop acute respiratory failure meeting the Berlin definition[14] of acute respiratory distress syndrome (ARDS): (1) acute hypoxemic respiratory failure, (2) onset within 7 days, (3) bilateral opacities on imaging, (4) cardiac failure not the primary cause of respiratory failure. Early in the pandemic, some observers suggested that COVID-19 pneumonia did not cause "typical" ARDS based on the observation of relatively well-preserved lung mechanics despite severe hypoxemia.[15,16] However, other observers noted that prepandemic ARDS also had patients with near-normal compliance despite hypoxemia. Instead of a different ARDS specific to COVID-19, there is rising recognition that ARDS per se exists along a physiologic continuum.[17] As a consequence, standard ARDS therapies remain a critical part of treatment for severely ill COVID-19 patients. Invasive mechanical ventilation is a common therapy used to sustain patients with respiratory failure. However, mechanical ventilation can both improve survival and cause further lung damage. To best optimize outcomes, low-tidal-volume ventilation should be used, targeting 6 mL/kg predicted body weight.[18,19] Additional mechanical ventilation therapies to prioritize include targeting higher rather than lower positive end-expiratory pressure and limiting plateau pressure to ≤30 cmH$_2$O.[18,20] Early prone positioning of intubated patients improves survival

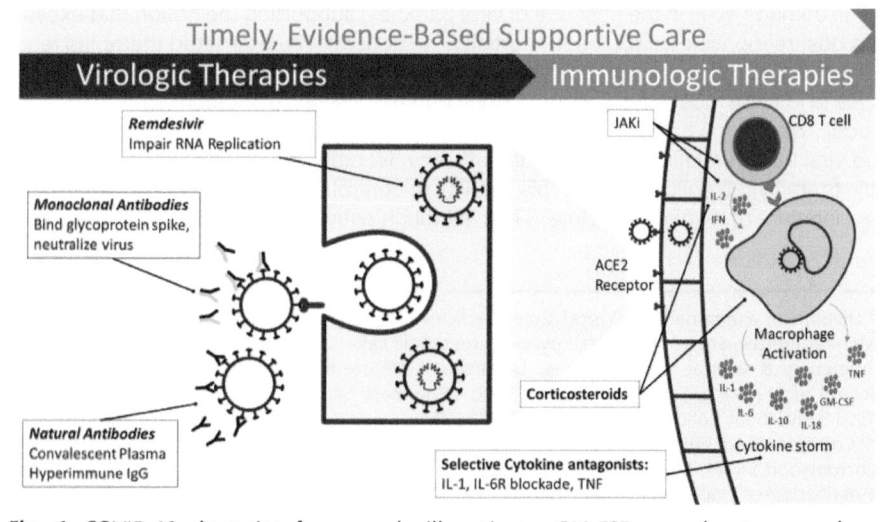

Fig. 1. COVID-19 therapies for severely ill patients. GM-CSF, granulocyte-macrophage colony-stimulating factor; IgG, immunoglobulin G; TNF, tumor necrosis factor. (*Courtesy of* Brandon Webb, MD, Intermountain Healthcare).

and has been an established therapy for patients with severe ARDS before the pandemic.[21] Although separate trials have not been performed in COVID-19 ARDS, prone positioning for patients with moderate to severe COVID-19 ARDS is in common use around the world. Restricted fluid management whereby fluid intake is limited and urinary output is increased also improves patient outcomes.[22,23]

The best noninvasive respiratory support strategy in patients not being treated with invasive mechanical ventilation remains unclear. The FLORALI trial, conducted before COVID-19, found significant mortality benefit from the use of high-flow nasal oxygen (HFNO) in patients with acute hypoxemic respiratory failure compared with standard oxygen or noninvasive ventilation.[24] However, the RECOVERY-RS trial in patients with COVID-19–related acute respiratory failure identified a significant decrease in intubation and mortality with the use of continuous positive airway pressure compared with HFNO or conventional oxygen.[25] Of note, RECOVERY-RS was not a study of the use of non-invasive ventilation for "rescue" of patients failing HFNO. Based on experience with intubated patients, many institutions have proposed prone positioning for nonintubated patients,[26,27] but data supporting this practice are controversial at best.[28–30] Although the role of extracorporeal membrane oxygenation (ECMO) in the treatment of ARDS remains unclear,[31] ECMO has been adopted as a rescue therapy option for management of severely ill COVID-19 patients at many institutions around the world.[32,33] This widespread adoption of ECMO has occurred without supporting trial evidence.

COVID-19–SPECIFIC THERAPIES

Pathophysiology of severe COVID-19 includes acute pneumonitis with extensive opacities, diffuse alveolar damage, and microthrombosis.[34] Additional host immune response is thought to play a role in perpetuating organ failure as evidenced by elevated inflammatory markers, such as ferritin, C-reactive protein, interleukin-1 (IL-1), and IL-6.[35,36] Early in the pandemic, therapeutic interventions targeting inflammatory organ injury were proposed, and the value of glucocorticoids was widely debated. Data regarding use of corticosteroids in viral respiratory infections before COVID-19 were mixed, and differing conclusions were drawn from meta-analysis.[37,38] GLUCO-COVID, an open-label trial, evaluated a 6-day course of methylprednisolone in 91 patients with SARS-CoV-2 receiving oxygen and evidence of systemic inflammation. This study suggested improved mortality but was severely underpowered.[39] More than 6000 patients were included in the RECOVERY trial, comparing up to 10 days of low-dose dexamethasone versus usual care. Dexamethasone was associated with decreased 28-day mortality among hospitalized patients, with the largest benefit in patients receiving supplemental oxygen and invasive mechanical ventilation (the trial did not distinguish conventional oxygen from HFNO).[40] A meta-analysis of other smaller trials suggested similar mortality benefit with glucocorticoids.[41] Therefore, glucocorticoids are now a mainstay of therapy for severely ill COVID-19 patients and is the only treatment with a strong recommendation in multiple international guidelines.[42–44]

The pathophysiology of severe COVID-19 plus the apparent benefit of glucocorticoids suggests that other immunomodulatory therapies may be beneficial. Tocilizumab is a recombinant anti-IL-6 receptor monoclonal antibody that inhibits the binding of IL-6 to receptors. Tocilizumab is licensed for autoimmune diseases, including cytokine release syndrome. Tocilizumab in COVID-19 has yielded strangely mixed results: placebo-controlled trials have been largely negative, whereas pragmatic unblinded trials suggested benefit in severe disease.[45–49] The largest trial included more than 4000 patients enrolled in the RECOVERY platform who were hospitalized and had evidence of systemic inflammation (C-reactive protein $\geq$75 mg/L). In this study, the addition of tocilizumab improved survival and other clinical outcomes, which persisted after control for level of respiratory support and concurrent systemic corticosteroids (82% of patients also received corticosteroids).[48] In addition, the pragmatic platform trial REMAP-CAP investigated both tocilizumab and sarilumab (another IL-6 receptor antagonist) in ~800 critically ill patients who were receiving organ support. IL-6 antagonists resulted in improved survival, increased organ support-free days, and other clinical outcomes. Nonetheless, several small to moderately sized randomized, placebo-controlled trials of hospitalized patients found no clinical benefit of tocilizumab.[46,47,50] Whether this discrepancy reflects type 2 error in the placebo-controlled trials, differences in target populations, or differences in therapeutic context is not clear. Given the lack of large safety signals, IL-6 antagonists may well be appropriate therapy for critically ill patients with COVID-19, particularly when started early in the course.

Remdesivir is a broad-spectrum antiviral with activity against coronaviruses. As a prodrug, it is converted to an adenosine analogue and acts as an inhibitor of the RNA polymerase found in SARS-CoV-2, which inhibits viral replication. Based on the PINETREE trial,[51] all major guidelines recommend remdesivir in nonsevere COVID-19 patients at high risk of hospitalization. Although the World Health Organization guidelines do not recommend remdesivir for hospitalized patients,[44] both the National Institutes of Health (NIH) and Infectious Diseases Society of America (IDSA) guidelines recommend the use of remdesivir for hospitalized patients receiving supplemental oxygen.[42,44,52] In patients receiving mechanical ventilation, the IDSA guidelines give a conditional recommendation against the routine initiation of remdesivir, whereas the NIH guidelines acknowledge differing opinions of panel members given the limited evidence. In 2 studies conducted predominantly in North America, remdesivir shortened the time to clinical improvement and reduced the likelihood for mechanical ventilation compared with placebo, with nonsignificant trends toward improved mortality.[53] However, improvement in mortality was not identified in international, pragmatic, open-label trials and one small, placebo-controlled trial conducted in China early in the pandemic.[54–56] Although most studies evaluated 10 days of therapy, 2 studies found comparable outcomes between patients randomized to 5 days or 10 days, and thus, many centers use shorter durations of therapy.[57,58] Earlier trials excluded patients with renal and hepatic dysfunction; however, the rate of renal and hepatic adverse events is low; effects are reversible, and observational studies support its use in these patient populations.[59] Although better data among critically ill patients would be useful, remdesivir appears reasonable to use, much as oseltamivir is commonly used in critically ill patients with influenza.

Janus kinase (JAK) 1 and 2 inhibit intracellular signaling pathways of cytokines, known to be elevated in COVID-19, act against the virus, and prevent viral cellular entry.[60–62] Baricitinib is an oral JAK 1 and 2 inhibitor, and, in combination with remdesivir, improves outcomes of hospitalized patients compared with remdesivir alone. In a multinational, double-blind, randomized, placebo-controlled trial, patients who received baricitinib and remdesivir had improved time to recovery, clinical status at 15 days, and mortality. This benefit was most notable in severely ill patients requiring high-flow nasal cannula and noninvasive ventilation.[63] Although in this trial corticosteroids were not administered for the treatment of COVID-19, another multicenter, double-blind, randomized, placebo-control trial found improved mortality when baricitinib was added to standard of care, which could include remdesivir (19% of participants) and dexamethasone (72% of participants).[64] Tofacitinib is another oral JAK inhibitor, which has been found in a multicenter, randomized placebo-control trial to lower risk of death or respiratory failure when given to hospitalized patients in addition to standard of care.[65] Overall, it appears that tofacitinib may have similar benefit to COVID-19 patients as baricitinib, although with the significantly smaller sample size, the level of certainty is lower.

Immune suppression with infliximab (a tumor necrosis factor inhibitor) and abatacept (a T-cell activation inhibitor) shows promising results in the randomized placebo-controlled ACTIV-1 trial. Compared with placebo, infliximab improved mortality with 40.5% lower adjusted odds of dying in patients hospitalized with COVID-19. Similarly, hospitalized patients receiving abatacept had 37.4% lower adjusted odds of dying compared with placebo.[66]

Serostatus, viral load, or both may be key factors contributing to efficacy of some therapies. Neutralizing monoclonal antibodies do not appear beneficial in "unselected" hospitalized patients.[8,67] However, increasing data suggest benefit in seronegative patients (ie, those who have not mounted their own humoral immune response). RECOVERY found seronegative hospitalized patients who received the REGEN-COV monoclonal antibody combination (casirivmab 4 g intravenously [IV] and imdevimab 4 g IV) plus usual care had improved mortality. This benefit was not seen in seropositive hospitalized patients.[68] Similarly, the ACTIV-3 bamlanivimab study group suggested difference in efficacy and safety of the monoclonal antibody bamlanivimab depending on serostatus and viral load, although the sample size was too small for definitive conclusions.[8] Based on available evidence, it seems wise to avoid administration of neutralizing monoclonal antibodies to seropositive inpatients. Where testing of serology is difficult to perform in a timely fashion, it may be difficult to administer such agents; valid point-of-care tests are an urgent priority.

Hypercoagulability together with severe inflammation related to COVID-19 infection is thought to contribute to multiorgan failure and death.[69] Thrombotic events are commonly reported in critically ill patients with COVID-19. Incidence ranges from about 22% to 60% in ICU patients, often despite use of standard prophylactic anticoagulation.[70–72] It is prudent to have a low threshold for evaluation for venous thromboembolism. Given the association of increased thrombotic risk in COVID-19, some early guidance recommended higher-dose anticoagulation for critically ill patients,[73] despite a lack of evidence at the time. A multiplatform, randomized clinical trial in hospitalized patients with COVID-19 compared therapeutic-dose heparin anticoagulation with usual care thromboprophylaxis. In noncritically ill patients, full-dose anticoagulation met its endpoint of more organ-support–free days, largely owing to a decrease in the use of HFNO.[74] However, full-dose anticoagulation was associated with a high likelihood of increased harm among critically ill patients receiving organ support.[75] In addition, intermediate-dose prophylaxis did not result in improved outcomes compared with standard-dose prophylaxis.[76] Therefore, based on the available evidence, standard thromboprophylaxis with diagnostic vigilance, rather than full-dose or intermediate-dose anticoagulation, should be used in critically ill patients with organ failure.

Limitations of all published studies include the constantly changing viral and therapeutic contexts of the pandemic, leading to a constantly changing standard of care (especially around immune suppression); limited data for most therapies in vaccinated patients; and a paucity of data for the most recent variants. Data suggest remdesivir maintains activity against Delta and Omicron[77]; however, as clinical disease varies, so may clinical effectiveness. Immunosuppressive agents are likely to remain effective across various strains; however, patient selection will remain critical to realize the intended benefits.

CRITICAL SHORTAGES

The COVID-19 pandemic has exposed critical supply shortages worldwide with a large influx of high-acuity patients requiring intensive care. The disruption in staff, equipment, and space contributes to complex interactions affecting patient care and outcomes.[78] Capacity strain includes patient census and volume, turnover, acuity, and workload.[78] Care of the critically ill patient requires a multidisciplinary team of clinicians, which can be challenging to replicate outside of traditional ICU settings when space becomes limited. Observational studies have demonstrated a relationship between strain on ICU resources and ICU patient outcomes. This can come in the form of ICU triage decisions,[79,80] adherence to guidelines,[81] timing of end-of-life discussions,[82] and mortality.[83] Despite the detrimental impact of strain and resource limitation, a counter-phenomenon is seen in the form of adaptation, whereby care and outcomes of patients improve over time through real-time learning.[78] This has been observed during the COVID-19 pandemic with decline in mortality over time, although population immunity and improved treatments also played a role in decreasing mortality over time.[84–86] As disruptions in availability of personnel, supplies, and space continue, health care systems will continue to find ways to mitigate the impact of capacity strain on care delivery and outcomes.

COMPLICATIONS

Patients with COVID-19 are at risk for invasive fungal diseases, such as aspergillus and mucor. COVID-19–associated pulmonary aspergillosis (CAPA) is seen in critically ill, mechanically ventilated patients and is associated with worse patient outcomes.[87,88] The European Confederation for Medical Mycology and the International Society for Human and Animal Mycology developed consensus criteria for the diagnosis of proven, probable, and possible CAPA, which relies on a combination of microbiology, imaging, and clinical data.[89] Of note, serum galactomannan alone is not reliable owing to low sensitivity, and radiographic imaging alone is not sufficient even in the presence of a halo sign. Recommended first-line treatment is either voriconazole or isavuconazole, with liposomal amphotericin B reserved for those with contraindications, poor response, or azole-resistant strains.

Another rare, poorly understood phenomenon is multisystem inflammatory syndrome in adults (MIS-A). Similar to multisystem inflammatory syndrome in children (MIS-C), key features include recent COVID-19 infection, often after a period of recovery; elevated inflammatory markers; and multisystem end-organ damage. Although differentiating between MIS-A and a biphasic presentation of acute COVID-19 remains a challenge, the Centers for Disease Control and Prevention (CDC) has developed diagnostic criteria.[90] The CDC's definition of MIS-A requires a fever plus rash with nonpurulent conjunctivitis or severe cardiac illness with additional clinical and laboratory criteria within the first 3 days of hospitalization. Patel and colleagues[91] have published the largest case series to date (>200 patients with MIS-A), of which more than half were admitted to the ICU and received vasoactive medication for severe hypotension. No clear treatment recommendations have been established in adults, but given the similarities with MIS-C, treatment recommendations by the American College of Rheumatology for MIS-C are often used, which includes IV immunoglobulin plus corticosteroids as the backbone with intensification of immunomodulatory treatments, such as anakinra and infliximab, for poor responders.[92]

SUMMARY

Since the beginning of the pandemic, COVID-19 treatment approaches have evolved substantially. Current standard of care for the COVID-19 patient in the ICU includes corticosteroids with or without remdesivir and secondary immunosuppression, in addition to high-quality supportive care. As scientific knowledge continues to grow, care of the critically ill patient with COVID-19 will continue to improve and evolve. Although there is still much to be learned about the optimal use of supportive care and COVID-19–specific therapies, it is a testament to modern medicine and the hard work of investigators around the world that treatment options are available.

CLINICS CARE POINTS

- COVID-19 therapies include virologic and immunologic therapies with anti-viral medications having most therapeutic impactful earlier in the course of illness. Glucocorticoids are an important immunologic therapy targeting inflammatory organ injury.
- Established acute respiratory distress syndrome therapies including lung protective ventilator management strategies, fluid management and prone positioning are important interventions.
- Based on available evidence, standard dose thromboprophylaxis, rather than full-dose or intermediate-dose anticoagulation, should be used along with diagnostic vigilance in critically ill patients with organ failure.

DISCLOSURE

Dr S.M. Brown reports royalties from Oxford University Press, research support from the National Institutes of Health, the Department of Defense, Faron, Sedana Medical, and Janssen, and payment for data safety monitoring board membership from New York University and Hamilton. Other authors report no conflicts of interest.

REFERENCES

1. McElvaney OJ, McEvoy NL, McElvaney OF, et al. Characterization of the Inflammatory Response to Severe COVID-19 Illness. Am J Respir Crit Care Med 2020; 202(6):812–21.
2. Du RH, Liu LM, Yin W, et al. Hospitalization and Critical Care of 109 Decedents with COVID-19 Pneumonia in Wuhan, China. Ann Am Thorac Soc 2020;17(7): 839–46.
3. Chalmers JD, Chotirmall SH. Rewiring the Immune Response in COVID-19. Am J Respir Crit Care Med 2020;202(6):784–6.
4. Dorward DA, Russell CD, Um IH, et al. Tissue-Specific Immunopathology in Fatal COVID-19. Am J Respir Crit Care Med 2021;203(2):192–201.
5. Gutmann C, Takov K, Burnap SA, et al. SARS-CoV-2 RNAemia and proteomic trajectories inform prognostication in COVID-19 patients admitted to intensive care. Nat Commun 2021;12(1):3406.
6. Bermejo-Martin JF, González-Rivera M, Almansa R, et al. Viral RNA load in plasma is associated with critical illness and a dysregulated host response in COVID-19. Crit Care 2020;24(1):691.
7. Fajnzylber J, Regan J, Coxen K, et al. SARS-CoV-2 viral load is associated with increased disease severity and mortality. Nat Commun 2020;11(1):5493.

8. Lundgren JD, Grund B, Barkauskas CE, et al. Responses to a Neutralizing Monoclonal Antibody for Hospitalized Patients With COVID-19 According to Baseline Antibody and Antigen Levels: A Randomized Controlled Trial. Ann Intern Med 2022;175(2):234–43.

9. Ram-Mohan N, Kim D, Zudock EJ, et al. SARS-CoV-2 RNAemia Predicts Clinical Deterioration and Extrapulmonary Complications from COVID-19. Clin Infect Dis 2022;74(2):218–26.

10. Angriman F, Scales DC. Estimating the Case Fatality Risk of COVID-19 among Mechanically Ventilated Patients. Am J Respir Crit Care Med 2021;203(1):3–4.

11. Lim ZJ, Subramaniam A, Ponnapa Reddy M, et al. Case Fatality Rates for Patients with COVID-19 Requiring Invasive Mechanical Ventilation. A Meta-analysis. Am J Respir Crit Care Med 2021;203(1):54–66.

12. Doidge JC, Gould DW, Ferrando-Vivas P, et al. Trends in Intensive Care for Patients with COVID-19 in England, Wales, and Northern Ireland. Am J Respir Crit Care Med 2021;203(5):565–74. https://doi.org/10.1164/rccm.202008-3212OC.

13. Churpek MM, Gupta S, Spicer AB, et al. Hospital-Level Variation in Death for Critically Ill Patients with COVID-19. Am J Respir Crit Care Med 2021;204(403–411): 403–11. https://doi.org/10.1164/rccm.202012-4547OC.

14. Ranieri VM, Rubenfeld GD, Thompson BT, et al. Acute respiratory distress syndrome: the Berlin Definition. JAMA 2012;307(23):2526–33. https://doi.org/10.1001/jama.2012.5669.

15. Gattinoni L, Coppola S, Cressoni M, et al. COVID-19 Does Not Lead to a "Typical" Acute Respiratory Distress Syndrome. Am J Respir Crit Care Med 2020;201(10): 1299–300. https://doi.org/10.1164/rccm.202003-0817LE.

16. Gattinoni L, Chiumello D, Rossi S. COVID-19 pneumonia: ARDS or not? Crit Care 2020;24(1):154.

17. Gattinoni L, Gattarello S, Steinberg I, et al. COVID-19 pneumonia: pathophysiology and management. Eur Respir Rev 2021;30(162). https://doi.org/10.1183/16000617.0138-2021.

18. Fan E, Del Sorbo L, Goligher EC, et al. An Official American Thoracic Society/European Society of Intensive Care Medicine/Society of Critical Care Medicine Clinical Practice Guideline: Mechanical Ventilation in Adult Patients with Acute Respiratory Distress Syndrome. Am J Respir Crit Care Med 2017;195(9): 1253–63.

19. ARDSNetwork. Ventilation with lower tidal volumes as compared with traditional tidal volumes for acute lung injury and the acute respiratory distress syndrome. The Acute Respiratory Distress Syndrome Network. N Engl J Med 2000; 342(18):1301–8.

20. Briel M, Meade M, Mercat A, et al. Higher vs lower positive end-expiratory pressure in patients with acute lung injury and acute respiratory distress syndrome: systematic review and meta-analysis. JAMA 2010;303(9):865–73.

21. Guérin C, Reignier J, Richard JC, et al. Prone positioning in severe acute respiratory distress syndrome. N Engl J Med 2013;368(23):2159–68.

22. Grissom CK, Hirshberg EL, Dickerson JB, et al. Fluid management with a simplified conservative protocol for the acute respiratory distress syndrome. Crit Care Med 2015;43(2):288–95.

23. Wiedemann HP, Wheeler AP, Bernard GR, et al. Comparison of two fluid-management strategies in acute lung injury. N Engl J Med 2006;354(24):2564–75.

24. Frat JP, Thille AW, Mercat A, et al. High-flow oxygen through nasal cannula in acute hypoxemic respiratory failure. N Engl J Med 2015;372(23):2185–96.

25. Perkins GD, Ji C, Connolly BA, et al. Effect of Noninvasive Respiratory Strategies on Intubation or Mortality Among Patients With Acute Hypoxemic Respiratory Failure and COVID-19: The RECOVERY-RS Randomized Clinical Trial. JAMA 2022; 327(6):546–58.

26. Taylor SP, Bundy H, Smith WM, et al. Awake Prone Positioning Strategy for Nonintubated Hypoxic Patients with COVID-19: A Pilot Trial with Embedded Implementation Evaluation. Ann Am Thorac Soc 2021;18(8):1360–8.

27. Klaiman T, Silvestri JA, Srinivasan T, et al. Improving Prone Positioning for Severe Acute Respiratory Distress Syndrome during the COVID-19 Pandemic. An Implementation-Mapping Approach. Ann Am Thorac Soc 2021;18(2):300–7.

28. Thompson AE, Ranard BL, Wei Y, et al. Prone Positioning in Awake, Nonintubated Patients With COVID-19 Hypoxemic Respiratory Failure. JAMA Intern Med 2020; 180(11):1537–9.

29. Rosén J, von Oelreich E, Fors D, et al. Awake prone positioning in patients with hypoxemic respiratory failure due to COVID-19: the PROFLO multicenter randomized clinical trial. Crit Care 2021;25(1):209.

30. Qian ET, Gatto CL, Amusina O, et al. Assessment of Awake Prone Positioning in Hospitalized Adults With COVID-19: A Nonrandomized Controlled Trial. JAMA Intern Med 2022;182(6):612–21.

31. Li X, Scales DC, Kavanagh BP. Unproven and Expensive before Proven and Cheap: Extracorporeal Membrane Oxygenation versus Prone Position in Acute Respiratory Distress Syndrome. Am J Respir Crit Care Med 2018;197(8):991–3.

32. Diaz RA, Graf J, Zambrano JM, et al. Extracorporeal Membrane Oxygenation for COVID-19-associated Severe Acute Respiratory Distress Syndrome in Chile: A Nationwide Incidence and Cohort Study. Am J Respir Crit Care Med 2021; 204(1):34–43.

33. Karagiannidis C, Strassmann S, Merten M, et al. High In-Hospital Mortality Rate in Patients with COVID-19 Receiving Extracorporeal Membrane Oxygenation in Germany: A Critical Analysis. Am J Respir Crit Care Med 2021;204(8):991–4.

34. Ackermann M, Verleden SE, Kuehnel M, et al. Pulmonary Vascular Endothelialitis, Thrombosis, and Angiogenesis in Covid-19. N Engl J Med 2020;383(2):120–8.

35. Ruan Q, Yang K, Wang W, et al. Clinical predictors of mortality due to COVID-19 based on an analysis of data of 150 patients from Wuhan, China. Intensive Care Med 2020;46(5):846–8.

36. Huang C, Wang Y, Li X, et al. Clinical features of patients infected with 2019 novel coronavirus in Wuhan, China. Lancet 2020;395(10223):497–506.

37. Russell CD, Millar JE, Baillie JK. Clinical evidence does not support corticosteroid treatment for 2019-nCoV lung injury. Lancet 2020;395(10223):473–5.

38. Shang L, Zhao J, Hu Y, et al. On the use of corticosteroids for 2019-nCoV pneumonia. Lancet 2020;395(10225):683–4.

39. Corral-Gudino L, Bahamonde A, Arnaiz-Revillas F, et al. Methylprednisolone in adults hospitalized with COVID-19 pneumonia: An open-label randomized trial (GLUCOCOVID). Wien Klin Wochenschr 2021;133(7–8):303–11.

40. Horby P, Lim WS, Emberson JR, et al. Dexamethasone in Hospitalized Patients with Covid-19. N Engl J Med 2021;384(8):693–704.

41. Sterne JAC, Murthy S, Diaz JV, et al. Association Between Administration of Systemic Corticosteroids and Mortality Among Critically Ill Patients With COVID-19: A Meta-analysis. JAMA 2020;324(13):1330–41.

42. Infectious Disease Society of America. IDSA Guidelines on the Treatment and Management of Patients with COVID-19. https://www.idsociety.org/practice-

guideline/covid-19-guideline-treatment-and-management/. Accessed 31 May 2022.

43. National Institutes of Health. Clinical Management Summary. Available at: https:// www.covid19treatmentguidelines.nih.gov/management/clinical-management/ clinical-management-summary/?utm_source=site&utm_medium=home&utm_ campaign=highlights. Accessed May 31, 2022.

44. World Health Organization. Therapeutics and COVID-19: living guideline. https:// www.who.int/publications/i/item/WHO-2019-nCoV-therapeutics-2022.3. Accessed 31 May 2022.

45. Salama C, Han J, Yau L, et al. Tocilizumab in Patients Hospitalized with Covid-19 Pneumonia. N Engl J Med 2021;384(1):20–30.

46. Rosas IO, Diaz G, Gottlieb RL, et al. Tocilizumab and remdesivir in hospitalized patients with severe COVID-19 pneumonia: a randomized clinical trial. Intensive Care Med 2021;47(11):1258–70.

47. Rosas IO, Bräu N, Waters M, et al. Tocilizumab in Hospitalized Patients with Severe Covid-19 Pneumonia. N Engl J Med 2021;384(16):1503–16.

48. Tocilizumab in patients admitted to hospital with COVID-19 (RECOVERY): a randomised, controlled, open-label, platform trial. Lancet 2021;397(10285):1637–45.

49. Gordon AC, Mouncey PR, Al-Beidh F, et al. Interleukin-6 Receptor Antagonists in Critically Ill Patients with Covid-19. N Engl J Med 2021;384(16):1491–502.

50. Stone JH, Frigault MJ, Serling-Boyd NJ, et al. Efficacy of Tocilizumab in Patients Hospitalized with Covid-19. N Engl J Med 2020;383(24):2333–44.

51. Gottlieb RL, Vaca CE, Paredes R, et al. Early Remdesivir to Prevent Progression to Severe Covid-19 in Outpatients. N Engl J Med 2022;386(4):305–15.

52. National Institutes of Health. COVID-19 Treatment Guidelines: Remdesivir. https:// www.covid19treatmentguidelines.nih.gov/therapies/antiviral-therapy/remdesivir/. Accessed May 31, 2022.

53. Beigel JH, Tomashek KM, Dodd LE, et al. Remdesivir for the Treatment of Covid-19 - Final Report. N Engl J Med 2020;383(19):1813–26.

54. Wang Y, Zhang D, Du G, et al. Remdesivir in adults with severe COVID-19: a randomised, double-blind, placebo-controlled, multicentre trial. Lancet 2020; 395(10236):1569–78.

55. Ader F, Bouscambert-Duchamp M, Hites M, et al. Remdesivir plus standard of care versus standard of care alone for the treatment of patients admitted to hospital with COVID-19 (DisCoVeRy): a phase 3, randomised, controlled, open-label trial. Lancet Infect Dis 2022;22(2):209–21.

56. Pan H, Peto R, Henao-Restrepo AM, et al. Repurposed Antiviral Drugs for Covid-19 - Interim WHO Solidarity Trial Results. N Engl J Med 2021;384(6):497–511.

57. Goldman JD, Lye DCB, Hui DS, et al. Remdesivir for 5 or 10 Days in Patients with Severe Covid-19. N Engl J Med 2020;383(19):1827–37.

58. Spinner CD, Gottlieb RL, Criner GJ, et al. Effect of Remdesivir vs Standard Care on Clinical Status at 11 Days in Patients With Moderate COVID-19: A Randomized Clinical Trial. JAMA 2020;324(11):1048–57.

59. van Laar SA, de Boer MGJ, Gombert-Handoko KB, et al. Liver and kidney function in patients with Covid-19 treated with remdesivir. Br J Clin Pharmacol 2021; 87(11):4450–4.

60. Stebbing J, Krishnan V, de Bono S, et al. Mechanism of baricitinib supports artificial intelligence-predicted testing in COVID-19 patients. EMBO Mol Med 2020; 12(8):e12697.

61. Sims JT, Krishnan V, Chang C-Y, et al. Characterization of the cytokine storm reflects hyperinflammatory endothelial dysfunction in COVID-19. J Allergy Clin Immunol 2021;147(1):107–11.

62. Hoang TN, Pino M, Boddapati AK, et al. Baricitinib treatment resolves lower-airway macrophage inflammation and neutrophil recruitment in SARS-CoV-2-infected rhesus macaques. Cell 2021;184(2):460–75, e21.

63. Kalil AC, Patterson TF, Mehta AK, et al. Baricitinib plus Remdesivir for Hospitalized Adults with Covid-19. N Engl J Med 2021;384(9):795–807.

64. Marconi VC, Ramanan AV, de Bono S, et al. Efficacy and safety of baricitinib for the treatment of hospitalised adults with COVID-19 (COV-BARRIER): a randomised, double-blind, parallel-group, placebo-controlled phase 3 trial. Lancet Respir Med 2021;9(12):1407–18.

65. Guimarães PO, Quirk D, Furtado RH, et al. Tofacitinib in Patients Hospitalized with Covid-19 Pneumonia. N Engl J Med 2021;385(5):406–15.

66. NCfAT Sciences. Immue Modulator Drugs Improved Survival for People Hospitalized with COVID-19. Available at: https://ncats.nih.gov/news/releases/2022/Immune-Modulator-Drugs-Improved-Survival-for-People-Hospitalized-with-COVID-19. Accessed June 9, 2022.

67. Efficacy and safety of two neutralising monoclonal antibody therapies, sotrovimab and BRII-196 plus BRII-198, for adults hospitalised with COVID-19 (TICO): a randomised controlled trial. Lancet Infect Dis 2021. https://doi.org/10.1016/s1473-3099(21)00751-9.

68. Casirivimab and imdevimab in patients admitted to hospital with COVID-19 (RECOVERY): a randomised, controlled, open-label, platform trial. Lancet 2022; 399(10325):665–76.

69. Panigada M, Bottino N, Tagliabue P, et al. Hypercoagulability of COVID-19 patients in intensive care unit: A report of thromboelastography findings and other parameters of hemostasis. J Thromb Haemost 2020;18(7):1738–42.

70. Klok FA, Kruip M, van der Meer NJM, et al. Incidence of thrombotic complications in critically ill ICU patients with COVID-19. Thromb Res 2020;191:145–7.

71. Middeldorp S, Coppens M, van Haaps TF, et al. Incidence of venous thromboembolism in hospitalized patients with COVID-19. J Thromb Haemost 2020;18(8): 1995–2002.

72. Nopp S, Moik F, Jilma B, et al. Risk of venous thromboembolism in patients with COVID-19: A systematic review and meta-analysis. Res Pract Thromb Haemost 2020;4(7):1178–91.

73. National Institute for Health and Care Excellence. Clinical Guidelines. *COVID-19 rapid guideline: reducing the risk of venous thromboembolism in over 16s with COVID-19*. London: National Institute for Health and Care Excellence (NICE) Copyright © NICE 2020.; 2020.

74. Lawler PR, Goligher EC, Berger JS, et al. Therapeutic Anticoagulation with Heparin in Noncritically Ill Patients with Covid-19. N Engl J Med 2021;385(9):790–802.

75. Goligher EC, Bradbury CA, McVerry BJ, et al. Therapeutic Anticoagulation with Heparin in Critically Ill Patients with Covid-19. N Engl J Med 2021;385(9):777–89.

76. Sadeghipour P, Talasaz AH, Rashidi F, et al. Effect of Intermediate-Dose vs Standard-Dose Prophylactic Anticoagulation on Thrombotic Events, Extracorporeal Membrane Oxygenation Treatment, or Mortality Among Patients With COVID-19 Admitted to the Intensive Care Unit: The INSPIRATION Randomized Clinical Trial. JAMA 2021;325(16):1620–30.

77. Pitts J, Li J, Perry JK, et al. Remdesivir and GS-441524 retain antiviral activity against Delta, Omicron, and other emergent SARS-CoV-2 variants. bioRxiv 2022;2022:479840.

78. Anesi GL, Kerlin MP. The impact of resource limitations on care delivery and outcomes: routine variation, the coronavirus disease 2019 pandemic, and persistent shortage. Curr Opin Crit Care 2021;27(5):513–9.

79. Anesi GL, Chowdhury M, Small DS, et al. Association of a novel index of hospital capacity strain with admission to intensive care units. Ann Am Thorac Soc 2020; 17(11):1440–7.

80. Anesi GL, Liu VX, Gabler NB, et al. Associations of intensive care unit capacity strain with disposition and outcomes of patients with sepsis presenting to the emergency department. Ann Am Thorac Soc 2018;15(11):1328–35.

81. Weissman GE, Gabler NB, Brown SE, et al. Intensive care unit capacity strain and adherence to prophylaxis guidelines. J Crit Care 2015;30(6):1303–9.

82. Hua M, Halpern SD, Gabler NB, et al. Effect of ICU strain on timing of limitations in life-sustaining therapy and on death. Intensive Care Med 2016;42(6):987–94.

83. Gabler NB, Ratcliffe SJ, Wagner J, et al. Mortality among patients admitted to strained intensive care units. Am J Respir Crit Care Med 2013;188(7):800–6.

84. Auld SC, Caridi-Scheible M, Robichaux C, et al. Declines in mortality over time for critically ill adults with COVID-19. Crit Care Med 2020;48(12):e1382.

85. Armstrong R, Kane A, Cook T. Outcomes from intensive care in patients with COVID-19: a systematic review and meta-analysis of observational studies. Anaesthesia 2020;75(10):1340–9.

86. Asch DA, Sheils NE, Islam MN, et al. Variation in US hospital mortality rates for patients admitted with COVID-19 during the first 6 months of the pandemic. JAMA Intern Med 2021;181(4):471–8.

87. White PL, Dhillon R, Cordey A, et al. A National Strategy to Diagnose Coronavirus Disease 2019-Associated Invasive Fungal Disease in the Intensive Care Unit. Clin Infect Dis 2021;73(7):e1634–44.

88. Permpalung N, Chiang TP, Massie AB, et al. Coronavirus Disease 2019-Associated Pulmonary Aspergillosis in Mechanically Ventilated Patients. Clin Infect Dis 2022;74(1):83–91.

89. Koehler P, Bassetti M, Chakrabarti A, et al. Defining and managing COVID-19-associated pulmonary aspergillosis: the 2020 ECMM/ISHAM consensus criteria for research and clinical guidance. Lancet Infect Dis 2021;21(6):e149–62.

90. Centers for Disease Control and Prevention. Multisystem Inflammatory Syndrome in Adults (MIS-A) Case Definition Information for Healthcare Providers. Available at: https://www.cdc.gov/mis/mis-a/hcp.html. Accessed May 31, 2022.

91. Patel P, DeCuir J, Abrams J, et al. Clinical Characteristics of Multisystem Inflammatory Syndrome in Adults: A Systematic Review. JAMA Netw Open 2021;4(9): e2126456.

92. Henderson LA, Canna SW, Friedman KG, et al. American College of Rheumatology Clinical Guidance for Multisystem Inflammatory Syndrome in Children Associated With SARS-CoV-2 and Hyperinflammation in Pediatric COVID-19: Version 3. Arthritis Rheumatol 2022;74(4):e1–20.

The Role of Long-Term Noninvasive Ventilation in Chronic Stable Hypercapnic Chronic Obstructive Pulmonary Disease

Madalina Macrea, MD, PhD, MPH[a,b,*], John M. Coleman III, MD[c]

KEYWORDS

- Chronic obstructive pulmonary disease • Chronic hypercapnia
- Non-invasive ventilation • Chronic obstructive pulmonary disease and obstructive sleep apnea overlap syndrome

KEY POINTS

- Noninvasive ventilation (NIV) should be considered for patients with severe stable chronic obstructive pulmonary disease (COPD) already on maximal pharmacotherapy who have evidence of chronic hypercapnia ($PaCO_2 > 52$ mm Hg).
- The initial assessment for home NIV use could be completed as outpatient, 2 to 4 weeks after the resolution of the acute-on-chronic hypercapnic respiratory failure episode rather than during in-hospital admission for the acute event.
- Questionnaire-based screening for obstructive sleep apnea (OSA) should be considered for patients with chronic stable hypercapnic COPD to evaluate for COPD–OSA overlap syndrome.
- The use of NIV in severe stable COPD is a covered benefit by the United States Center for Medicare and Medicaid Services when certain criteria are met.
- The NIV management for severe stable COPD is complex and assistance from a pulmonary or sleep specialist is often required.

Despite improvements in pharmacotherapy, pulmonary rehabilitation and campaigns for smoking cessation, chronic obstructive pulmonary disease (COPD) remains a major cause of disability and the third leading cause of death in the United States.[1] Noninvasive ventilation (NIV) has the potential to improve clinical outcomes in a

[a] Division of Pulmonary and Sleep Medicine, Salem Veterans Affairs Medical Center, 1970 Roanoke Boulevard, Salem, VA 24153, USA; [b] Department of Medicine, University of Virginia, Charlottesville, VA 22913, USA; [c] Division of Pulmonary and Critical Care Medicine, Department of Neurology, Northwestern University Feinberg School of Medicine, 676 North St. Clair, Arkes Pavilion, Suite 1400, Chicago, IL 60611, USA
* Corresponding author.
E-mail address: Madalina.Macrea@va.gov

Med Clin N Am 106 (2022) 961–969
https://doi.org/10.1016/j.mcna.2022.07.004
0025-7125/22/Published by Elsevier Inc.
medical.theclinics.com

subcategory of COPD patients with severe disease and chronic stable hypercapnic respiratory [3]failure.

INTRODUCTION

The use of NIV in patients with acute hypercapnic respiratory failure during a COPD exacerbation is supported by strong evidence and currently accepted as the standard of care. In contrast, the evidence for the benefit of NIV in patients with COPD and chronic hypercapnic respiratory failure is more heterogenous and yet to be widely translated in clinical practice. In select patients, NIV has the potential to improve physiologic parameters (lung function, gas exchange), clinical symptoms (functional capacity, dyspnea, quality of life), and outcomes (hospital readmission, survival).[2] When considering data from current trials, it is important to delineate the COPD phenotype that would benefit most from NIV. This review will focus on the evidence for NIV use in the following groups of patients with severe COPD: those with chronic stable hypercapnic respiratory failure, those who recover from an episode of acute-on-chronic hypercapnic respiratory failure, and those with obstructive sleep apnea (OSA) disease (COPD–OSA overlap syndrome). In addition, there will be an overview of the 2 major categories of NIV devices, a summary of the current clinical practice guidelines on this topic, and answers to common clinical practice questions.

NATURE OF THE PROBLEM
Chronic Hypercapnic Respiratory Failure

Chronic hypercapnic respiratory failure, or chronic hypercapnia is common in severe COPD with a reported prevalence ranging from 23% to 38%. The optimal definition of "stable chronic hypercapnia" is still unclear. Most frequently, it is defined as a $PaCO_2$ above 45 mm Hg either chronically or after a minimum period of 2 to 4 weeks following a COPD exacerbation.[4] The mechanisms underlying the development of chronic hypercapnia in COPD are several and frequently overlap. Mechanical inefficiencies, gas exchange imbalances, and expiratory flow limitation are a few of the etiologies that contribute to increased work of ventilation in this population.[5] The relative importance of these specific pathophysiologic derangements on the development of chronic hypercapnia are not yet clearly delineated.[6] Despite that, the prognostic implications of chronic hypercapnia are well acknowledged and include impaired health-related quality of life,[7] increased COPD exacerbations and hospitalizations, and poorer survival. Conceptually, the goal of NIV in COPD is to unload respiratory muscles for prolonged periods of time, typically during sleep and reduce chronic hypercapnia through decreased mechanical load/capability imbalances.[8] With the introduction of high-intensity NIV, which is defined as specific settings aimed at achieving normocapnia or the lowest $PaCO_2$ values possible, both physiologic and clinical benefits of long-term NIV have been shown in chronic hypercapnic COPD.[8]

Chronic Obstructive Pulmonary Disease Exacerbations and Hospitalizations

In the United States, acute exacerbations of COPD (AECOPD) account for more than 10 million unscheduled visits per year with associated direct costs exceeding 16 billion dollars per year.[9] AECOPD have a direct effect on the disease progression and outcomes, including accelerated lung function decline, reduced health-related quality of life, and mortality. The survival rate following AECOPD requiring hospitalizations is significantly decreased, as 8% of these patients are dying during the hospital stay and another 23% are dying within the first year after hospitalization. Long-term use of oral corticosteroids, higher $PaCO_2$, and older age are identified as risk factors associated with higher mortality.[10] Moreover, the number of acute COPD exacerbations could predict the future long-term rate of exacerbations and risk of death. In a large population-based study of patients with COPD with up to 10 years of follow-up (mean, 4.9 years), 2 or more moderate AECOPD were associated with an increased risk of death in a graduated fashion, ranging from 10% (for 2 moderate AECOPDs) to 57% higher (for 5 or more moderate AECOPDs), compared with those with no AECOPDs at baseline.[11] These disappointing outcomes raised the question of whether and when long-term NIV should be initiated after an admission to the hospital due to AECOPD.[2]

Chronic Obstructive Pulmonary Disease– Obstructive Sleep Apnea Overlap Syndrome

Obstructive sleep apnea (OSA) is a disease characterized by repetitive episodes of upper airway closure during sleep. The COPD–OSA overlap syndrome (OS) had been reported in up to 65% in a pulmonary rehabilitation population with moderate to severe COPD (mean FEV1, 42%; 39% on long-term oxygen therapy).[12] However, the true OS prevalence in those with severe COPD (ie, those most likely to qualify for NIV) is not exactly known. During sleep, patients with OS have higher frequency of nocturnal oxygen desaturations and longer total sleep time with hypoxemia and hypercapnia than patients with OSA alone. These pathophysiologic features increase the risks of arrhythmias, pulmonary hypertension, and right-sided heart failure.[13–15] A landmark trial showed that, after a median follow-up of over 9 years, all-cause and cardiovascular mortality was higher in the untreated OS group (42.2%) (no continuous positive airway pressure therapy, CPAP) than in the COPD-only group (24.2%).[16] Therefore, patients with COPD ideally would undergo questionnaire-based screening for OSA because, if present, treatment with CPAP is associated with improved outcomes.[4]

A BRIEF DESCRIPTION OF HOW NONINVASIVE VENTILATION WORKS

NIV is a form of mechanical ventilation support that does not require an artificial airway (ie, endotracheal tube or tracheostomy). It is used with an interface that provides ventilation support through either the nose or nose and mouth.[17] The device provides a positive inspiratory pressure to assist during inhalation, commonly called the inspiratory positive airway pressure (IPAP) and an expiratory pressure during exhalation, commonly called the expiratory positive airway pressure (EPAP). This type of NIPPV is commonly called bilevel ventilation or BPAP. The difference between the IPAP and the EPAP is known as pressure support (PS). The larger the PS, the more augmented the inhaled tidal volume.[18]

Bilevel NIPPV can be divided into two large categories, spontaneous (BPAP-S) and spontaneous-timed (BPAP-ST). Spontaneous modes do not have a back-up rate and the device only provides support on breaths initiated by the patient. If there is no drive to breathe, the machine is ineffective. Spontaneous-timed modes do include a back-up breath rate and will augment breaths triggered by the patient and when breath is absent, provide more consistent full ventilation support.[19] Volume assured pressure support (VAPS) is a type of spontaneous-timed ventilation, by which PS is adjusted to achieve a previously determined respiratory target, either tidal volume or alveolar ventilation (18).

When discussing NIV, it is important to delineate the differences between modes of ventilation (BPAP-S, BPAP-ST, VAPS) and devices that deliver these modes. There are two major categories of NIV devices: respiratory assist devices (RAD) and home mechanical ventilators (HMV). RAD devices are more common and can be used for CPAP and BPAP (S and ST). These devices can only have one active mode of ventilation, they need to be plugged into a wall for power, and there is a limit to the amount of allowed pressure. HMV devices have an internal battery because they are life-sustaining devices, thus there are multiple options for active modes and there is no limit for pressure. Both devices can provide NIV, but the documentation required to obtain both under insurance are quite different.[20]

CURRENT CLINICAL PRACTICE GUIDELINES

The available evidence for the use of NIV in stable patients with COPD and chronic hypercapnia (FEV_1/FVC < 0.70 and resting $PaCO_2$ > 45 mm Hg; not during exacerbation) has been summarized in a recently published American Thoracic Society (ATS) Clinical Practice Guideline. This ATS guideline focused on delineating the subgroups who might benefit from NIV therapy, along with the optimal timing, location, and settings for NIV initiation. The equally recent "European Respiratory Society Guideline on Long-term Home Non-Invasive Ventilation for Management of Chronic Obstructive Pulmonary Disease" provided additional information related to the factors that could impact NIV effectiveness and adherence, including patients' baseline comorbidities and discomfort with NIV equipment.[21]

The available data on NIV use in patients with COPD and chronic hypercapnia are clinically heterogeneous, and include a wide range of baseline disease severity and interventions (use of oxygen therapy in the control groups) and diverse modes of ventilation and pressure settings. Thus, the certainty of evidence for the data included in the 2020 ATS Clinical Practice Guideline entitled "Long-Term Noninvasive Ventilation in Chronic Stable Hypercapnic Chronic Obstructive Pulmonary Disease" was mostly low, and as such, the recommendations were "conditional." For clinicians, this implies that "different choices are likely to be appropriate for different patients and that therapy should be tailored to the individual patient's circumstances."[19]

Recommendations Regarding the Use of Nocturnal Non-invasive Ventilation in Addition to Usual Care in Patients with Chronic Stable Hypercapnic Chronic Obstructive Pulmonary Disease

Pooled analyses have shown that NIV use resulted in a 14% decrease in the mortality risk compared with those receiving usual care (RR, 0.86; 95% CI, 0.6 to 1.3) as well as reductions in hospitalizations (MD, 1.26 fewer; 95% CI, 2.6 fewer to 0.1 more hospitalizations). There were consistent improvements in the quality of life (standard MD [SMD], 0.48; 95% CI, 0.1 to 0.9) and dyspnea (SMD, 20.51; 95% CI, 21 to 20) with NIV use. No serious adverse events were found. However, if NIV with targeted normalization of $PaCO_2$ is implemented, then the potential negative effects on cardiac hemodynamics (decreased perfusion) need to be considered, given the use of high inspiratory pressures and higher-than-baseline respiratory rates.[22]

Recommendations Regarding the Location and Timing of Non-invasive Ventilation Initiation After an Episode of Acute-on-Chronic Hypercapnic Respiratory Failure

In 2 landmark studies, respiratory support in COPD after acute exacerbation (RESCUE)[23] and home oxygen therapy–home mechanical ventilation (HOT-HMV),[24] up to 21% of patients who were hypercapnic at hospital discharge were no longer hypercapnic after 2 to 4 weeks. In addition, Duiverman and colleagues[25] showed that the home initiation of NIV in stable hypercapnic COPD patients was cost-effective and noninferior to in-hospital initiation. These data favor the location and timing of the assessment for home NIV use as outpatient, 2 to 4 weeks after the resolution of the acute-on-chronic hypercapnic respiratory failure episode, rather than during in-hospital admission for the acute event.

Recommendations Regarding Screening for Obstructive Sleep Apnea and In-Laboratory Overnight Polysomnography Titration Before Initiation of Long-Term Non-invasive Ventilation in Patients with Chronic Stable Hypercapnic Chronic Obstructive Pulmonary Disease

Benefits of screening using a highly sensitive test (the STOP-Bang questionnaire)[26] likely outweigh the harms in a population in which the prevalence of severe OSA is 10%. This approach is especially advised for patients with COPD who are overweight (BMI > 25 kg/m^2) and have cardiovascular disease, due to their higher risk of COPD–OSA OS. Although in-laboratory overnight NIV titration was not suggested for all patients with chronic stable hypercapnic COPD, the COPD–OSA OS was considered to be an exception. These patients often require NIV titration to determine the optimal end expiratory airway pressure needed to eliminate the obstructive events. However, the certainty of these recommendations was very low, given the limited data from randomized controlled trials or trials in the target population of COPD–OSA OS.

COMMON CLINICAL QUESTIONS
How to Document the Need for Home Non-invasive Ventilation in a Patient with Chronic Obstructive Pulmonary Disease and Stable Chronic Hypercapnia

The use of NIV in severe stable COPD is a covered benefit by the United States Center for Medicare and Medicaid Services (CMS).[27] The current guidelines that define the requirements to qualify for home support with NIV by RAD are based on the data by Meecham Jones and colleagues,[28] which showed significant improvements in daytime arterial PaO$_2$ and PaCO$_2$, total sleep time, sleep efficiency, and overnight PaCO$_2$ after 3 months of oxygen plus NIV (BPAP S device) as compared with oxygen alone. The PaCO$_2$ level of 52 mm Hg was chosen based on the lower range of the enrolled patients (52–65 mm Hg) and thus, it is higher and more restrictive than 45 mm Hg, the PaCO$_2$ cutoff selected by the 2020 ATS Clinical Practice Guidelines.

In summary, both hypoxemia and hypercapnia are required, but demonstration of obstructive lung disease by spirometry is not. To qualify for home NIV, *all* the following criteria need to be satisfied:

- Arterial blood gas (ABG) while awake and on supplemental oxygen (if prescribed) demonstrating a PaCO$_2 \geq$ 52 mm Hg.
- Overnight oxygen saturation $\leq$ 88% for over 5 minutes, with a minimum of 2 hours of nocturnal recording on 2 liters per minute (LPM) supplemental oxygen or the patient's prescribed level, whichever is higher.
- OSA and CPAP treatment have been considered and ruled out (formal testing is not required—this only requires clinical documentation).

Currently, the requirements to qualify for an HMV for NIV are less stringent and have led to increased prescribing. To order an HMV, there just needs to be evidence of chronic hypercapnic respiratory failure with a PaCO$_2$ >52 mm Hg (most durable medical equipment [DMEs] will accept either an arterial blood gas or venous blood gas [VBG]). This requires significantly less testing and documentation and has contributed to the significant increase in HMV for COPD.[29]

How to Evaluate a Patient with Stable Chronic Obstructive Pulmonary Disease for Home Non-invasive Ventilation

NIV should only be considered for patients with severe stable COPD already on maximal pharmacotherapy who have evidence of stable chronic hypercapnia

(PaCO$_2$ > 52 mm Hg). If hypercapnia is present, the next step is to evaluate for hypoxia with an overnight oximetry, defined as an SaO$_2$ < 88% for 5 minutes (not continuous) while on supplemental O$_2$ at 2 LPM or the patient's prescribed O$_2$ if higher than 2 LPM. If this is present, then the patient will meet criteria for a RAD without a back-up rate.[30]

Alternatively, patients who fail to meet these criteria may undergo a diagnostic polysomnography to evaluate for sleep apnea to confirm OS. If sleep apnea is present with an apnea–hypopnea index (AHI) greater than 5 events per hour, a trial of CPAP therapy can be attempted, which may help patients with COPD–OSA OS. This option however does not provide NIV support to treat hypercapnia, but treatment of COPD–OSA OS may improve clinical symptoms.[31]

If a patient does not meet any of the previous criteria and there is evidence of chronic hypercapnia and increased rates of acute exacerbations of COPD requiring hospitalizations, certain insurance companies will cover the cost of an HMV rather than a RAD device.[31]

Despite clearly defined criteria to qualify a patient for NIV with severe COPD, the practice of navigating the most efficient method to initiate therapy continues to be challenging, especially as changes to the current coverage determination for this population are discussed. To help navigate this process, we recommend a pragmatic treatment algorithm to help initiate the referral process for NIV for patients with severe COPD and chronic hypercapnia (**Fig. 1**).

How to Refer Stable Patients with Severe Chronic Obstructive Pulmonary Disease and Chronic Hypercapnia for Home Non-invasive Ventilation

Although NIV for severe stable COPD is beneficial in select patients, its management is complex and assistance from a pulmonary or sleep specialist is often required. Depending on their underlying training, many of these specialists may not be familiar with the modes or devices used for NIV in chronic stable hypercapnic respiratory failure associated with COPD. Ultimately, these patients may require referral to a university medical center that may have physicians with unique training in pulmonary and sleep medicine, who can navigate the specific needs and hurdles for the use of NIV.

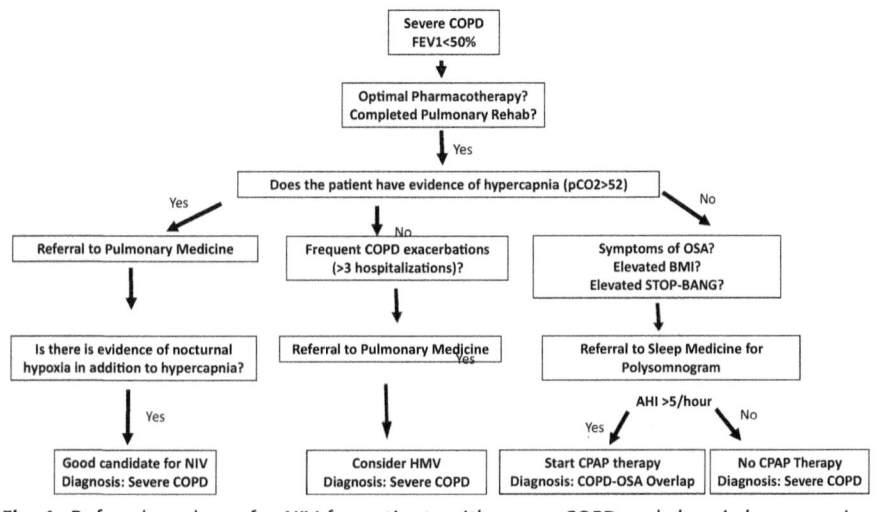

Fig. 1. Referral roadmap for NIV for patients with severe COPD and chronic hypercapnia.

What is the Relationship Between the Home-Non-invasive Ventilation Adherence and Efficacy?

Adherence to therapy has a key role in the efficacy of home NIV in stable patients with severe COPD and chronic hypercapnia. That there is a linear relationship between the number of hours of use per night and the outcomes is yet to be determined.[21] A meta-analysis by Struik and colleagues[32] showed that a minimum use of 5 hours per night resulted in a significant change in $PaCO_2$ after 3 months of treatment. It is worth mentioning that NIV adherence in excess of 9 hours a day may signal increased dependence on NIV due to the worsening of the patient status.[31]

SUMMARY

COPD remains a leading cause for increased hospitalizations and mortality despite improvements in pharmacotherapy, pulmonary rehabilitation, and campaigns for smoking cessation. Despite the heterogeneity of data on the role of NIV in severe stable COPD with chronic hypercapnia, the current evidence supports the use of NIV in select populations and phenotypes. The current CMS reimbursement criteria are complex, and the practice of navigating the most efficient method to initiate NIV therapy continues to be challenging, especially as changes to the current coverage determination for this population are discussed. These patients require referral to a university medical center that have physicians with specific training in pulmonary and sleep medicine, who can navigate the specific needs for the use of NIV.

CLINICS CARE POINTS

- NIV should be considered for patients with severe stable COPD already on maximal pharmacotherapy who have evidence of chronic hypercapnia ($PaCO_2$ >52 mm Hg).
- The initial assessment for home NIV use could be completed as outpatient, 2 to 4 weeks after the resolution of the acute-on-chronic hypercapnic respiratory failure episode, rather than during in-hospital admission for the acute event.
- Questionnaire-based screening for OSA should be considered for patients with chronic stable hypercapnic COPD to evaluate for COPD–OSA OS.
- The use of NIV in severe stable COPD is a covered benefit by the US CMS, when certain criteria are met.
- The NIV management for severe stable COPD is complex and assistance from a pulmonary or sleep specialist is often required.

FUNDING ACKNOWLEDGMENT

Dr M. Macrea's work was supported by the Department of Veterans Affairs, Veterans Health Administration, Rehabilitation Research and Development Service, Grant/Award Number: Career Development Award, 1IK2RX003535-01A2.

DISCLOSURE

The authors have nothing to disclose.

REFERENCES

1. May SM, Li JT. Burden of chronic obstructive pulmonary disease: healthcare costs and beyond. Allergy Asthma Proc 2015;36:4–10.

2. Macrea M, Oczkowski S, Rochwerg B, et al. Long-term noninvasive ventilation in chronic stable hypercapnic chronic obstructive pulmonary disease. an official american thoracic society clinical practice guideline. Am J Respir Crit Care Med 2020;202:e74–87.

3. Dreher M, Neuzeret PC, Windisch W, et al. Prevalence of chronic hypercapnia in severe chronic obstructive pulmonary disease: data from the HOmeVent registry. Int J Chron Obstruct Pulmon Dis 2019;14:2377–84.

4. Ergan B, Scala R, Windisch W. Defining "stable chronic hypercapnia" in patients with COPD: the physiological perspective. Eur Respir J 2020;55:1902365.

5. Loring SH, Garcia-Jacques M, Malhotra A. Pulmonary characteristics in COPD and mechanisms of increased work of breathing. J Appl Physiol (1985) 2009; 107:309–14.

6. Matthews AM, Wysham NG, Xie J, et al. Hypercapnia in advanced chronic obstructive pulmonary disease: a secondary analysis of the National Emphysema Treatment Trial. Chronic Obstr Pulm Dis 2020;7:336–45.

7. Budweiser S, Hitzl AP, Jorres RA, et al. Health-related quality of life and long-term prognosis in chronic hypercapnic respiratory failure: a prospective survival analysis. Respir Res 2007;8:92.

8. van Dijk M, Gan CT, Koster TD, et al. Treatment of severe stable COPD: the multidimensional approach of treatable traits. ERJ Open Res 2020;6:00322–2019.

9. Mannino DM, Braman S. The epidemiology and economics of chronic obstructive pulmonary disease. Proc Am Thorac Soc 2007;4(7):502–6.

10. Groenewegen KH, Schols AM, Wouters EF. Mortality and mortality-related factors after hospitalization for acute exacerbation of COPD. Chest 2003;124:459–67.

11. Rothnie KJ, Müllerová H, Smeeth L, et al. Natural History of Chronic Obstructive Pulmonary Disease Exacerbations in a General Practice-based Population with Chronic Obstructive Pulmonary Disease. Am J Respir Crit Care Med 2018;198: 464–71.

12. Soler X, Gaio E, Powell FL, et al. High prevalence of obstructive sleep apnea in patients with moderate to severe chronic obstructive pulmonary disease. Ann Am Thorac Soc 2015;12:1219–25.

13. Chaouat A, Weitzenblum E, Krieger J, et al. Association of chronic obstructive pulmonary disease and sleep apnea syndrome. Am Rev Respir Dis 1995; 151:82–6.

14. Weitzenblum E, Krieger J, Apprill M, et al. Daytime pulmonary hypertension in patients with obstructive sleep apnea syndrome. Am Rev Respir Dis 1988;138: 345–9.

15. Bradley TD, Rutherford A, Grossmann RF, et al. Role of daytime hypoxemia in the pathogenesis of right heart failure in the obstructive sleep apnea syndrome. Am Rev Respir Dis 1985;131:835–9.

16. Marin JM, Soriano JB, Carrizo SJ, et al. Outcomes in patients with chronic obstructive pulmonary disease and obstructive sleep apnea: the overlap syndrome. Am J Respir Crit Care Med 2010;182(3):325–31.

17. British Thoracic Society Standards of Care Committee, Non-invasive ventilation in acute respiratory failure. Thorax 2002;57(3):192–211.

18. Selim BJ, Wolfe L, Coleman JM 3rd, et al. Initiation of noninvasive ventilation for sleep related hypoventilation disorders: advanced modes and devices. Chest 2018;153:251–65.

19. Guyatt GH, Oxman AD, Kunz R, et al. GRADE Working Group. Going from evidence to recommendations. BMJ 2008;336:1049–51.

20. Centers for Medicare & Medicaid Services. Noninvasive positive pressure ventilation in the home. Available at. https://www.cms.gov/medicare-coverage-database/view/technology assessments.aspx?TAId=108&bc=AAAIAAAAAAAA. Accessed May 23rd, 2022.
21. Ergan B, Oczkowski S, Rochwerg B, et al. Respiratory Society guidelines on long-term home non-invasive ventilation for management of COPD. Eur Respir J 2019; 54:1901003.
22. Duiverman ML, Maagh P, Magnet FS, et al. Impact of high-intensity-NIV on the heart in stable COPD: a randomised cross-over pilot study. Respir Res 2017; 18:76.
23. Struik FM, Sprooten RT, Kerstjens HA, et al. Nocturnal non-invasive ventilation in COPD patients with prolonged hypercapnia after ventilatory support for acute respiratory failure: a randomised, controlled, parallel-group study. Thorax 2014; 69:826–34.
24. Murphy PB, Rehal S, Arbane G, et al. Effect of home noninvasive ventilation with oxygen therapy vs oxygen therapy alone on hospital readmission or death after an acute COPD exacerbation: a randomized clinical trial. JAMA 2017;317: 2177–86.
25. Duiverman ML, Vonk JM, Bladder G, et al. Home initiation of chronic non-invasive ventilation in COPD patients with chronic hypercapnic respiratory failure: a randomised controlled trial. Thorax 2020;75:244–52.
26. Chung F, Abdullah HR, Liao P. STOP-bang questionnaire: a practical approach to screen for obstructive sleep apnea. Chest 2016;149(3):631–8.
27. Centers for Medicare & Medicaid Services. Local Coverage Determination (LCD): Respiratory Assist Devices (L33800). Available at: https://www.cms.gov/medicare-coverage-database/view/lcd.aspx?lcdid=33800&ver=26&TAId=108&NCAId=243&NCDId=226&ncdver=3&SearchType=Advanced&CoverageSelection=Both&NCSelection=NCA%7cCAL%7cNCD%7cMEDCAC%7cTA%7cMCD&ArticleType=Ed%7cKey%7cSAD%7cFAQ&PolicyType=Final&s=5%7c6%7c66%7c67%7c9%7c38%7c63%7c41%7c64%7c65%7c44&KeyWord=Home+Oxygen&KeyWordLookUp=Doc&KeyWordSearchType=And&kq=true&bc=IAAAABAAAAAA&=. Accessed May 2nd, 2022.
28. Meecham Jones DJ, Paul EA, Jones PW, et al. Nasal pressure support ventilation plus oxygen compared with oxygen therapy alone in hypercapnic COPD. Am J Respir Crit Care Med 1995;152:538–44.
29. U.S. Department of Health and Human Services, Office of Inspector General. Escalating Medicare billing for ventilators raises concerns. HHS OIG Brief OEI-12-15-00370. Available at: Escalating Medicare Billing for Ventilators Raises Concerns (OEI-12-15-00370) 09-22-2016 (hhs.gov). Accessed May 27th, 2022.
30. Coleman JM 3rd, Wolfe LF, Kalhan R. Noninvasive Ventilation in Chronic Obstructive Pulmonary Disease. Ann Am Thorac Soc 2019;16:1091–8.
31. Borel JC, Pepin JL, Pison C, et al. Long-term adherence with non-invasive ventilation improves prognosis in obese COPD patients. Respirology 2014;19:857–65.
32. Struik FM, Lacasse Y, Goldstein RS, et al. Nocturnal noninvasive positive pressure ventilation in stable COPD: a systematic review and individual patient data meta-analysis. Respir Med 2014;108:329–37.

Advances in Evaluation and Treatment of Severe Asthma (Part One)

Christopher H. Fanta, MD

KEYWORDS

- Severe asthma • Diagnosis • Systematic assessment
- Allergic bronchopulmonary aspergillosis
- Eosinophilic granulomatosis with polyangiitis • Pulmonary function testing • Allergy
- Aspirin-exacerbated respiratory disease

KEY POINTS

- Patients with poorly controlled asthma despite inhaled corticosteroids and long-acting bronchodilators pose a particular challenge for their medical providers.
- A systematic approach to their management includes ensuring the correct diagnosis; reducing exposure to stimuli that incite airway inflammation; modifying comorbid conditions that aggravate asthma; and emphasizing medication adherence and, for inhaled medications, proper technique for delivery to the airways.
- Syndromes that may complicate asthma and make it difficult to control include aspirin-exacerbated respiratory disease, allergic bronchopulmonary aspergillosis, and eosinophilic granulomatosis with polyangiitis.
- Blood studies, pulmonary function testing, chest imaging, and sputum analysis are appropriate in the evaluation of most patients; additional specialized testing may be needed, depending on the initial assessment.

The last 30 years have seen major progress in our understanding and treatment of asthma. Perhaps the most important single advance was the recognition that a chronic, often eosinophilic, airway inflammation exists in the bronchi and bronchioles of persons with asthma, regardless of disease severity[1–3]; and that suppression of that airway inflammation can lead to fewer symptoms, improved lung function, and reduced risk of exacerbations, including the severe exacerbations that can lead to hospitalization and death from asthma.[4–6] In the United States, the incidence of hospitalizations and deaths from asthma had been steadily rising through the decades of the 1970s and 1980s. Beginning in the early 1990s, coincident with the release of widely disseminated recommendations from the National Asthma Education

Partners Asthma Center, Pulmonary and Critical Care Medicine Division, Brigham and Women's Hospital, Harvard Medical School, PBB – Clinics 3, 75 Francis Street, Boston, MA 02115, USA
E-mail address: cfanta@bwh.harvard.edu

Med Clin N Am 106 (2022) 971–986
https://doi.org/10.1016/j.mcna.2022.08.003
0025-7125/22/© 2022 Elsevier Inc. All rights reserved.

Program[7] to treat persistent asthma with regular inhaled anti-inflammatory corticosteroids (in preference to adding the long-acting bronchodilator, theophylline), rates for hospitalizations and deaths from asthma have been steadily decreasing, despite continued high disease prevalence.[8]

Another major step forward in treating asthma that is more than mild in severity was the introduction of long-acting beta-agonist bronchodilators, beginning with salmeterol (approved for use in the United States in 1994).[9] The combination of an inhaled corticosteroid (ICS) and inhaled long-acting beta-agonist (LABA) proved highly effective for symptom control and prevention of exacerbations, more so than regular ICS use alone.[10] Salmeterol was initially released as a single-drug inhaler and could be taken alone, without an accompanying ICS. Shortly thereafter, concern was raised about increased near-fatal and fatal asthma attacks in association with salmeterol use,[11] and a "black-box" warning was issued by the Food and Drug Administration in 2003 that was applied to all LABAs when prescribed to treat asthma. Only after the publication of three large-scale, randomized, controlled clinical trials that documented the safety and efficacy of LABAs when administered in combination with an ICS[12–14] was the "black-box" warning removed from ICS/LABA combination inhalers in 2017. These combination ICS/LABA inhalers, administered once or twice daily, are currently recommended by national and international expert panels[15,16] for the treatment of moderate and severe asthma.

Nonetheless, there remains a portion of patients with asthma, perhaps 15% to 20% of the total asthmatic population, that continues symptomatic despite being prescribed a combination ICS/LABA inhaler to be taken daily.[17] These patients have uncontrolled severe asthma, with frequent, perhaps daily symptoms of cough, chest tightness, wheeze, and shortness of breath; they suffer frequent exacerbations of asthma, prompting courses of systemic corticosteroids and urgent care or hospital-based care; and some are prescribed long-term, daily oral corticosteroids in an effort to prevent a recurring pattern of exacerbations and brief steroid "pulses." Their lives are disrupted; employment may suffer; families are burdened by their uncontrolled illness. It is said that the per-person medical costs of poorly controlled asthma are comparable to those of type 2 diabetes and emphysema.[18]

It is this group of patients with severe asthma that is the focus of this review, which is presented in two parts, exploring the definition and evaluation of severe asthma in Part One, then treatment of severe asthma in Part Two. Exciting advances in our understanding of the pathobiology of asthma have led to the discovery of highly targeted drug therapies newly available to treat severe asthma. We have progressed beyond the paradigm: bronchodilators to treat bronchoconstriction, and corticosteroids to treat asthmatic airway inflammation. Identification of specific cellular and molecular pathways driving severe asthma has made possible the development of novel monoclonal antibody therapies, heralding an era of "precision medicine" for the management of severe asthma.[19]

DEFINITION

National and international societies along with various research consortia have offered definitions of severe asthma for the purpose of epidemiologic classification of a subgroup of patients with asthma—a disease phenotype based on disease severity.[20–22] For example, the European Respiratory Society/American Thoracic Society Task Force on severe asthma defined it as follows: "asthma that requires treatment with high dose inhaled corticosteroids plus a second controller and/or systemic corticosteroids to prevent it from becoming "uncontrolled" or that remains "uncontrolled" despite this therapy."[20] The first half of this definition includes patients who require high-dose ICS/LABA combination to maintain good asthma control, Step 5 of the step-care approach to asthma treatment based on disease severity of the National Asthma Education and Prevention Program[15] (and ICD-10 diagnosis code J45.50 of the International Classification of Diseases). It is the latter half of the definition, focusing on those who fail to achieve good asthma control despite high-dose ICS/LABA combination, that pertains to the current discussion.

Poor control can take various forms. It may manifest as frequent cough, wheezing, exercise limitation, and nocturnal awakenings due to asthma. It may cause frequent exacerbations, necessitating oral corticosteroids (and their attendant side effects) and urgent medical care. Patients with uncontrolled severe asthma are at increased risk for exacerbations that necessitate hospitalization, respiratory failure requiring intensive care unit stay, and death from asthma. Some patients suffer persistent airflow obstruction, akin to chronic obstructive pulmonary disease (COPD), limiting exercise and sometimes causing chronic dyspnea on exertion. Goals for the treatment of uncontrolled severe asthma therefore include the following: improved symptoms/quality of life; fewer exacerbations; reduced need for systemic corticosteroids; and improved lung function.

DIFFERENTIAL DIAGNOSIS

Although an ~~older~~ adult newly presenting with shortness of breath and wheezing may have a new onset of asthma, it is worth remembering that most asthma begins in early childhood[23] and that shortness of breath and wheezing in an adult may have many potential causes other than asthma. It is possible that a patient's failure to improve despite intensive anti-asthmatic therapy reflects not refractory, severe asthma but an alternative diagnosis mimicking asthma. Myriad other diseases can manifest with cough, wheeze, and shortness of breath (**Box 1**). The following two case examples illustrate this point.

Case example 1: A 27-year-old man presented with a persistent cough and mild shortness of breath. He recalled frequent bronchitis as a child and teenager in El Salvador, but his symptoms worsened and became more severe in the 2 years since immigrating to the U.S. He tried albuterol and fluticasone inhalers without relief. His history was notable for a productive cough on a daily basis. Chest auscultation was

---

Box 1
Differential diagnosis of wheezing and shortness of breath in the adult

Upper and central airway diseases
    Vocal fold movement disorder (Vocal cord dysfunction)
    Tracheobronchomalacia
    Focal airway narrowing due to endobronchial obstruction or extrinsic compression

Other intrathoracic airway diseases
    Chronic obstructive pulmonary disease
    Bronchiolitis
    Bronchiectasis

Other diseases manifesting with airflow obstruction
    Congestive heart failure
    Sarcoidosis
    Chronic oropharyngeal aspiration
    Lymphangioleiomyomatosis

remarkable for scattered low-pitched expiratory wheezes ("rhonchi") and distant heart sounds over the left precordium. A chest X-ray and ultimately a chest computed tomogram (CT) were obtained (**Fig. 1**A, B). Sputum culture was positive for Hemophilus influenzae.

A diagnosis of bronchiectasis due to primary ciliary dyskinesia was made, and his treatment focused on rotating antibiotics and airway clearance maneuvers.

Case example 2: A 56-year-old woman was referred for refractory asthma. Despite treatment with ICS/LABA, a leukotriene modifier, and daily prednisone at 30 mg/day, she presented with loud wheezing audible without a stethoscope. Her past medical history included an episode of respiratory distress for which emergency department records were available: immediately before intubation her arterial blood gases breathing supplemental oxygen at 2 L/min revealed a $PaO_2 = 115$ mm Hg, $PaCO_2 = 31$ mm Hg, and pH 7.48. On auscultation, she had high-pitched expiratory wheezing loudest over the neck and upper chest and distant-sounding over the lower lung fields bilaterally.

A diagnosis of paroxysmal vocal fold movement disorder (vocal cord dysfunction)[24] was suspected and later confirmed on direct laryngoscopy. Her arterial blood gases

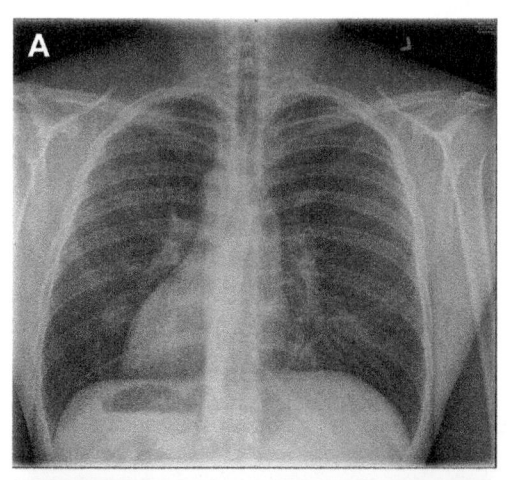

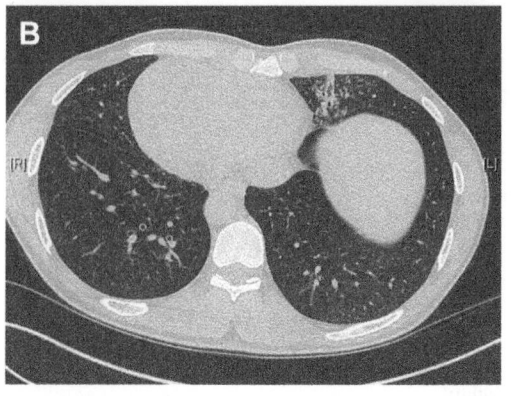

Fig. 1. Chest X-ray (*A*) and CT scan (*B*) in a patient with bronchiectasis due to primary ciliary dyskinesia. (*A*) Showing dextrocardia and possible increased lung markings at the left lung base medially. (*B*) Confirming the presence of bronchiectasis in the inferior portion of the lingula.

reflected hyperventilation rather than the alveolar hypoventilation (with hypercapnia and respiratory acidosis) encountered in life-threatening asthma attacks. Therapy focused on steroid dose reduction, speech therapy, and psychological counseling.

APPROACH TO THE PATIENT WITH DIFFICULT-TO-CONTROL ASTHMA

Managing a patient whose asthma fails to improve despite the prescription of appropriate and intensive therapy can be daunting. Asthma may be difficult to control not because of the intrinsic severity of the disease but because of complicating factors. A systematic approach to evaluation, implementing the following four areas of exploration, can be helpful. In some studies, more than 50% of patients presenting with severe, uncontrolled asthma had control of their asthma achieved by application of a structured approach such as described here.[25,26]

1. *Do I have the correct diagnosis?* As noted above, patients with diseases mimicking asthma may have limited or no response to anti-asthmatic medications. It is imperative to confirm the initial suspicion of severe asthma (that was based on history and physical examination) with pulmonary function tests that document variable airflow obstruction over time or in response to a bronchodilator.[27] Airflow obstruction is defined on spirometry by a reduced ratio of the one-second forced expiratory volume (FEV_1) to the forced vital capacity (FVC). Variability in FEV_1 (more than can be attributed to variability of the measurement from repeat testing alone) has traditionally been defined as a 12% change with at least 200-mL change in absolute volume.

   Bronchoprovocation testing, such as a methacholine challenge, is rarely necessary for severe asthma. It requires cessation of anti-asthmatic medications before testing (a risky intervention in someone with potentially severe asthma) and is usually performed in persons with normal or near-normal lung function. In a patient in whom a diagnosis of severe asthma is doubted, tapering or cessation of medications followed by spirometry would likely suffice to confirm or refute the diagnosis. Occasionally, a patient's main complaint is exercise-induced wheezing and shortness of breath despite maximal anti-asthmatic medications, including a rapid-acting bronchodilator before exercise. In that circumstance, an exercise challenge with spirometry pre- and postexercise may be helpful and can be performed with the patient taking all medications on the day of testing. If performed with the patient taking anti-asthmatic medications, a negative exercise challenge (failure of the FEV_1 to decline by 10% following exercise) does not exclude a diagnosis of asthma but does rule out exercise-induced bronchoconstriction due to inadequately controlled asthma as the cause of the patient's exercise-induced symptoms.

2. *Are there persistent triggers/inciters of asthma?* It may be possible to improve asthma control without additional medications by reducing a patient's exposure to the triggers that provoke asthmatic attacks and the inciters of persistent severe airway inflammation. Allergic and irritant exposures in the home or work environment should be sought.[28] Ask about exposure to common aeroallergens that can elicit an allergic response in the airways, especially the indoor allergens: animal danders, mold, dust, cockroaches, and mice. Confirmation of allergic sensitization can be obtained by blood testing of antigen-specific immunoglobulin E (IgE) (often referred to as RAST tests, after a previous method of measurement called radioallergosorbent tests). For instance, one can order IgE specific for cat dander, dog dander, aspergillus, cockroach, mouse urine, and *Dermatophagoides pteronyssinus* and *D. farinae* (for dust mite antigen). Alternatively, allergists will perform skin

testing (prick and selective intradermal tests) to a large panel of common environmental allergens.

Allergen remediation or avoidance can improve asthma control[29]; and even a cat lover may be willing to find another home for a pet cat rather than face another hospitalization with a frightening attack of asthma. In general, allergen desensitization injections ("allergy shots") are not recommended to treat severe asthma, because of their uncertain benefit and the risk of inducing a life-threatening asthmatic attack or anaphylaxis in response to the small amount of antigen administered subcutaneously in a highly allergic patient.[30]

Potentially remediable chronically inhaled irritants include cigarette smoking, secondhand (passive) smoke exposure, vaping, and marijuana smoking; wood-burning fireplaces and stoves; and exposure to workplace chemicals, airborne particulates, and fumes. Similarly, air pollution can worsen asthma control and disproportionately affects poor and inner-city residents.[31,32]

3. *Are medical comorbidities contributing to poor asthma control?* Symptoms of cough, chest congestion, and shortness of breath are made worse by comorbid rhinosinusitis. The symptoms of nasal congestion and consequent mouth-breathing, sinus pressure, postnasal drip, and possible anosmia from chronic rhinosinusitis with or without nasal polyps can all impair the quality of life of persons with asthma; and the inflammatory mediators released in the upper airway may aggravate the underlying asthmatic diathesis.[33]

Likewise, gastroesophageal reflux can cause cough, chest tightness, and breathlessness. Lay persons often confuse the term "heartburn" with the symptom of (epigastric) dyspepsia, so one should inquire specifically about retrosternal burning and the sensation of liquid regurgitating up toward the throat. Gastroesophageal reflux to the level of the throat ("laryngo-pharyngeal reflux") can lead to aspiration of stomach acid and digestive enzymes, aggravating airway inflammation; and it has been speculated that gastric reflux into the lower esophagus worsens asthma via vagally mediated reflex pathways. Effective treatment of symptomatic reflux improves chest symptoms in persons with asthma.[34] However, empiric treatment of severe asthma with proton-pump inhibitors on the speculation that "silent reflux" is worsening asthma control is ineffective.[35,36]

Obesity frequently contributes to exertional dyspnea and nocturnal respiratory symptoms. It may also contribute to worsened airway inflammation via pro-inflammatory mediators released from adipocytes and from changes in the gut microbiome associated with obesity.[37] Exercise capacity typically improves with weight reduction; and limited studies point to improved asthma control following successful bariatric surgery.[38]

Like the general population, persons with asthma who smoke as much as a pack of cigarettes per day for 20 or more years can develop COPD and acquire a condition referred to as asthma-COPD overlap.[39,40] As a result, they will often have persistent exercise limitation due to a component of irreversible airflow obstruction from their COPD. Their maximal achievable lung function will not be the normal predicted value for someone of the same age, height, and sex; their target peak expiratory flow (PEF) or FEV_1 needs to be adjusted accordingly. Other interventions, including smoking cessation, outpatient pulmonary rehabilitation, and occasionally home supplemental oxygen may be applicable, as well as their intensive anti-asthma therapies.

Besides addressing chronic rhinosinusitis, gastroesophageal reflux disease, obesity, and asthma-COPD overlap, consider medications that may be aggravating the patient's asthma, particularly beta-blockers. Nonselective beta-blockers, including the nonspecific beta-blocker eyedrop, timolol, are contraindicated in severe, poorly controlled asthma[41]; and beta-1 selective beta-blockers should be used only in low doses. Measurement of lung function before and after administration of the initial dose of a beta-1 selective beta-blocker may be a useful precaution to ensure its safety in persons with severe asthma.

4. *Is the patient adherent to the prescribed therapy?* Medication non-adherence is common in many chronic diseases; and asthma poses unique challenges because most of the routine medications used to treat asthma are delivered by inhalation rather than swallowed as a tablet or capsule. Proper inhalation technique is not intuitive, and inhalers do not fit into the 7-day pill box organizers that some patients use to remember their regular medications. It is worth routinely inquiring (nonjudgmentally) about medication use in severe asthma, reviewing the proper technique for inhaling medication from each device that the patient is using (which may include a metered-dose inhaler, a dry-powder inhaler, and a soft-mist inhaler), and exploring barriers to daily use. Common barriers include cost of medication, lack of perceived benefit, fear of long-term harm or dependency, comorbid mental health issues, including depression or alcoholism, and medication side effects.[42]

A particularly common and frustrating side effect of the inhaled steroids is dysphonia.[43] The hoarseness is often intermittent, and it may interfere with professional or avocational activities like speaking on the telephone, lecturing, or singing. Sometimes changing the specific steroid medication, changing the delivery system (metered-dose inhaler vs dry-powder inhaler), or use of a valved-holding chamber ("spacer") with the metered-dose inhaler may help.

"ASTHMA PLUS"

There are three disorders, unique to persons with asthma, that on occasion complicate their disease and may make it difficult-to-control: aspirin-exacerbated respiratory disease (AERD); allergic bronchopulmonary aspergillosis (ABPA); and eosinophilic granulomatosis with polyangiitis (EGPA).

AERD: It has been recognized since the beginning of the twentieth century that some patients with asthma develop worsened asthmatic symptoms following ingestion of aspirin. In 1968 Dr. Max Samter published a case series of patients with asthma, aspirin intolerance, and associated nasal polyposis,[44] subsequently described as Samter's triad and now referred to as AERD. In parts of the world, it is called nonsteroidal anti-inflammatory drug (NSAID)-exacerbated respiratory disease, in recognition of the fact that not only aspirin but any inhibitor of the enzyme cyclooxygenase-1 will trigger symptoms in this patient population.

It is estimated that 5% to 10% of adults with asthma will develop aspirin/NSAID intolerance, which is frequently associated with nasal polyposis.[45] A disproportionate percentage of patients with AERD have severe, refractory asthma. It is rare in children, typically developing in early adulthood; it is not an inherited disorder. Although the precise disease mechanism is unknown, it is thought to represent a biochemical abnormality involving metabolism of arachidonic acid via the cyclooxygenase and lipoxygenase pathways, with overproduction of cysteinyl leukotrienes even in the absence of aspirin stimulation.[46] Treatment of this distinct asthma endotype involves strict aspirin/NSAID avoidance; trial of leukotriene modifying drugs; and in some patients, monoclonal antibody therapy targeting both asthma and nasal polyposis. Patients who might need aspirin as an important part of their treatment (eg, following myocardial infarction or stroke) can undergo an oral aspirin desensitization regimen followed by daily aspirin ingestion without exacerbation of their respiratory disease.[47]

ABPA: Many atopic patients with asthma are allergic to molds, including aspergillus. However, a small percentage of asthmatic patients (probably fewer than 1%) develop an unusually intense immune response to aspergillus, characterized by eosinophilia and very high circulating levels of IgE (often greater than 1000 IU/mL).[48] Aspergillus persists in airway mucus and can often be identified in expectorated sputum. However, it is the immune response to aspergillus rather than an invasive infection that causes the airway damage, manifesting as bronchiectasis. Bronchiectasis involving the central bronchi in a person with asthma (**Fig. 2**) is pathognomonic of ABPA, but more peripheral bronchiectasis is also common in ABPA. Patients may experience regular expectoration of purulent-appearing sputum (typical of bronchiectasis) and sometimes large tubular (worm-like) plugs of dark mucus (**Fig. 3**), reflecting the bronchiectasis of larger, central airways.

Treatment of ABPA focuses on suppression of the intense immune response to aspergillus, typically with systemic corticosteroids. Anti-fungal therapy with modern oral azoles is adjunctive therapy, allowing dose reduction of oral corticosteroids and reducing the frequency of disease relapses.[49,50] Reports of case series suggest potential benefit from monoclonal antibodies that target IgE or eosinophils.[51,52] Avoidance of mold-rich substances with the potential for aerosolization, like garden mulch, should be part of the treatment plan.

EGPA: Asthma, an airway disease, may on rare occasion be complicated by systemic eosinophilic inflammation and eosinophilic vasculitis. First described by Drs. Jacob Churg and Lotte Strauss in 1951,[53] this syndrome presents not only with severe asthma but also eosinophilic tissue infiltration at multiple sites, commonly manifesting with rashes, rhinosinusitis, pneumonia, cardiomyopathy, colitis, and neuropathy (mononeuritis multiplex). Pathology reveals a small- and medium-sized vessel vasculitis with eosinophilia and granuloma formation. Laboratory data that provide a clue to the presence of EGPA include an elevated erythrocyte sedimentation rate (ESR) and C-reactive protein (CRP) and, in up to 50% of cases, the presence of circulating antineutrophil cytoplasmic antibodies (ANCA).[54]

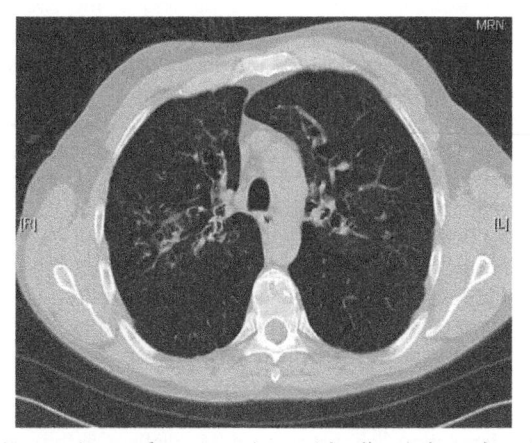

Fig. 2. Transaxial CT scan image from a patient with allergic bronchopulmonary aspergillosis. This transaxial chest CT image at the level of the aortic arch shows bilateral upper lobe cystic bronchiectasis, most notable for its location in central bronchi, characteristic of allergic bronchopulmonary aspergillosis.

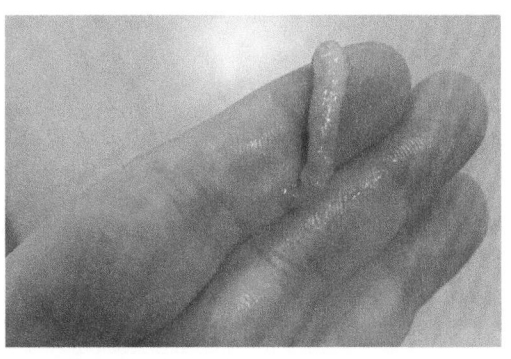

Fig. 3. Large sputum plug expectorated by a patient with allergic bronchopulmonary aspergillosis.

In the late 1990s, not long after the introduction of the leukotriene receptor antagonists, montelukast and zafirlukast, case series described the onset of EGPA in the days and weeks following initiation of treatment of asthma with these medications.[55] It is thought that the association was in most cases mediated by the concurrent withdrawal of chronically administered oral corticosteroids, rather than any unique effect of this class of medication.

Treatment of EGPA has traditionally necessitated high doses of systemic corticosteroids, with addition of alternative immunosuppressive agents (such as azathioprine, mycophenalate, or rituximab) for refractory disease or disease requiring maintenance prednisone at high doses. More recently, the anti-interleukin-5 monoclonal antibody, mepolizumab (administered subcutaneously once monthly at a high dose) has for many patients proven an effective alternative with infrequent side effects.[56]

DIAGNOSTIC TESTING IN SEVERE, REFRACTORY ASTHMA

Diagnostic testing in severe asthma is designed to confirm the diagnosis of asthma, assess for comorbid or complicating illnesses, and characterize specific endotypes that can direct the choice of advanced biologic therapies, if needed. No single algorithm is appropriate for all patients; and there is no set of tests that has been validated by prospective analysis as the most cost-effective. History and physical examination, together with the results of initial diagnostic testing, will guide the choice of more detailed investigations in individual patients. A basic approach likely appropriate for most patients will include some combination of blood studies, pulmonary function testing, and chest imaging (**Box 2**).[57,58]

Blood tests. A complete blood count with differential will help to identify patients with eosinophilic asthma (>300 eosinophils/uL), who are then potential candidates for certain targeted biologic therapies. Because systemic corticosteroids are highly effective in clearing peripheral blood eosinophils, confirmation of the endotype of eosinophilic asthma typically requires blood testing at a time when the patient is not taking any systemic corticosteroid and may require a retrospective review of prior blood test results. On the contrary, a striking neutrophilia may point to a bacterial infection or systemic inflammatory process contributing to the patient's respiratory symptoms.

Similarly, identifying an elevated total serum IgE level points to an allergic (atopic) predisposition and potential candidacy for anti-IgE monoclonal antibody therapy. The current indication for anti-IgE monoclonal antibody therapy includes evidence

---

Box 2
Diagnostic testing in severe asthma

Tests useful in most patients:
  Blood:
    Complete blood count (CBC) with differential
    Total immunoglobulin E (IgE)
    Antigen-specific IgE (also called RAST) for common environmental allergens, such as
    Dermatophagoides farina, Dermatophagoides pteronyssinus, cat dander, dog dander,
    aspergillus, mouse antigen, and cockroach
  Sputum (if expectorated):
    Cytology (to assess for eosinophilia)
  Pulmonary function testing:
    Spirometry
    Exhaled nitric oxide (if available)
  Radiology:
    Chest radiograph

Additional testing in some patients:
  Blood:
    Serum immunoglobulins
    Erythrocyte sedimentation rate, C-reactive protein
    Antineutrophil cytoplasmic antibody (ANCA)
    Alpha-1 antitrypsin level
  Sputum:
    Microbiology (routine and fungal cultures)
  Pulmonary function testing:
    Lung volumes and diffusion capacity
    Bronchoprovocation challenge (eg, with exercise)
  Radiology:
    Chest computed tomography (CT)
    Sinus CT
    Tracheal imaging (chest CT with inspiratory and dynamic expiratory images)
    Videofluoroscopic swallowing study
  Other testing:
    Allergy skin testing
    24-h pH monitoring
    Esophageal manometry
    Laryngoscopy
    Bronchoscopy
    Aspirin challenge

---

for allergic sensitization to one or more perennial environmental aeroallergens. Allergic sensitization can be tested by measurement of antigen-specific IgE blood tests or allergy skin tests, as discussed above.

In patients with manifestations of asthma and multisystem involvement, such as sinusitis, skin rashes, renal dysfunction, cardiomyopathy, gastroenteritis, and neuropathy, measurement of the ESR, CRP, and ANCA should be performed to assess for evidence of systemic vasculitis. In patients with persistent airflow obstruction on pulmonary function testing even when they are at their best, measurement of alpha-1 antitrypsin level is appropriate, especially in nonsmokers.

Pulmonary function tests. Spirometry is indicated in all patients with difficult-to-control asthma. It has the following advantages over peak flow measurement alone: it may reveal significant airflow obstruction even when the peak flow is normal; it can distinguish a pattern of obstruction (as expected in asthma) from one of restriction (raising concern for an alternative diagnosis); and on the flow-volume display of test results, it may identify patients with upper airway obstruction, mimicking or complicating asthma.

If the patient's chest X-ray is normal, full pulmonary function tests with measurement of lung volumes (ie, total lung capacity, functional residual capacity, and residual volume) are rarely needed. These additional pulmonary function tests can be useful when the vital capacity measurement on spirometry is disproportionately low or if a concomitant restrictive disease such as heart failure or respiratory muscle weakness is suspected. Likewise, measurement of the diffusion capacity for carbon monoxide (DL_{CO}) can be reserved for patients in whom the alternative or comorbid diagnosis of emphysema or pulmonary hypertension is suspected.

Measurement of the concentration of nitric oxide in the exhaled breath, referred to as the fractional exhaled nitric oxide or F_ENO, is a clinically useful marker of eosinophilic airway inflammation in asthma.[59] Compact equipment is commercially available that scrubs ambient nitric oxide during inhalation and then measures in the exhaled breath (in the phase that reflects lower airways) the concentration of nitric oxide. Patients are coached to exhale at a steady flow; and the results, reported in parts per billion, are immediately available. An elevated F_ENO results from upregulation of inducible nitric oxide synthase in airway epithelium and correlates with unchecked eosinophilia of the airways.[60–62] Treatment with ICSs effectively suppresses F_ENO in most patients. An elevated F_ENO (>40 ppb) that persists despite treatment with ICSs may indicate refractory airway eosinophilia, a potential target for modern biologic therapy for asthma, or possibly medication nonadherence.

Chest imaging. Although the chest radiograph in most patients with asthma will be normal, in those with severe, refractory disease it is an important part of the diagnostic evaluation. It is indicated to assess for comorbid illnesses (eg, eosinophilic pneumonia, bronchiectasis with mucoid impaction) or alternative diagnoses (eg, sarcoidosis, heart failure). In many instances, additional chest imaging with computed tomography (CT) is warranted, particularly in patients with daily or near-daily sputum production or persistent airflow obstruction. Even in the presence of a normal chest X-ray, the chest CT scan may detect, among other relevant findings, bronchiectasis, cystic lung disease, extrinsic airway compression, and emphysema, thereby influencing patient management.[63]

Additional radiographic studies may be appropriate in selected patients. In a patient with a deep, bark-like cough, inability fully to clear airway secretions for days and weeks after a chest cold, and wheezing that seems to emanate from the upper airways, a chest CT scan with inspiratory and dynamic expiratory imaging may identify tracheobronchomalacia.[64] In a patient with recurrent sinus infections or symptoms of chronic nasal congestion and sinus pressure, sinus CT imaging may help guide therapy and perhaps indicate the need for otolaryngologic consultation. And in the patient at risk for oropharyngeal aspiration, as suggested by history or underlying neurologic disease, a videofluoroscopic swallowing study is warranted.

Sputum analysis. Patients with chronic production of purulent-appearing sputum may have underlying bronchiectasis. Sputum should be sent for routine bacterial and fungal cultures, the latter to evaluate for aspergillus colonization or infection. More often, sputum in patients with severe asthma is mucoid. To characterize patient endotype, especially with an eye toward potential biologic therapy for eosinophilic asthma, it is helpful to evaluate sputum for the presence of eosinophils, reflective of airway eosinophilia. A limited number of specialized research laboratories are equipped to do sputum total and differential cell counts.[65] However, many clinical cytology laboratories will provide a qualitative assessment of sputum eosinophilia, reporting "no," "few," "moderate," or "numerous" eosinophils in expectorated sputum. Remember that the distinction between mucoid and purulent-appearing sputum is subjective, and that sputum may appear thick and yellow when loaded with eosinophils.

Specialized diagnostic testing. Evaluation of the patient with severe, refractory asthma often requires an interdisciplinary team approach. When esophageal reflux is thought to be a contributing factor, the gastroenterologist may undertake 24-h pH monitoring and esophageal manometry to assess for the presence of acid and nonacid reflux and its correlation to respiratory symptoms.[66] When vocal fold movement disorder is thought to complicate or mimic severe asthma, the otolaryngologist will be involved to perform laryngoscopy, and speech therapists may be called upon to provide therapy. Allergists may be requested to perform detailed assessment of allergic sensitivities (allergen skin testing); and when a history of aspirin/NSAID intolerance is ambiguous, oral aspirin challenge. In general, fiberoptic bronchoscopy as a diagnostic technique is reserved for research studies. It may prove useful in routine clinical practice when focal bronchial narrowing (bronchial stenosis or localized extrinsic compression) or dynamic expiratory airway collapse of the trachea and main bronchi is suspected.

SUMMARY

In approaching the patient with severe asthma poorly responsive to conventional therapy, it is helpful to ask: what makes this patient different from the vast majority of patients with asthma who can achieve good control with ICSs and long-acting bronchodilators? A systematic approach includes the following: (1) Is asthma the correct diagnosis? (2) Are there modifiable inciting stimuli in the home or work/school environment that are driving persistent airway inflammation? (3) Are there treatable medical comorbidities that are intensifying the symptoms of asthma? (4) Is the patient suffering from a unique asthma-associated condition, such as AERD, ABPA, or EGPA? (5) Is the patient adherent to prescribed medications?

No single set of diagnostic tests is appropriate for all patients with severe asthma. Spirometry, chest imaging, and testing for certain asthma endotypes (with measurement of blood eosinophils, total serum IgE, and allergen sensitization, as well as F_ENO and sputum eosinophilia where available) are appropriate for all patients. Additional testing is guided by the individual patient's unique medical presentation and often benefits from a multidisciplinary approach, with help from allergy, pulmonology, otolaryngology, gastroenterology, and other subspecialists.

CLINICS CARE POINTS

- Exclude alternative diagnoses, such as chronic obstructive pulmonary disease, bronchiectasis, tracheomalacia, and vocal fold movement disorder.
- Minimize patient exposures to the inciters of airway inflammation, such as aeroallergens, cigarette smoke, and air pollutants.
- Modify to the extent possible accompanying comorbidities, such as chronic rhinosinusitis, gastroesophageal reflux, and obesity.
- Review obstacles to regular medication adherence and reinforce proper inhaler technique.
- Consider "asthma plus" syndromes, such as aspirin-exacerbated respiratory disease, allergic bronchopulmonary aspergillosis, and eosinophilic granulomatosis with polyangiitis.
- Use blood and pulmonary function studies to assess for allergic/eosinophilic asthmatic inflammation.

DISCLOSURE

The author has nothing to disclose.

REFERENCES

1. Laitinen LA, Heino M, Laitinen A, et al. Damage of airway epithelium and bronchial reactivity in patients with asthma. Am Rev Respir Dis 1985;131:599–606.
2. Djukanovic R, Roche WR, Wilson JW, et al. Mucosal inflammation in asthma. Am Rev Respir Dis 1990;142:434–57.
3. Haley KJ, Sunday ME, Wiggs BR, et al. Inflammatory cell distribution within and along asthmatic airways. Am J Respir Crit Care Med 1998;158:565–72.
4. Haahtela T, Jarvinen M, Kava T, et al. Comparison of a β_2-agonist, terbutaline, with an inhaled corticosteroid, budesonide, in newly detected asthma. N Engl J Med 1991;325:388–92.
5. Donahue JG, Weiss ST, Livingston JM, et al. Inhaled steroids and the risk of hospitalization for asthma. J Amer Med Assoc 1997;277:877–91.
6. Suissa S, Ernst P, Benayoun S, et al. Low-dose inhaled corticosteroids and the prevention of death from asthma. N Engl J Med 2000;343:332–6.
7. Sheffer AL, Bailey WC, Bleecker ER, et al. Guidelines for the diagnosis and management of asthma: National Heart, Lung and Blood Institute. National Asthma Education Program - Expert Panel Report. J Allergy Clin Immunol 1991;88:425–534.
8. Pate CA, Zahran HS, Qin X, et al. Asthma Surveillance — United States, 2006–2018. MMWR Surveill Summ 2021;70(No. SS-5):1–32.
9. Pearlman DS, Chervinsky P, LaForce C, et al. A comparison of salmeterol with albuterol in the treatment of mild-to-moderate asthma. N Engl J Med 1992;327:1420–5.
10. Pauwels RA, Löfdahl C-G, Postma DS, et al. Effect of inhaled formoterol and budesonide on exacerbations of asthma. N Engl J Med 1997;337:1405–11.
11. Nelson HS, Weiss ST, Bleecker ER, et al. The Salmeterol Multicenter Asthma Research Trial: a comparison of usual pharmacotherapy for asthma or usual pharmacotherapy plus salmeterol. Chest 2006;129:15–26.
12. Stempel DA, Raphiou IH, Kral KM, et al. Serious asthma events with fluticasone plus salmeterol versus fluticasone alone. N Engl J Med 2016;374:1822–30.
13. Peters SP, Bleecker ER, Canonica GW, et al. Serious asthma events with budesonide plus formoterol vs. budesonide alone. N Engl J Med 2016;375:850–60.
14. Weinstein CLJ, Ryan N, Shekar T, et al. Serious asthma events with mometasone furoate plus formoterol compared with mometasone furoate. J Allergy Clin Immunol 2019;143:1395–402.
15. Expert Panel Working Group of the National Heart, Lung, and Blood Institute (NHLBI) administered and coordinated National Asthma Education and Prevention Program Coordinating Committee (NAEPPCC). 2020 Focused Updates to the Asthma Management Guidelines: A Report from the National Asthma Education and Prevention Program Coordinating Committee Expert Panel Working Group. J Allergy Clin Immunol 2020;146:1217–70.
16. Global Initiative for Asthma. Global strategy for asthma management and prevention. 2021. Available at: www.ginasthma.org. Accessed July 20, 2022.
17. Bateman ED, Boushey HA, Bousquet J, et al. Can guideline-defined asthma control be achieved? The Gaining Optimal Asthma Control study. Am J Respir Crit Care Med 2004;170:836–44.

18. O'Neill S, Sweeney J, Patterson CC, et al. The cost of treating severe refractory asthma in the UK: an economic analysis from the British Thoracic Society Difficult Asthma Registry. Thorax 2015;70:376–8.

19. Israel E, Reddel HK. Severe and difficult-to-treat asthma in adults. N Engl J Med 2017;377:965–76.

20. Chung KF, Wenzel SE, Brozek JL, et al. International ERS/ATS guidelines on definition, evaluation and treatment of severe asthma. Eur Respir J 2014;43:343–73.

21. American Thoracic Society. Proceedings of the ATS workshop on refractory asthma: current understanding, recommendations, and unanswered questions. Am J Respir Crit Care Med 2000;162:2341–51.

22. Wang E, Wechsler ME, Tran TN, et al. Characterization of severe asthma worldwide: data from the International Severe Asthma Registry. Chest 2020;157:790–804.

23. Yunginger JW, Reed CE, O'Connell EJ, et al. A community-based study of the epidemiology of asthma: incidence rates, 1964-1983. Am Rev Respir Dis 1992;146:888–94.

24. Matrka L. Paradoxic vocal fold movement disorder. Otolaryngol Clin North Am 2014;47:135–46.

25. Heaney LG, Conway E, Kelly C, et al. Predictors of therapy resistant asthma: outcome of a systematic evaluation protocol. Thorax 2003;58:561–6.

26. Robinson DS, Campbell DA, Durham SR, et al. Systematic assessment of difficult-to-treat asthma. Eur Respir J 2003;22:478–83.

27. Aaron SD, Vandemheen KL, FitzGerald JM, et al. Reevaluation of diagnosis in adults with physician-diagnosed asthma. J Amer Med Assoc 2017;317:269–79.

28. Rosenstreich DL, Eggleston P, Kattan M, et al. The role of cockroach allergy and exposure to cockroach allergen in causing morbidity among inner-city children with asthma. N Engl J Med 1997;336:1356–63.

29. Morgan WJ, Crain EF, Gruchalla RS, et al. Results of a home-based environmental intervention among urban children with asthma. N Engl J Med 2004;351:1068–80.

30. Epstein TG, Murphy-Berendts K, Liss GM, et al. Risk factors for fatal and nonfatal reactions to immunotherapy (2008-2018): postinjection monitoring and severe asthma. Ann Allergy Asthma Immunol 2021;127:64–9.

31. Balmes JR, Earnest G, Katz PP, et al. Exposure to traffic: lung function and health status in adults with asthma. J Allergy Clin Immunol 2009;123:626–31.

32. Thurston GD, Balmes JR, Garcia E, et al. Outdoor air pollution and new-onset airway disease. An official American Thoracic Society workshop report. Ann Am Thorac Soc 2020;17:387–98.

33. Laidlaw TM, Mullol J, Woessner KM. Chronic rhinosinusitis with nasal polyps and asthma. J Allergy Clin Immunol Pract 2021;9:1133–41.

34. McCallister JW, Parsons JP, Mastronarde JG. The relationship between gastroesophageal reflux and asthma: an update. Ther Adv Respir Dis 2011;5:143–50.

35. American Lung Association Clinical Research Centers, Mastronarde JG, Anthonisen NR, et al. Efficacy of esomeprazole for treatment of poorly controlled asthma. N Engl J Med 2009;360:1487–99.

36. Zheng Z, Luo Y, Gao J. Randomised trials of proton pump inhibitors for gastro-oesophageal reflux disease in patients with asthma: an updated systematic review and meta-analysis. BMJ Open 2021;11:e043860.

37. Dixon AE, Que LG. Obesity and asthma. Semin Respir Crit Care Med 2022. https://doi.org/10.1055/s-0042-1742384.

38. Chaaban TA. Bariatric surgery: a potential cure for asthma? Eur Respir Rev 2019; 28:190003.
39. Hardin M, Cho M, McDonald M-L, et al. The clinical and genetic features of COPD-asthma overlap syndrome. Eur Respir J 2014;44:343–50.
40. Postma DS, Rabe KF. The asthma-COPD overlap syndrome. N Engl J Med 2015; 373:1241–9.
41. Odeh M, Oliven A, Bassan H. Timolol eyedrop-induced fatal bronchospasm in an asthmatic patient. J Fam Pract 1991;32:97–8.
42. Amin S, Soliman M, McIvor A, et al. Understanding patient perspectives on medication adherence in asthma: a targeted review of qualitative studies. Patient Prefer Adherence 2020;14:541–51.
43. Spantideas N, Drosou E, Bougea A, et al. Inhaled corticosteroids and voice problems. What is new? J Voice 2017;31:384.e1–7.
44. Samter M, Beers RF Jr. Concerning the nature of intolerance to aspirin. J Allergy 1967;40:281–93.
45. White AA, Stevenson DD. Aspirin-exacerbated respiratory disease. N Engl J Med 2018;379:1060–70.
46. Laidlaw TM, Boyce JA. Aspirin-exacerbated respiratory disease – new prime suspects. N Engl J Med 2016;374:484–8.
47. Stevens WW, Jerschow E, Baptist AP. The role of aspirin desensitization followed by oral aspirin therapy in managing patients with aspirin-exacerbated respiratory disease: a work group report from the rhinitis, rhinosinusitis and ocular allergy committee of the American Academy of Allergy, Asthma & Immunology. J Allergy Clin Immunol 2021;147:827–44.
48. Patel G, Greenberger PA. Allergic bronchopulmonary aspergillosis. Allergy Asthma Proc 2019;40:421–4.
49. Stevens DA, Schwartz HJ, Lee JY, et al. A randomized trial of itraconazole in allergic bronchopulmonary aspergillosis. N Engl J Med 2000;342:756–62.
50. Agarwal R, Muthu V, Sehgal IS, et al. A randomized trial of prednisolone versus prednisolone and itraconazole in acute-stage allergic bronchopulmonary aspergillosis complicating asthma. Eur Respir J 2022;59:2101787.
51. Schleich F, Vaia E-S, Pilette C, et al. Mepolizumab for allergic bronchopulmonary aspergillosis: report of 20 cases from the Belgian severe asthma registry and review of the literature. J Allergy Clin Immunol Pract 2020;8:2412–3.e2.
52. Li J-X, Fan L-C, Li M-H, et al. Beneficial effects of omalizumab therapy in allergic bronchopulmonary aspergillosis: a synthesis review of published literature. Respir Med 2017;122:33–42.
53. Churg J, Strauss L. Allergic granulomatosis, allergic angiitis, and periarteritis nodosa. Am J Pathol 1951;27:277–301.
54. Berti A, Boukhlal S, Groh M, et al. Eosinophilic granulomatosis with polyangiitis: the multifaceted spectrum of clinical manifestations at different stages of disease. Expert Rev Clin Immunol 2020;16:51–61.
55. Wechsler ME, Drazen JM. Zafirlukast and Churg-Strauss syndrome. Chest 1999; 116:266–7.
56. Wechsler ME, Akuthota P, Jayne D, et al. Mepolizumab or placebo for eosinophilic granulomatosis with polyangiitis. N Engl J Med 2017;376:1921–32.
57. Wenzel S. Severe asthma in adults. Am J Respir Crit Care Med 2005;172:149–60.
58. Long AA, Fanta CH. Assessment and management of difficult asthma: part 1. Allergy Asthma Proc 2012;33:305–12.

59. Dweik RA, Boggs PB, Erzurum SC, et al. An official ATS clinical practice guideline: interpretation of exhaled nitric oxide levels (FE_{NO}) for clinical applications. Am J Respir Crit Care Med 2011;184:602–15.
60. Khatri SB, Iaccarino JM, Barochia A, et al. Use of fractional exhaled nitric oxide to guide the treatment of asthma: an official American Thoracic Society clinical practice guideline. Am J Respir Crit Care Med 2021;204:e97–109.
61. Schleich FN, Seidel L, Sele J, et al. Exhaled nitric oxide thresholds associated with a sputum eosinophil count >3% in a cohort of unselected patients with asthma. Thorax 2010;65:1039–44.
62. Jeppegaard M, Veidal S, Sverrild A, et al. Validation of ATS clinical practice guideline cut-points for FeNO in asthma. Respir Med 2018;144:22–9.
63. Zamarron E, Romero D, Fernández-Lahera J, et al. Should we consider paranasal and chest computed tomography in severe asthma patients? Respir Med 2020; 169:106013.
64. Carden KA, Boiselle PM, Waltz DA, et al. Tracheomalacia and tracheobronchomalacia in children and adults: an in-depth review. Chest 2005;127:984–1005.
65. Hargreave FE. Induced sputum for the investigation of airway inflammation: evidence for its clinical application. Can Respir J 1999;6:169–74.
66. Gyawali CP, Kahrilas PJ, Savarino E, et al. Modern diagnosis of GERD: the Lyon consensus. Gut 2018;67:1351–62.

Advances in Evaluation and Treatment of Severe Asthma (Part Two)

Christopher H. Fanta, MD

KEYWORDS

- Severe asthma • Monoclonal antibodies • Biologics • SMART therapy
- Leukotriene modifiers • Long-acting muscarinic antagonists
- Bronchial thermoplasty

KEY POINTS

- Traditional medical therapies available to treat therapy-resistant asthma include high-dose inhaled corticosteroids, inhaled corticosteroid/formoterol combination as maintenance and rescue, long-acting muscarinic antagonists, and a lipoxygenase inhibitor.
- Targeted monoclonal antibodies have been developed that block key components of the inflammatory cascade in asthma and can be life changing for the treatment of severe asthma.
- The bronchoscopy-based treatment of thermal energy applied to airway walls via a special catheter, bronchial thermoplasty, remains controversial and recommended only in special circumstances.
- Extra care is needed to protect patients with severe asthma from life-threatening asthma attacks; a patient "survival toolkit" is recommended.

Despite confirmation of the correct diagnosis, reduction or elimination of factors inciting airway inflammation, appropriate treatment of comorbidities that may be aggravating asthma, and confirmation of medication adherence, some patients with asthma will remain symptomatic from uncontrolled asthma. These patients have exercise limitation, troublesome cough, sleep disturbance, and/or recurrent exacerbations requiring repeated courses of oral corticosteroids despite appropriate use of high-dose inhaled corticosteroids (ICSs), long-acting beta-agonist (LABA) bronchodilators, and leukotriene modifiers. They have true therapy-resistant severe asthma. In the past, often the only option available to them was long-term oral corticosteroids, with myriad attendant adverse side effects (iatrogenic Cushing syndrome). Now, alternative treatments have become available that successfully control the vast majority of such patients with severe, refractory asthma. Part 2 of this discussion of "Advances in

Pulmonary and Critical Care Medicine Division, Partners Asthma Center, Brigham and Women's Hospital, Harvard Medical School, PBB – Clinics 3, 75 Francis Street, Boston, MA 02115, USA
E-mail address: cfanta@bwh.harvard.edu

Med Clin N Am 106 (2022) 987–999
https://doi.org/10.1016/j.mcna.2022.08.004
medical.theclinics.com
0025-7125/22/

Evaluation and Treatment of Severe Asthma" focuses on approaches to intensify treatment of patients with severe asthma who have failed to achieve good asthma control despite treatment with combination ICS/LABA and a leukotriene receptor antagonist (Step 4) in the Asthma Management Guidelines.[1,2]

CONVENTIONAL DRUG THERAPIES

High-dose ICSs: ICSs when used in combination with LABAs prove more effective than ICSs alone as maintenance therapy for moderate and severe asthma (**Box 1**). The safety of the ICS/LABA combination inhalers has been confirmed in multiple large-scale clinical trials, exonerating LABAs from any drug class-associated effect causing near-fatal or fatal asthma attacks.[3–5] For severe asthma, evidence from randomized clinical trials supports increasing the dose of ICSs in combination ICS/LABA inhalers to the highest corticosteroid concentration.[6,7] With once or twice daily dosing, patients can receive 1000 µg/d of fluticasone propionate or the equivalent.

At these high doses, ICSs are to some extent systemically absorbed and with long-term use can manifest with side effects commonly associated with oral corticosteroids: glaucoma,[8] cataracts,[9] skin thinning with ecchymoses, and accelerated bone loss.[10] Periodic eye examinations and bone densitometry (dual-energy X-ray absorptiometry scans) are indicated, with therapeutic options available to maintain bone health. It is worth remembering that the purpose of prescribing high-dose ICSs is to reduce the need for oral corticosteroids, with their far more severe side effect profile.

As-needed ICS together with albuterol or levalbuterol: In patients prone to recurrent asthma exacerbations, an effective preventive strategy is the administration of an ICS with each as-needed use of quick-reliever medication.[11] For instance, patients using albuterol by metered-dose inhaler or nebulizer can be advised to use a separate inhaler containing an ICS with each use of their albuterol taken as needed for relief of symptoms. It is likely that in the near future combination inhalers containing both an ICS and albuterol will become available in the United States, as are currently marketed in other parts of the world.[12]

ICS-formoterol combination: Alternatively, the LABA bronchodilator, formoterol, has a rapid onset of action similar to that of the short-acting beta-agonist (S albuterol.[13] Formoterol is available combined with an ICS, either budesonide or mometasone. A strategy that has been proved effective in reducing asthma exacerbations, including severe exacerbations requiring oral corticosteroids or urgent care, is use of a combination formoterol/ICS inhaler taken both twice daily for asthma control and as needed for rescue therapy, an approach referred to as SMART (single inhaler for maintenance

---

Box 1
Conventional drug therapies

- ICS/LABA combination inhaler at highest corticosteroid dose.
- ICS as needed together with albuterol or levalbuterol.
- ICS/formoterol combination inhaler as maintenance and rescue therapy.
- Inhaled LAMA bronchodilator.
- Lipoxygenase inhibitor, zileuton.
- Ultra-high doses of ICS.

LAMA, long-acting muscarinic antagonist.

and rescue therapy).[14,15] In this strategy, formoterol replaces albuterol or other short-acting beta-agonist bronchodilators as the quick-reliever medication. This approach has strong supportive evidence and is recommended in their guidelines by national and international asthma expert panels.[1,2]

Both the aforementioned treatment strategies (as-needed ICS administered together with a short-acting beta-agonist bronchodilator and ICS-formoterol combination used for acute relief of asthma symptoms) can be referred to as *anti-inflammatory rescue* or *AIR*. The concept is that anti-inflammatory corticosteroids should be part of the treatment of acute asthma symptoms and that the more frequent the symptoms, the larger the dose of inhaled steroids that will be administered in a timely fashion. We are in a period of transition in asthma practice, and increasingly, AIR, although not yet approved by the US Food and Drug Administration (FDA), is being recommended by expert opinion for asthma of all degrees of severity.

Anticholinergic bronchodilators: For many years the long-acting anticholinergic bronchodilators, referred to as long-acting muscarinic antagonists (LAMAs), had been reserved for treatment of chronic obstructive pulmonary disease (COPD). In patients with asthma, the short-acting anticholinergic bronchodilator, ipratropium, is less potent and has a slower onset of action than albuterol; in COPD it has comparable bronchodilator activity with the advantage of less sympathomimetic stimulation. However, as maintenance therapy, where the rapidity of onset of action is less important, LAMAs provide long-lasting bronchodilation in asthma comparable to LABAs,[16] and combining these 2 types of long-acting bronchodilators offers additive benefit. In a study of patients with severe asthma symptomatic despite high-dose ICS and LABA bronchodilators, adding the LAMA, tiotropium, resulted in improved lung function and prolongation of the time to the first exacerbation of asthma.[17] This approach has been simplified with development of a 3 (medications)-in-1 inhaler approved for use in asthma that combines an ICS (fluticasone furoate), a LABA (vilanterol), and a LAMA (umeclidinium).[7]

Lipoxygenase inhibitor: Most patients with severe, refractory asthma will receive a trial of a leukotriene receptor antagonist (montelukast or zafirlukast) added to their ICS/LABA combination, although evidence in support of an additive benefit is lacking; some caution is indicated because of occasional medication-induced depression and suicidal ideation associated with montelukast.[18] In some patients an alternative leukotriene modifier, the lipoxygenase inhibitor zileuton, has proved to be particularly effective. Anecdotally, zileuton has occasionally been dramatically helpful in patients with aspirin-intolerant asthma (aspirin-exacerbated respiratory disease), an asthma endotype that is characterized by overproduction of leukotrienes at baseline as well as in response to aspirin/nonsteroidal anti-inflammatory drug ingestion.[19]

Ultra-high-dose ICS: Some asthma specialists have used ultra-high doses of ICSs for treatment of severe, refractory asthma, prescribing up to 2000 μg/d. As an example, this approach might include fluticasone/salmeterol combination inhaler 500/50 μg per inhalation taken 1 inhalation twice daily plus as a separate inhaler, fluticasone propionate 220 μg/puff, 2 puffs twice daily. Alternatively, in an approach particularly suited to patients who have difficulty coordinating medication delivery from metered-dose or dry-powder inhalers, additional ICS can be administered by nebulizer, in the form of budesonide unit-dose vials, 500 μg or 1000 μg/vial, twice daily. However, recent analysis using adrenal suppression as a marker of systemic absorption suggests that most of the benefit from ultra-high doses of ICS derives from systemic absorption and systemic delivery of medication to the airways,[20] raising the possibility that this strategy may be of little benefit beyond daily administration of oral corticosteroids.

Theophylline: Finally, addition of the long-acting bronchodilator, theophylline, is notably absent from this list of conventional drug therapies used to treat severe, refractory asthma. Alternative long-acting bronchodilators are equally or more effective,[21] and the frequency of adverse side effects and the potential for life-threatening complications from theophylline overdose outweigh its limited potential additive benefit.

TARGETED MONOCLONAL ANTIBODIES

In recent years scientific advances into the pathobiology of asthma have revealed key metabolic pathways and cellular components important in driving true therapy-resistant severe asthma.[22] These discoveries were closely followed by the development of directed therapies that can block crucial components of these pathways without the many off-target side effects of systemic corticosteroids[23] (**Table 1**). For many patients with severe asthma who had until now been "therapy resistant," these

Table 1
Monoclonal antibodies for severe asthma

Generic Name	Brand Name	Route of Administration	Dosing Frequency	Patient Selection in Asthma	Other Related Indications
Omalizumab	Xolair	Subcutaneous	Every 2–4 wk depending on dose	IgE 30–700 IU/L and sensitization ≥1 perennial aeroallergen	Chronic idiopathic urticaria, nasal polyposis
Mepolizumab	Nucala	Subcutaneous	Every 4 wk	Peripheral blood eosinophilia	Nasal polyposis, EGPA, hypereosinophilic syndrome
Benralizumab	Fasenra	Subcutaneous	Every 4 wk for 3 doses, then every 8 wk	Peripheral blood eosinophilia	None
Reslizumab	Cinqair	Intravenous	Every 4 wk	Peripheral blood eosinophilia	None
Dupilumab	Dupixent	Subcutaneous	Every 2 wk	Peripheral blood eosinophilia; steroid-dependent asthma	Nasal polyposis, atopic dermatitis, eosinophilic esophagitis
Tezepelumab	Tezspire	Subcutaneous	Every 4 wk	Severe asthma regardless of peripheral blood eosinophil number	None

Abbreviation: EGPA, Eosinophilic granulomatosis with polyangiitis.

monoclonal antibody therapies, often referred to as "biologics," have been dramatically effective, described by some patients as "life-altering." Their most consistent benefit has been a significant reduction in the frequency of steroid-requiring exacerbations of asthma. Often, monoclonal antibody therapies have also permitted dose reduction or elimination of daily oral corticosteroids, improved asthma control and asthma quality of life, and to a small extent increased lung function (see **Table 1**).

Mepolizumab is a monoclonal antibody that binds to and interferes with the functioning of interleukin-5 (IL-5). IL-5 is an important driver of eosinophilia in asthma, promoting eosinophil maturation, activation, survival, and migration from the bloodstream into the airways. An early trial of mepolizumab in patients with moderate asthma, still symptomatic despite regular use of ICSs, found mepolizumab no better than placebo in achieving good asthma control.[24] However, multiple subsequent studies have found mepolizumab to be highly effective when used to treat the subset of patients with severe asthma who demonstrate significant blood eosinophilia (generally defined as $\geq$300 eosinophils/μL).[25,26] These observations epitomize the concept of personalized or precision medicine, in which a subpopulation of patients can be identified as most likely to benefit from a therapy based on a certain characteristic or "biomarker" of their disease.

The biomarkers used to identify patients with severe asthma as favorable candidates for monoclonal antibody therapy are blood eosinophilia, elevated total serum immunoglobulin E (IgE), and an exhaled breath nitric oxide concentration that remains elevated despite ICS use. Taken together, these biomarkers identify a characteristic pattern of inflammation in asthma, referred to as type-2 or "type-2 high" inflammation. This inflammation is distinguished from type-1 or "type-2 low" inflammation, in which airways may demonstrate predominantly neutrophilic inflammation, mixed eosinophilic and neutrophilic inflammation, or few inflammatory cells (paucigranulocytic inflammation).[27] Fortunately, most patients with severe therapy-resistant asthma seem to have type-2 high airway inflammation[28] and can benefit from currently available monoclonal antibody therapies. The high cost of these medications makes them inappropriate for treatment of patients with type-2 high inflammation who have mild-to-moderate disease or even severe asthma that can be well controlled by conventional therapies.

All but 1 of the monoclonal antibodies for asthma are administered as subcutaneous injection; the exception (reslizumab) is given as an intravenous infusion. Given their excellent safety profile, home administration is available for most of the agents, facilitated by their preparation in prefilled syringes and autoinjector pens. Dosing intervals vary between every 2 and every 4 weeks and in 1 case (benralizumab) every 8 weeks (after the initial 3 months of monthly dosing). It is often possible to reduce the intensity of conventional therapies (inhaled steroids, LABAs bronchodilators, LAMAs, and leukotriene modifiers), although in most instances patients are encouraged to continue at least a low dose of ICS with or without a LABA bronchodilator. The duration of treatment seems now to be indefinite; to date there is no evidence that these therapies induce disease remission, and therefore relapsed symptoms are anticipated if the monoclonal antibody is stopped.[29] The safety of the monoclonal antibody therapies for asthma administered during pregnancy is uncertain. Many providers choose not to initiate therapy during pregnancy but recommend continuing therapy that has been proved to be effective, weighing the benefits of keeping asthma well controlled during pregnancy over the uncertainty of potential harmful effects on the course of pregnancy or on the fetus.

The first of the biologics for asthma, omalizumab, was introduced in 2003. Omalizumab is an anti-IgE monoclonal antibody that binds to circulating IgE at the site along its Fc region that normally binds to the high-affinity IgE receptor on mast cells. IgE-anti-

IgE complexes can no longer participate in antigen-mediated activation of mast cells. Omalizumab effectively reduces the level of free circulating IgE in the peripheral blood to less than 10% of initial values.[30,31] Commercially available IgE assays cannot distinguish between free IgE and IgE bound to omalizumab; therefore, it is not possible to monitor blood (unbound) IgE levels in response to treatment. In adults omalizumab is approved for use in severe asthma characterized by a peripheral blood IgE level of 30 to 700 IU/mL together with evidence for sensitization (by blood or skin test) to at least 1 perennial aeroallergen (such as dust mite, animal dander, cockroach, mouse, or mold). Because of rare delayed anaphylactic-type reactions to omalizumab, patients are asked to carry with them an epinephrine prefilled syringe for the 24 hours following omalizumab administration.[32] Dosing is adjusted according to total blood IgE level and body weight and, depending on dose, is administered once every 2 or 4 weeks. Other approved indications for omalizumab include chronic idiopathic urticaria and nasal polyposis.

The monoclonal antibodies targeting IL-5 are mepolizumab, benralizumab, and reslizumab. Mepolizumab and reslizumab bind directly to IL-5; benralizumab binds to the alpha-subunit of the IL-5 receptor and activates cell-mediated eosinophil apoptosis.[33] Fixed dosing is used for mepolizumab and benralizumab; the dosing of reslizumab is adjusted according to patient weight, a potential advantage in the morbidly obese patient. These medications achieve rapid reduction of peripheral blood eosinophils, typically within days following the initial injection.[34] In the absence of parasitic infection, this reduction seems not to have harmful consequences. On the other hand, in a person with asthma, eosinophilia, and a history of residence in or travel to areas with endemic parasitic infections, it seems prudent to check blood for evidence of strongyloides infection (strongyloides antibody in peripheral blood) before initiating therapy. Side effects are few but include generalized arthralgias and myalgias. Anti-IL-5 monoclonal antibody therapies may be associated with cases of reactivated herpes zoster infection (shingles),[35] and the author has encouraged his patients to obtain recombinant zoster vaccine when receiving IL-5-targeted antibody therapies. There does not seem to be any increased risk of coronavirus disease 2019 (COVID-19) infection or heightened COVID-19 disease severity with any of the biologics used to treat asthma, nor do the biologics blunt the immune response to severe acute respiratory syndrome coronavirus 2 vaccines. Mepolizumab has also been approved for the treatment of chronic rhinosinusitis with nasal polyps, eosinophilic granulomatosis with polyangiitis, and certain types of hypereosinophilic syndrome.

By binding to the alpha subunit of the IL-4 receptor, dupilumab blocks the activity of both IL-4 and IL-13, 2 cytokines important in type-2 airway inflammation.[36] IL-4 promotes B-cell production of IgE, and IL-13 stimulates airway hyperresponsiveness, mucus production, and airway remodeling. Like the monoclonal antibodies targeting IL-5, dupilumab is indicated for severe asthma with eosinophilia.[37] Dupilumab has also been shown to be effective in achieving steroid dose reduction in patients on daily oral corticosteroids and is approved for the treatment of steroid-dependent asthma.[38] Dupilumab was the first monoclonal antibody approved for the treatment of nasal polyposis, and it seems particularly effective in patients with asthma, aspirin-exacerbated respiratory disease, and nasal polyps.[39] Uncommon side effects include conjunctivitis and hair loss.[40] A transient increase in peripheral blood eosinophils, potentially lasting up to several weeks, is seen in approximately 10% of patients. Dupilumab is also approved for the treatment of atopic dermatitis and eosinophilic esophagitis.

Tezepelumab is the most recently approved monoclonal antibody for the treatment of severe asthma; it inhibits the activity of thymic stromal lymphopoietin, one of the cytokines released from airway epithelial cells (referred to as alarmins) and important in driving cellular function toward type-2 high inflammation, beginning with antigen-presenting dendritic cells.[41] Tezepelumab stands unique among the biologics used to treat severe asthma in that although it is most effective in patients with peripheral blood eosinophilia, it also reduces exacerbations and improves symptoms in patients with less than 150 eosinophils/μL. Adverse side effects of tezepelumab were no more frequent than placebo in phase 3 clinical trials. Given its recent development, with approval by the FDA in December 2021, "real-world" experience with tezepelumab outside of clinical trials is largely lacking at the time of this writing.

Bronchial thermoplasty: A tantalizing alternative approach to therapy-resistant severe asthma, one that does not involve long-term administration of injections or intravenous infusions, is the procedural intervention, bronchial thermoplasty. Using a specially designed catheter that can be passed through a conventional bronchoscope, thermal energy (at approximately 150°F) is applied to the walls of medium-sized and large bronchi. The operator, typically an interventional pulmonologist, can treat approximately one-third of accessible bronchi in a single, hour-long session. The procedure is repeated twice at 3-week intervals to target the remaining bronchi. The mechanism by which this procedure might be beneficial is uncertain, with speculation including thinning of hypertrophied airway smooth muscle,[42] interruption of neural pathways important in bronchoconstriction, and alteration of proinflammatory epithelial function.[43]

This technique was evaluated in a double-blind, sham-controlled Asthma Intervention Research trial, called AIR2, involving 288 persons with asthma still symptomatic despite high-dose ICS and LABA bronchodilator (with forced expiratory volume in the first second of expiration [FEV_1] at least 60% of predicted).[44] The primary end point, an improved score on the Asthma Quality of Life Questionnaire, was achieved in those randomized to the active intervention. In addition, over the ensuing 12 months, those treated with bronchial thermoplasty had fewer severe asthma exacerbations, unscheduled medical office visits, emergency department visits, and hospitalizations compared with the sham-treated control group. Observational follow-up of patients 5 and 10 years after bronchial thermoplasty (without a comparator control group) have reported enduring benefit (compared with before bronchial thermoplasty) and the absence of the emergence of any harmful sequelae (such as airway stenoses or bronchiectasis).[45]

Bronchoscopy and catheter deployment in patients with severe asthma are not without risks. In the AIR2 trial, adverse respiratory events were common during the 3 procedures, including 1 episode of major hemoptysis and the need for hospitalization for asthma in 8% of the study population during the 6 weeks following bronchial thermoplasty.[44] In their *2020 Focused Updates to the Asthma Management Guidelines*, the Expert Panel of the National Asthma Education and Prevention Program did not endorse bronchial thermoplasty for most persons with severe asthma, finding on review of available evidence that "the benefits are small, the risks are moderate, and the long-term outcomes are uncertain."[1]

Off-label therapy: Until now, specialized treatment options for patients with type-2 low severe therapy-resistant asthma have been few or nonexistent. The availability of tezepelumab, as described earlier, may change that deficiency, given its efficacy in patients with normal peripheral blood eosinophils and in those with the absence of allergic sensitization to perennial allergens. However, the benefits of tezepelumab in patients with normal peripheral blood eosinophils and low exhaled nitric oxide concentration proved to be minimal in seminal phase 3 studies.[41]

Off-label therapies worth briefly mentioning for this asthma endotype (type-2 low) are azithromycin and imatinib. In one study of patients with severe uncontrolled asthma, including noneosinophilic asthma, azithromycin 500 mg administered 3 days per week for 48 weeks resulted in fewer exacerbations and improved quality of life compared with placebo.[46] Safety concerns include hearing loss, life-threatening cardiac arrhythmias due to QT interval prolongation, and the emergence of resistant organisms.

Mast cells are centrally important in mediating airway inflammation in asthma. Stem cell factor and its receptor, a receptor tyrosine kinase called c-Kit, promote mast cell development and survival in tissues. A 6-month, placebo-controlled trial of the c-Kit inhibitor, imatinib, in patients with severe asthma found decreases in airway hyperresponsiveness and increases in lung function in the imatinib-treated group, with the greatest improvements in lung function found in those with type-2 low disease.[47] Imatinib is one of the drugs now being studied in the National Institutes of Health-sponsored Precision Interventions for Severe and/or Exacerbation-Prone Asthma (PrecISE) trial.[48] Gastrointestinal upset, liver function abnormalities, and electrolyte disturbances are among the common side effects of imatinib.

PROTECTION AGAINST LIFE-THREATENING ASTHMA ATTACKS

Patients with severe, poorly controlled asthma are at increased risk for severe asthma attacks, including those that cause respiratory failure, intensive care unit admission, and death. In particular, any patient who has previously required intensive care unit care for asthma should be flagged as being vulnerable to a repeat life-threatening event, and every effort should be made to protect the patient from a recurrent attack of such severity.[49] The cause of death due to asthma is virtually always asphyxia due to severe airways obstruction.[50] Interrupting and reversing an asthma attack before it becomes life threatening is possible, especially when efforts are initiated early in the course of an exacerbation. Management of any patient with asthma, but especially those with severe asthma, should include discussion of how to recognize a severe asthma attack, actions that the patient can take to reverse the attack, and when and how to get medical help if initial actions are ineffective (**Box 2**).

Some patients, particularly those who do not develop wheezing with worsened airways obstruction, may have difficulty recognizing that they are experiencing an asthma attack. Others may be in denial or confuse their symptoms with a chest cold. A peak flow meter or home spirometer can help patients identify worsened lung function and gauge its severity; it is also a useful tool when communicating with the health care provider, as a thermometer is when discussing a fever. A plan that details how the patient should adjust medications when an asthma attack develops (an asthma action plan) can be designed based on symptoms that the patient is experiencing or peak flow or FEV_1 measurements made by the patient (with reference to baseline values recorded when well).

Rapid-acting inhaled beta-agonist bronchodilators (albuterol, levalbuterol, or formoterol) can be taken with increased frequency (up to every 20–30 minutes initially during a severe attack) and at higher-than-usual doses (4–6 puffs) in an acute crisis, ideally with use of a valved holding chamber (spacer) to improve medication delivery. Because patient technique for inhaling medication from metered-dose inhalers is often less than optimal, many patients benefit from having a hand-held nebulizer to deliver beta-agonist bronchodilator during an attack. Portable, battery-operated nebulizers are available for use outside of the home. In patients with a history of severe asthma attacks of sudden and rapid onset, mimicking (or representing) anaphylaxis, a prefilled epinephrine syringe for self-administration can be lifesaving.

Box 2
Severe asthma survival toolkit

- Peak flow meter or home spirometer
- Asthma action plan
- Hand-held nebulizer and rapid-acting beta-agonist bronchodilator solution
- Epinephrine prefilled syringe
- Oral corticosteroids available at home
- Rapid medical access

Treatment with systemic corticosteroids can also begin at home. Because the response to systemic steroids is typically not observed for 6 or more hours after administration,[51] early administration in a severe attack is often crucially important. Responsible patients can be given a supply of prednisone or methylprednisolone to have at home,[52] available to begin without the delay of having to contact a provider, having a prescription sent to a pharmacy, and then obtaining the medication from a pharmacy, all during their asthma attack.

Finally, patients experiencing an asthma attack, especially those as discussed in this article who are at risk for a severe, life-threatening attack, should have rapid access to medical advice and emergency medical treatment. A health care provider accessible 24 hours a day for medical guidance is ideally part of the care of the patient with severe asthma. In addition, asthma action plans need to include a "red zone," where patients experiencing a severe attack (eg, peak flow or FEV_1 <50% of personal best value; shortness of breath at rest or with minimal activity) are advised to seek emergency help. Early initiation of treatment in the home is not meant to substitute for hospital-based care, if needed.

SUMMARY

Two important developments have transformed our treatment approach to severe asthma. One is the emerging novel strategy that encourages use of an inhaled steroid with each administration of a quick-acting bronchodilator taken for relief of asthmatic symptoms (referred to as *anti-inflammatory rescue* or AIR).[53] This strategy can use a separate corticosteroid inhaler with each administration of a short-acting beta-agonist (eg, albuterol) inhaler (or nebulizer), or it can employ a combination ICS/LABA inhaler in which the LABA, specifically formoterol, has a rapid onset of action. The latter approach has the advantage of requiring only a single inhaler, one that can be used for both daily maintenance therapy and acute symptom relief. It has the disadvantages of cost, limited accessibility depending on health insurance coverage, and lack of FDA approval (and therefore an off-label use).

The other transformative development has been the discovery and commercialization of targeted monoclonal antibodies that block type-2 asthmatic inflammation at crucial steps along the immune cascade, before the formation and release of proinflammatory chemical mediators. In patients with severe, therapy-resistant asthma who have evidence of (1) allergic sensitivities (high IgE level and sensitization to at least 1 perennial aeroallergen by skin test or antigen-specific IgE blood test), (2) peripheral blood eosinophilia (generally ≥300 eosinophils/μL), and/or (3) an elevated exhaled nitric oxide value despite inhaled steroid therapy (generally ≥40 ppb) indicative of persistent airway eosinophilia, appropriate monoclonal antibody therapies can decrease symptoms, reduce the frequency of asthmatic exacerbations, permit steroid dose reduction, and to some extent improve lung function. The monoclonal antibody most recently approved for treatment of severe asthma, tezepelumab, has proved to be effective in clinical trials even in patients with low peripheral blood eosinophils and normal serum IgE. Most of these monoclonal antibodies are given as subcutaneous injections every 2 to 8 weeks and can be self-administered by patients at home. Negative aspects of their use are their high cost and the indefinite (possibly lifelong) duration of therapy. With these novel therapies, the number of patients requiring daily oral steroids for asthma control continues to decline rapidly toward zero.

CLINICS CARE POINTS

- In the patient with severe uncontrolled asthma despite ICSs and LABA bronchodilator, do not assume that chronic oral steroids are needed for long-term asthma control.
- Evaluate patients with therapy-resistant severe asthma for type-2 asthmatic inflammation by measuring total serum immunoglobulin E, blood and/or sputum eosinophils, and exhaled nitric oxide concentration.
- Optimize medical treatment with high-dose inhaled steroids, dual long-acting bronchodilators, inhaled steroids paired to rescue bronchodilator, and occasionally a lipoxygenase inhibitor (zileuton).
- Identify candidates for targeted monoclonal antibodies (biologics); their use in appropriate patients can be life changing.
- Give patients with severe asthma extra instruction in the prevention of asthma attacks, including identification of worsening airflow obstruction, initial home management, and options for acute medical care in the absence of improvement at home.

DISCLOSURE

The author has nothing to disclose.

REFERENCES

1. Expert Panel Working Group of the National Heart, Lung, and Blood Institute (NHLBI) administered and coordinated National Asthma Education and Prevention Program Coordinating Committee (NAEPPCC). 2020 Focused Updates to the Asthma Management Guidelines: A Report from the National Asthma Education and Prevention Program Coordinating Committee Expert Panel Working Group. J Allergy Clin Immunol 2020;146:1217–70.
2. Global Initiative for Asthma. Global strategy for asthma management and prevention. 2022. Available at: www.ginasthma.org. Accessed July 20, 2022.
3. Stempel DA, Raphiou IH, Kral KM, et al. Serious asthma events with fluticasone plus salmeterol versus fluticasone alone. N Engl J Med 2016;374:1822–30.
4. Peters SP, Bleecker ER, Canonica GW, et al. Serious asthma events with budesonide plus formoterol vs. budesonide alone. N Engl J Med 2016;375:850–60.
5. Weinstein CLJ, Ryan N, Shekar T, et al. Serious asthma events with mometasone furoate plus formoterol compared with mometasone furoate. J Allergy Clin Immunol 2019;143:1395–402.
6. Bateman ED, Boushey HA, Bousquet J, et al. Can guideline-defined asthma control be achieved? The Gaining Optimal Asthma Control study. Am J Respir Crit Care Med 2004;170:836–44.

7. Lee LA, Bailes Z, Barnes N, et al. Efficacy and safety of once-daily single-inhaler triple therapy (FF/UMEC/VI) versus FF/VI in patients with inadequately controlled asthma (CAPTAIN): a double-blind, randomised, phase 3A trial. Lancet Respir Med 2021;9:69–84.

8. Garbe E, LeLorier J, Boivin JF, et al. Inhaled and nasal glucocorticoids and the risk of ocular hypertension or open-angle glaucoma. JAMA 1997;277:722–7.

9. Cumming RG, Mitchell P, Leeder SR. Use of inhaled corticosteroids and the risk of cataracts. N Engl J Med 1997;337:8–14.

10. Israel E, Banerjee TR, Fitzmaurice GM, et al. Effects of inhaled glucocorticoids on bone density in premenopausal women. N Engl J Med 2001;345:941–7.

11. Israel E, Cardet J-C, Carroll JK, et al. Reliever-triggered inhaled glucocorticoid in Black and Latinx adults with asthma. N Engl J Med 2022;386:1505–18.

12. Papi A, Chipps BE, Beasley R, et al. Albuterol-budesonide fixed-dose combination rescue inhaler for asthma. N Engl J Med 2022. https://doi.org/10.1056/NEJMoa2203163.

13. Ringdal N, Derom E, Wåhlin-Boll E, et al. Onset and duration of action of single doses of formoterol inhaled via Turbulaler. Respir Med 1998;92:1017–21.

14. O'Byrne PM, Bisgaard H, Godard PP, et al. Budesonide/formoterol combination therapy as both maintenance and reliever medication in asthma. Am J Respir Crit Care Med 2005;171:129–36.

15. Sobieraj DM, Weeda ER, Nguyen E, et al. Association of inhaled corticosteroids and long-acting ß-agonists as controller and quick relief therapy with exacerbations and symptom control in persistent asthma: a systematic review and meta-analysis. JAMA 2018;319:1485–96.

16. Peters SP, Kunselman SJ, Icitovic N, et al. Tiotropium bromide step-up therapy for adults with uncontrolled asthma. N Engl J Med 2010;363:1715–26.

17. Kerstjens HAM, Engel M, Dahl R, et al. Tiotropium in asthma poorly controlled with standard combination therapy. N Engl J Med 2012;367:1198–207.

18. U.S. Food and Drug Administration. FDA requires Boxed Warning about serious mental health side effects for asthma and allergy drug montelukast (Singulair); advises restricting use for allergic rhinitis. FDA Drug Safety Communication (March 4, 2020). Available at. https://www.fda.gov/drugs/drug-safety-and-availability/fda-requires-boxed-warning-about-serious-mental-health-side-effects-asthma-and-allergy-drug. Accessed July 20, 2022.

19. Dahlen B, Nizankowska E, Szczeklik A, et al. Benefits from adding the 5-lipoxygenase inhibitor zileuton to conventional therapy in aspirin-intolerant asthmatics. Am J Respir Crit Care Med 1998;157:1187–94.

20. Maijers I, Kearns N, Harper J, et al. Oral steroid-sparing effect of high-dose inhaled corticosteroids in asthma. Eur Respir J 2020;55:1901147.

21. Tee A, Koh MS, Gibson PG, et al. Long-acting beta2-agonists versus theophylline for maintenance treatment of asthma. Cochrane Database Syst Rev 2007;(3): CD001281. https://doi.org/10.1002/14651858.CD001281.pub2.

22. Wenzel SE. Severe adult asthmas: integrating clinical features, biology, and therapeutics to improve outcomes. Am J Respir Crit Care Med 2021;203:809–21.

23. Israel E, Reddel HK. Severe and difficult-to-treat asthma in adults. N Engl J Med 2017;377:965–76.

24. Flood-Page P, Swenson C, Faiferman I, et al. A study to evaluate safety and efficacy of mepolizumab in patients with moderate persistent asthma. Am J Respir Crit Care Med 2007;176:1062–71.

25. Ortega HG, Liu MC, Pavord ID, et al. Mepolizumab treatment in patients with severe eosinophilic asthma. N Engl J Med 2014;371:1198–207.

26. Bel EH, Wenzel SE, Thompson PJ, et al. Oral glucocorticoid-sparing effect of me-polizumab in eosinophilic asthma. N Engl J Med 2014;371:1189–97.
27. Hamilton D, Lehman H. Asthma phenotypes as a guide for current and future bio-logic therapies. Clin Rev Allergy Immunol 2020;59:16–74.
28. Fahy JV. Type 2 inflammation in asthma — present in most, absent in many. Nat Rev Immunol 2015;15:57–65.
29. Moore WC, Kornmann O, Humbert M, et al. Stopping *versus* continuing long-term mepolizumab treatment in severe eosinophilic asthma (COMET study). Eur Respir J 2022;59:2100396.
30. Fahy JV, Fleming E, Wong HH, et al. The effect of an anti-IgE monoclonal antibody on early- and late-phase responses to allergen inhalation in asthmatic subjects. Am J Respir Crit Care Med 1997;155:1828–34.
31. Hanania NA, Alpan O, Hamilos DL, et al. Omalizumab in severe allergic asthma inadequately controlled with standard therapy: a randomized trial. Ann Intern Med 2011;154:573–82.
32. Lieberman PL, Jones I, Rajwanshi R, et al. Anaphylaxis associated with omalizu-mab administration: risk factors and patient characteristics (Letter to the Editor). J Allergy Clin Immunol 2017;140:1734–6.
33. Tan LD, Bratt JM, Godor D, et al. Benralizumab: a unique IL-5 inhibitor for severe asthma. J Asthma Allergy 2016;9:71–81.
34. Pham T-H, Damera G, Newbold P, et al. Reductions in eosinophil biomarkers by benralizumab in patients with asthma. Respir Med 2016;111:21–9.
35. Mishra AK, Sahu KK, James A. Disseminated herpes zoster following treatment with benralizumab. Clin Respir J 2019;13:189–91.
36. Harb H, Chatila T. Mechanisms of dupilumab. Clin Exp Allergy 2020;50:5–14.
37. Castro M, Corren J, Pavord ID, et al. Dupilumab efficacy and safety in moderate-to-severe uncontrolled asthma. N Engl J Med 2018;378:2486–96.
38. Rabe KF, Nair P, Brusselle G, et al. Efficacy and safety of dupilumab in glucocorticoid-dependent severe asthma. N Engl J Med 2018;378:2475–85.
39. Bavaro N, Gakpo D, Mittal A, et al. Efficacy of dupilumab in patients with aspirin-exacerbated respiratory disease and previous inadequate response to anti-IL-5 or anti-IL5Ralpha in a real-world setting. J Allergy Clin Immunol Pract 2021;9:2910–2.e1.
40. Kychygina A, Cassagne M, Tauber M, et al. Dupilumab-associated adverse events during treatment of allergic diseases. Clin Rev Allergy Immunol 2022. https://doi.org/10.1007/s12016-022-08934-0.
41. Menzies-Gow A, Corren J, Bourdin A, et al. Tezepelumab in adults and adoles-cents with severe, uncontrolled asthma. N Engl J Med 2021;384:1800–9.
42. Goorsenberg AWM, d'Hooghe JNS, Srikanthan K, et al. Bronchial thermoplasty induced airway smooth muscle reduction and clinical response in severe asthma. The TASMA randomized trial. Am J Respir Crit Care Med 2021;203:175–84.
43. Pretolani M, Bergqvist A, Thabut G, et al. Effectiveness of bronchial thermoplasty in patients with severe refractory asthma: clinical and histopathologic correla-tions. J Allergy Clin Immunol 2017;139:1176–85.
44. Castro M, Rubin AS, Laviolette M, et al. Effectiveness and safety of bronchial ther-moplasty in the treatment of severe asthma: a multicenter, randomized, double-blind, sham-controlled clinical trial. Am J Respir Crit Care Med 2010;181:116–24.
45. Chaudhuri R, Rubin A, Sumino K, et al. Safety and effectiveness of bronchial ther-moplasty after 10 years in patients with persistent asthma (BT10+): a follow-up of three randomised controlled trials. Lancet Respir Med 2021;9:457–66.

46. Gibson PG, Yang IA, Upham JW, et al. Effect of azithromycin on asthma exacerbations and quality of life in adults with persistent uncontrolled asthma (AMAZES): a randomised, double-blind, placebo-controlled trial. Lancet 2017; 390:659–68.
47. Cahill KN, Katz HR, Cui J, et al. KIT inhibition by imatinib in patients with severe refractory asthma. N Engl J Med 2017;376:1911–20.
48. Israel E, Denlinger LC, Bacharier LB, et al. PrecISE: Precision medicine in severe asthma: an adaptive platform trial with biomarker ascertainment. J Allergy Clin Immunol 2021;147:1594–601.
49. Marquette CH, Saulnier F, Leroy O, et al. Long-term prognosis of near-fatal asthma. A 6-year follow-up study of 145 asthmatic patients who underwent mechanical ventilation for a near-fatal attack of asthma. Am Rev Respir Dis 1992; 146:76–81.
50. Molfino NA, Nannini LJ, Martelli AN, et al. Respiratory arrest in near-fatal asthma. N Engl J Med 1991;324:285–8.
51. Fanta CH, Rossing TH, McFadden ER Jr. Glucocorticoids in acute asthma. A critical controlled trial. Am J Med 1983;74:845–51.
52. Mayo PH, Richman J, Harris HW. Results of a program to reduce admissions for adult asthma. Ann Intern Med 1990;112:864–71.
53. Papi A, Blasi F, Canonica GW, et al. Treatment strategies for asthma: reshaping the concept of asthma management. Allergy Asthma Clin Immunol 2020;16:75.

Cystic Fibrosis
Highly Effective Targeted Therapeutics and the Impact on Sex and Racial Disparities

Kristina Montemayor, MD, MHS[a], Raksha Jain, MD, MSc[b],*

KEYWORDS

- Cystic fibrosis
- Cystic fibrosis transmembrane conductance regulator (CFTR) modulators
- Sex disparity • Gonadal hormones • Estrogen • Racial disparities

KEY POINTS

- Most of the people with cystic fibrosis (CF) live longer and healthier lives secondary to advances in therapies, including cystic fibrosis transmembrane conductance regulator (CFTR) modulators.
- Although the overall life expectancy of people with CF has improved, multiple epidemiologic studies show that women have worse outcomes than men, and people of Hispanic ethnicity have poorer outcomes than non-Hispanics.
- Whether CFTR modulators will change the disparities in outcomes in people with CF will likely depend on the overall contribution of CFTR function to the mechanism behind the disparities and the distribution of mutation variants in differing populations.

INTRODUCTION

People with cystic fibrosis (CF) are living longer and healthier lives due to advances in therapies, aimed at targeting the underlying pathophysiology and more recently at the underlying genetic defects. Based on US CF Foundation patient registry data from 2020, the median predicted survival for a person born with CF is 59 years of age.[1] There has been a steady improvement in survival over the past 3 decades, with the median life expectancy predicted to be in the late 20s in 1990, in the mid-30s in 2000, and in the late 30s in 2010.[1] The recent jump in predicted life expectancy is largely due to the availability of small molecule therapies that target the underlying genetic defect in CF, called cystic fibrosis transmembrane conductance regulator (CFTR) modulators. These agents are not gene therapy but instead work to stabilize or make the CFTR protein more effective. CFTR

[a] Department of Medicine, Johns Hopkins University, 1830 E. Monument Street 5th Floor, Baltimore, MD 21205, USA; [b] Department of Medicine, University of Texas Southwestern, 5323 Harry Hines Boulevard, Dallas, TX 75390-8558, USA
* Corresponding author.
E-mail address: raksha.jain@utsouthwestern.edu

Med Clin N Am 106 (2022) 1001–1012
https://doi.org/10.1016/j.mcna.2022.07.005
0025-7125/22/© 2022 Elsevier Inc. All rights reserved.

medical.theclinics.com

modulator therapies are now available for almost 90% of people with CF and has improved quantity as well as quality of life.[2,3] Pulmonary disease is the primary cause of mortality in people with CF, though with considerable variability in severity and progression from person to person. Differences in phenotype despite similar genotypes can be attributed to a variety of factors including race and ethnicity as well as sex among a number of other variables.[4,5] Despite this overall improvement in the health, disparities in outcomes exist, with minority populations such as Hispanics and African Americans demonstrating poorer outcomes despite accounting for nearly 15% of the US population with CF.[1,6–8] In addition, women with CF have a shorter life expectancy than men; this is opposed to the typical female versus male life expectancy in the general US population.[9] Whether or not these disparities will narrow in the coming years will depend on the mechanisms driving these differences and the relative contribution of CFTR to the cause.

PATHOPHYSIOLOGY AND EPIDEMIOLOGY OF CYSTIC FIBROSIS

CF is an autosomal recessive life-limiting genetic disease caused by mutations in CFTR. The CFTR protein regulates movement of chloride, sodium as well as bicarbonate across epithelial cell membranes. Dysfunction of the ion transporter, CFTR, classically leads to dehydrated, viscous, and acidic secretions on the surface of epithelial cells in tissues and organs throughout the body.[10] In the airways, CFTR dysfunction leads to thick secretions, impaired mucociliary clearance, chronic respiratory infections, and progressive airflow obstruction that commonly results in early mortality. Other common manifestations include pancreatic insufficiency from blocked pancreatic ducts, intestinal obstruction from dehydrated stool, and infertility in men secondary to obliterated vas deferens in utero as well as many other features.

CF is the most common genetic disorder in people of Northern European descent, with a prevalence of 1 in 3000 in North America and a carrier frequency of 1 in 25.[10] Importantly, people of all races and ethnicities are affected including Hispanics, Asians, and Africans. The Hispanic population makes up 9.6% of people in the United States with CF, whereas African Americans account for 4.7%, and the minority populations are growing.[1] Unfortunately, these populations are commonly diagnosed late and often have worse overall outcomes than non-Hispanic white people.[6,7,11,12] In addition, given the autosomal pattern of inheritance, CF is equally present in men and women, but multiple epidemiologic studies indicate worse outcomes in women for unclear reasons.[9,13,14] CF was historically described as disease of children, but with the advent of new therapies, there are now more adults with CF than children. What was once thought of as an illness of children is now affecting more adults, and the prevalence is expected to increase, as the median predicted survival is now well greater than 50 years of age. However, there are vulnerable populations that may not improve to the same degree as the overall population.

THERAPEUTIC ADVANCES IN CYSTIC FIBROSIS

Since the discovery of the CFTR gene in 1989, the race for a genetic cure has been on full throttle. However, the use of gene therapy has still not reached people with CF.[15] Instead, however, therapeutics targeting the underlying pathophysiology and now CFTR protein function have made a significant impact to the lives of people with CF (**Fig. 1**). In the 1930s, people with CF were not predicted to live past a few years of age, largely driven by nutritional deficiencies and failure to thrive. With the use of pancreatic replacement enzymes in the 1940s to help with digestion, life expectancy improved. The focus then shifted to chronic respiratory disease, where people with CF were experiencing significant morbidity and mortality from chronic airway infections,

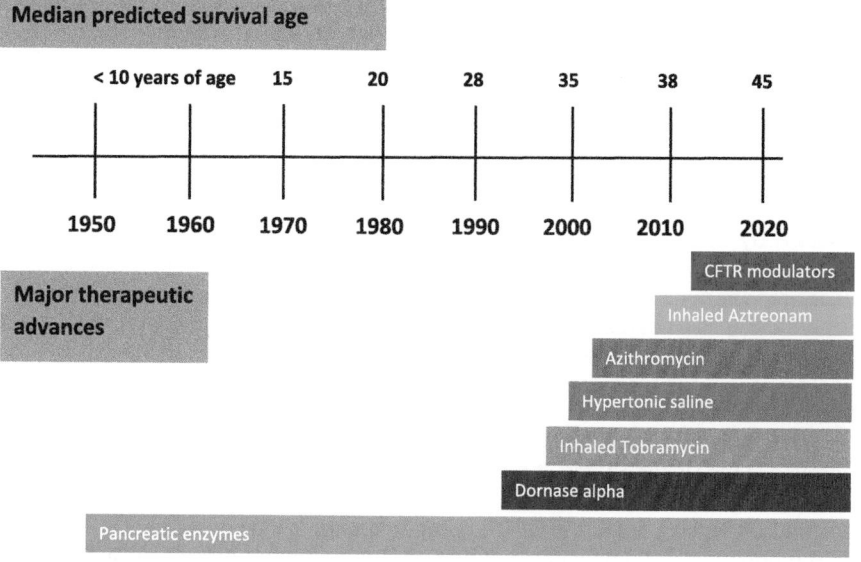

Fig. 1. Therapeutic advances for people with CF over time. Timeline of major therapeutic advances in CF.

inflammation, and scarring, leading to progressive obstructive lung disease. A number of therapies targeting the underlying pathophysiology were developed over the following 4 decades including airway clearance therapy, dornase alfa, hypertonic saline, inhaled antibiotics such as tobramycin and aztreonam, and antiinflammatories such as azithromycin.[16] Airway clearance therapy devices such as the chest vest and vibratory positive expiratory pressure devices aided in clearance of thick secretions from the lungs. The first nebulized drug therapy available to people with CF was dornase alfa. This agent thins respiratory secretions in people with CF by cleaving the DNA released from neutrophils and reducing mucous viscosity.[17] Hypertonic saline is another mucolytic agent that was later shown to be effective in CF.[18] The hypertonic solution works to draw water out of the epithelial cells and rehydrate the mucus. The thick secretions in the CF airway have long been a nidus for infections such as *Pseudomonas aeruginosa* and *Staphylococcus aureus*. *P aeruginosa* is associated with increased pulmonary exacerbations, a more rapid lung function decline, and earlier mortality in CF.[19] Therefore, nebulized antibiotics such as inhaled tobramycin aimed at suppressing *P aeruginosa* and improving lung function were next added to the repertoire of therapies in the late 1990s along with nebulized aztreonam in 2009; both antibiotics resulted in improvement in symptoms associated with CF.[20,21] Antiinflammatory agents, such as orally available ibuprofen and azithromycin, also decreased rates of pulmonary exacerbations (PEx) and improved lung function in people with CF.[22,23] The combination of these advances moved the median predicted survival for people with CF into the 30s but were focused on treating the pathophysiologic respiratory complications of CF rather than correcting the underlying genetic defect.

Cystic Fibrosis Transmembrane Conductance Regulator Modulator Therapy

Mutations in CFTR result in deficient or dysfunctional CFTR protein, which decreases the amount of protein able to reach the cell surface and impairs the ability of the CFTR channels at the cell surface to remain open.[24] CFTR modulators are the first oral therapies for people with CF that aim to correct these defects (**Table 1**). The first CFTR modulator, ivacaftor, was released in the United States in 2012 and subsequently in other countries. Ivacaftor works on CFTR variants known as gating mutations, in which the chloride channel is present on the epithelial cell surface, but does not open properly.[24,25] Ivacaftor, referred to as a potentiator, works by increasing the time that activated CFTR channels at the cell surface remain open. Clinical trials showed that use of ivacaftor increased pulmonary function as measured by percent predicted FEV1 (ppFEV1) by 10.6 percentage points after 24 weeks of use, and these results were sustained through week 48. In addition, ivacaftor resulted in improvements in patient-reported respiratory symptoms, increased weight, and decreased pulmonary exacerbations.[24] Ivacaftor is intended for use in those with CF who have gating mutations, of which *G551D* is the most prevalent example. As these mutations are relatively uncommon, only approximately 5% of all patients with CF in the United States were eligible for therapy.

In 2015, a 2-drug combination, lumacaftor/ivacaftor (lum/iva), was developed and approved in the United States. It is indicated for people with CF who are homozygous for the F508del mutation, the most common CFTR mutation.[26] This combination targets the 2 underlying defects in CFTR, greatly expanding the pool of people eligible for CFTR modulators.[25] Lumacaftor, referred to as a corrector, enhances CFTR protein folding, resulting in increased amounts of protein able to reach the cell surface. Combined with the potentiator ivacaftor, the activated CFTR channels of the larger quantity reaching the surface were able to stay open longer, resulting in improved chloride transport. While expanding the pool of those eligible, the improvement in lung function from this combination was more modest, with a mean absolute improvement in ppFEV1 ranging from 2.6 to 4.0 percentage points.[26]

Two additional CFTR modulator combination therapies have subsequently become widely available. In 2018, tezacaftor/ivacaftor (tez/iva), another corrector and potentiator combination, was approved for people with CF homozygous for F508del mutation. Use of tez/iva resulted in a decrease in pulmonary exacerbation rates by 35% and in modest improvements in lung function, weight gain, and respiratory symptoms.[27] In 2019, a triple combination therapy was approved, combining the corrector elexacaftor with tezacaftor/ivacaftor. Elexacaftor/tezacaftor/ivacaftor (ETI) use caused robust improvements in lung function as well as a 63% lower rate of PEx over a 24-week study period.[28,29] ETI is now approved for people with CF ages 6 years and older with at least one copy of the F508del mutation, making CFTR modulators available for approximately 90% of the CF population.

FACTORS KNOWN TO AFFECT SURVIVAL IN CYSTIC FIBROSIS

The global increase in median age of survival associated with medical advances has not been uniform. Research has shown several key variables that affect survival in people with CF.

Nonmodifiable risk factors identified in studies of survival in CF include female sex and Hispanic ethnicity.[6,13] Additional factors associated with worse survival in CF are severely decreased lung function (ppFEV1 <30%), pancreatic insufficiency, CF-related diabetes (CFRD), and infection with certain bacterial pathogens including *P aeruginosa*, *Burkholderia cepacia* complex, and methicillin-resistant *S aureus*.[30–32] In addition, Stephenson and colleagues[30] demonstrated that modifiable risk factors including malnutrition and PEx increased the risk of death in a contemporary cohort of people with CF in Canada. Furthermore, they also demonstrated an interaction

Table 1

Cystic fibrosis transmembrane conductance regulator modulator therapies available in the United States

Therapy	Type of Modulator	Mechanism of Action	Availability	Indication
Ivacaftor (VX-770)	Potentiator	Increases channel opening	Ivacaftor 2012	Gating mutations
Lumacaftor (VX-809)	Corrector	Moves defective CFTR protein to proper place in cell membrane and improves chloride channel function;	Lumacaftor + Ivacaftor 2015	F508del/F508del
Tezacaftor (VX-661)	Corrector		Tezacaftor + Ivacaftor 2018	F508del/F508del
Elexacaftor (VX-445)	Corrector	Increases mature protein at cell surface (folding, processing, trafficking)	Elexacaftor + Tezacaftor + Ivacaftor 2019	Single copy of F508del

between sex and CFRD, with an increased prevalence of CFRD in women and a higher mortality in women with CFRD compared with men.

RACIAL AND ETHNIC DISPARITIES IN PEOPLE WITH CYSTIC FIBROSIS

CF was long thought of as a disease of people of Northern European ancestry with an incidence of approximately 1 in 3000. The incidence is thought to be 1 in 9200 in individuals of Hispanic descent and 1 in 15,000 in African Americans.[7] The most common allelic variant, F508del, likely originated 11,000 to 34,000 years ago in Europe and spread beyond.[33] There are now more than 2000 known disease-causing CFTR mutations, and the incidence of the disease as well as the frequency of specific mutations probably reflect ancient migratory patterns, genetic drift, and possibly a selective advantage of heterozygous carriers (protective against death from cholera).[33]

In the United States, every state has a newborn screening (NBS) program to help identify babies born with CF early to enable early intervention. Members of minority groups are more likely to be diagnosed later secondary to missed diagnosis with traditional genetic panels and the methods used in state newborn screening.[11,12] Most state NBS protocols rely on detecting pancreatic insufficiency via measurement of immunoreactive trypsinogen. Elevated levels are commonly the trigger for CFTR mutation panel testing. Importantly, almost 75% of non-Hispanic White people with CF have class I to III mutations (typically resulting in pancreatic insufficiency), compared with approximately 50% of Black, Hispanic, and people of other races with CF.[33] Approximately 25% of Black, Hispanic, and people of other minorities have unclassified CFTR mutations, compared with only 11% of non-Hispanic White people with CF.[33] In addition, only 3% of non-Hispanic White people with CF do not have 2 identified CFTR mutations, whereas 8% to 10% of Black, Hispanic, and members of other minority groups have at least one CFTR mutation that has not been not identified.[33] As a result, more members of minority groups are missed on NBS and are diagnosed later in life, putting them at risk of experiencing significant malnutrition and pulmonary damage before diagnosis.

In the United States, multiple studies have shown that racial and ethnic minorities also have increased morbidity and mortality from CF compared with people of non-Hispanic White background, even when controlling for socioeconomic status.[6,8] Hispanic people with CF in the United States have an increased risk of mortality compared with non-Hispanic White people and die at an earlier age.[6,34] Hispanic people with CF are at increased risk of acquiring pulmonary infections and acquiring them at a younger age compared with non-Hispanic White people with CF.[12] Both Hispanic and Black people with CF have lower pulmonary function compared with non-Hispanic White people with CF.[7,8] Differences in morbidity or mortality have not yet been investigated specifically in Asian or Native American people with CF in the United States, and limited data in those groups from outside of the United States make it difficult to compare racial and ethnic outcomes.

Finally, because of differences in CFTR mutation frequency, fewer members of racial and ethnic minorities qualify for CFTR modulators. Although greater than 90% of non-Hispanic White people with CF in the United States have CFTR mutations that qualify for a CFTR modulator, only 70% of American Black, 75% of Hispanic, and 80% of other racial minorities with CF have qualifying mutations.[35] This lower frequency of mutation responsive to current CFTR modulators may compound the racial disparity already present in CF. However, racial/ethnic differences in CFTR mutations are not the only explanation for disparities in CFTR modulator use. Even among people with a G551D mutation allele qualifying for the highly effective modulator, ivacaftor, its use has been found to be significantly lower in Hispanic and non-White adults than in white, non-Hispanics.[36] The cause of this difference is unclear and may be due to a number of factors, including provider bias, lack of awareness or interest in these therapies among minority patients, cultural biases, and barriers with cost. Regardless of cause, ethnic and racial disparities exist in the diagnosis and outcomes of people with CF, a disparity that may potentially grow with fewer minority group members receiving CFTR modulator therapy. Approaches to disparity reduction will need to be multipronged. Improvement in diagnostic and screening methods in minority populations are needed, such as CFTR mutation sequencing. Cultural barriers need to be addressed, including, but not limited to, increased patient education on CF, expanded non-English language material, and addressing medication affordability.

Sex Disparity in Outcomes of People with Cystic Fibrosis

Another area of disparity in CF that affects half of the population is that of sex. Although an autosomal recessive inherited disease with similar male and female prevalence, females with CF have worse clinical outcomes, including survival.[9] First reported by Rosenfeld and colleagues in 1997,[13] female sex was shown to be independently associated with risk of death, and women had a decrease in median life expectancy compared with men[13]; this was corroborated by Demko and colleagues,[14] who showed an earlier acquisition of *P aeruginosa* in women that was associated with increased mortality. Although survival has increased in both sexes over the years with advances in therapies, large registry analysis continue to show that female sex is associated with an increased risk of death, with a median life expectancy nearly 3 years shorter than men.[9] However, the long-term impact of CFTR modulators on the sex disparity in CF is not yet known.

Various mechanisms have been explored in an effort to understand the observed sex disparity in CF (**Fig. 2**). Differences in anatomy, microbial acquisition, immune-mediated effects, variations in endogenous sex hormones, and CFTR function itself are considered plausible biological mechanisms. Women have smaller lungs at birth and maintain smaller conducting airways into adulthood, possibly leading to impaired mucociliary clearance and increased susceptibility to pulmonary infections.[37] Women acquire *P aeruginosa* earlier than men, and this pathogen has been associated with a

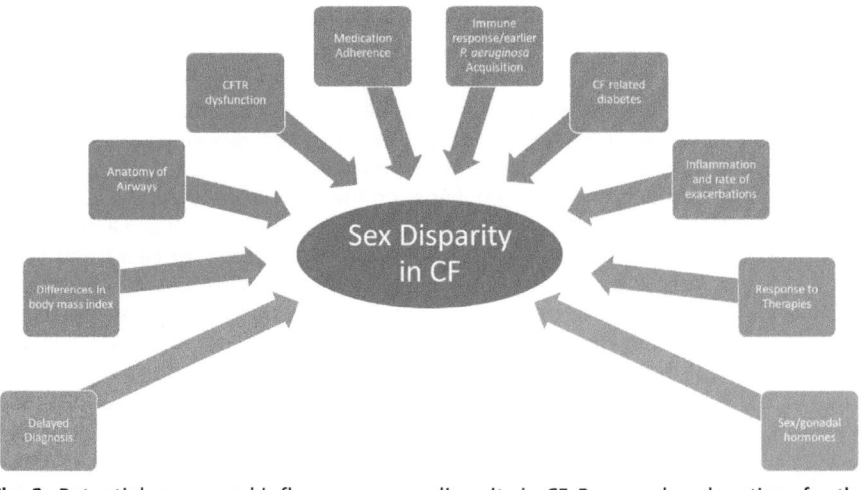

Fig. 2. Potential causes and influences on sex disparity in CF. Proposed explanations for the disparity in outcomes between men and women with CF.

2.6 times higher risk of death in people with CF as well as independently associated with an increased rate of lung function decline.[38] In addition to *P aeruginosa*, researchers demonstrated earlier acquisition of other pathogens including methicillin-resistant *S aureus*, *Achromobacter xylosoxidans*, *Burkholderia cepacia*, *Aspergillus species*, and nontuberculous mycobacterium infections in women with CF.[9]

In addition to increased mortality, women with CF are disproportionately affected by PEx and have worse clinical outcomes. PEx, commonly defined as an acute worsening of pulmonary symptoms and/or decrease in lung function requiring treatment with antibiotics, remain common occurrences in people with CF despite recent advances.[1] Women have more PEx per year compared with men, and women are less likely to return to baseline lung function following PEx treatment.[9,39,40] Women are also more likely to require retreatment within 30 days of initial PEx treatment.[9,39,40] Female sex has also been independently associated with a higher rate of treatment days with intravenous antibiotics. Despite receiving longer treatment, women reported worse respiratory symptoms as the end of intravenous treatment compared with men.[41]

Researchers have also shown that women with CF have a significantly higher rate of PEx beginning after puberty, suggesting female sex hormones may affect respiratory health.[42] Animal models demonstrate that estrogen affects mucous cell hyperplasia and upregulates mucous production while inhibiting chloride secretion, resulting in disturbances in mucociliary clearance.[43] Chotirmall and colleagues showed that in vitro exposure of *P aeruginosa* to 17β-estradiol was associated with mucoid colony formation and proposed that estradiol levels correlated with PEx in women with CF. Importantly, they observed that PEx occurred less frequently in women taking hormonal contraceptive pills (which suppress endogenous 17β-estradiol)[44]; this was corroborated by work that showed increased inflammatory markers and serine proteases including neutrophil elastase in the sputum of women with CF at times of ovulation (high estrogen) relative to menses (low estrogen) and that the markers of inflammation were attenuated with use of oral hormone contraception.[45] Additional work including studies in mouse models supports these studies.[46,47] Wang and colleagues studied the effects of exogenous estrogen treatment by infecting male mice with a mucoid *P aeruginosa* isolate. Their data showed higher levels of inflammation including neutrophilic infiltration and higher levels of inflammatory markers in the lung tissue and bronchial alveolar fluid in the estrogen-treated groups.[46] Furthermore, Abid and colleagues[47] used a CF murine model infected with a nonmucoid *P aeruginosa* strain and similarly showed that estrogen-treated ovariectomized female mice had more lung inflammation with higher levels of inflammatory markers and decreased survival. Both animal and human data suggest that estrogen contributes to a dysregulated inflammatory response; further work is needed to consider targeted therapies based on sex to improve the outcomes in all people with CF.

The long-term impact of CFTR modulators on the sex disparity in CF is unknown, but understanding sex-specific differences in CFTR function as well as CFTR modulator response is essential. Data from the International Society of Heart and Lung Transplantation (ISHLT) database of men and women lung transplant recipients with CF show that despite women being transplanted at a younger age, there is no difference in survival posttransplant or time to bronchiolitis obliterans syndrome[48]; this was true regardless of the sex of the donor and suggests that CFTR dysfunction in the lungs of people with CF may affect survival differences before lung transplantation.[48] Recent data suggest sex differences in CFTR modulator response based on sweat chloride levels. A study by Secunda and colleagues[49] using data from a multicenter study of people with CF started on ivacaftor showed that women had a significant decrease in sweat chloride levels at 3 months compared with men (55.5 mEq/L vs

48.8 mEq/L, respectively; p = 0.045). The investigators also demonstrated that sweat chloride response was correlated with body weight. Although there were no differences in lung function as measured by ppFEV1, women had a greater decline in PEx despite having a higher baseline rate of PEx.[33] In a study of lum/iva by Aalbers and colleagues,[50] the investigators also reported a greater decline in sweat chloride in women, but no correlation with the change in sweat chloride and changes in lung function or body mass index in those treated with lum/iva for at least 6 months. Given the shorter follow-up time in this study, changes in PEx rate were not able to be evaluated.[50] Data thus far suggest that sweat chloride levels do not correlate well with clinical outcomes in CF.[51,52] These studies, however, collectively describe some of the first epidemiologic evidence describing a differential response to CFTR modulators by sex. Given the widespread use of ETI, further studies evaluating sex differences in ETI response is a field of active study.

SUMMARY AND FUTURE CARE CONSIDERATIONS IN PEOPLE WITH CYSTIC FIBROSIS

Improved therapies have led to better outcomes and an increased life expectancy in the population of people with CF as a whole. With the advent of CFTR modulators targeting underlying genetic defects, the CF community has moved to personalized medicine. Yet there is much still to be learned about sex as well as about racial and ethnic differences in response to CF-specific therapies. Studies evaluating differences in pharmacokinetics of therapies in CF by sex, race, or ethnicity are limited, and learning whether these differences exist is needed to help improve outcomes. We have learned that genotype does not always lead to the same phenotype. There is a growing minority population among those with CF whose outcomes are lagging behind those of non-Hispanic white people. Biases in diagnosis and treatment of underrepresented people with CF remain to be addressed. Improved diagnostic protocols including NBS and educational efforts to support minority populations is still needed. Furthermore, there are robust data suggesting a sex disparity in CF that may be driven by gonadal hormones such as estrogen. A number of questions about future outcomes in women with CF remain to be answered. Understanding if clinical outcomes improve as women with CF age into menopause and estrogen levels decline remains a priority. The association of gonadal hormones with respiratory health remains an active area of research within CF, and future targeted therapies may be possible to eliminate differences. Finally, as more people identify as a gender that is not congruent with their sex assigned at birth and consider gender transition, the impact of gender-affirming hormone therapies on lung health is critical to understand. Although the health of people with CF has dramatically improved over the past few decades, we have to consider genotype and phenotype as we aim for personalized medicine approaches in CF care.

CLINICS CARE POINTS

- Advances in therapies with CF have transformed it from a pediatric illness to an illness of adults and even older adults.
- The multisystem nature of CF in a life-long illness will require a number of specialists to become well versed in the disease.
- Disparities in outcomes in people with CF when it comes to race and sex disparities need to be addressed.

DISCLOSURE

K. Montemayor receives funding from the CF Foundation (MONTEMQ020), none of which is related to the content of this article. R. Jain receives consulting fees from Boehringer Ingelheim, Gilead Sciences, and Vertex Pharmaceuticals, none of which are related to the content of this article.

REFERENCES

1. Cystic Fibrosis Foundation Patient Registry. 2020 Annual Data Report. 2021. https://www.cff.org/sites/default/files/2021-11/Patient-Registry-Annual-Data-Report.pdf. Online.
2. Balfour-Lynn IM, King JA. CFTR modulator therapies - Effect on life expectancy in people with cystic fibrosis. Paediatr Respir Rev 2020;42:3–8.
3. Bierlaagh MC, Muilwijk D, Beekman JM, et al. A new era for people with cystic fibrosis. Eur J Pediatr 2021;180(9):2731–9.
4. Schechter MS. Non-genetic influences on cystic fibrosis lung disease: the role of sociodemographic characteristics, environmental exposures, and healthcare interventions. Semin Respir Crit Care Med 2003;24(6):639–52.
5. Wolfenden LL, Schechter MS. Genetic and non-genetic determinants of outcomes in cystic fibrosis. Paediatr Respir Rev 2009;10(1):32–6.
6. Rho J, Ahn C, Gao A, et al. Disparities in mortality of hispanic patients with cystic fibrosis in the united states. A national and regional cohort study. Am J Respir Crit Care Med 2018;198(8):1055–63.
7. Hamosh A, FitzSimmons SC, Macek M Jr, et al. Comparison of the clinical manifestations of cystic fibrosis in black and white patients. J Pediatr 1998;132(2):255–9.
8. McGarry ME, Neuhaus JM, Nielson DW, et al. Pulmonary function disparities exist and persist in Hispanic patients with cystic fibrosis: a longitudinal analysis. Pediatr Pulmonol 2017;52(12):1550–7.
9. Harness-Brumley CL, Elliott AC, Rosenbluth DB, et al. Gender differences in outcomes of patients with cystic fibrosis. J Womens Health (Larchmt) 2014;23(12):1012–20.
10. O'Sullivan BP, Freedman SD. Cystic fibrosis. Lancet 2009;373(9678):1891–904.
11. Pique L, Graham S, Pearl M, et al. Cystic fibrosis newborn screening programs: implications of the CFTR variant spectrum in nonwhite patients. Genet Med 2017;19(1):36–44.
12. Watts KD, Layne B, Harris A, et al. Hispanic Infants with cystic fibrosis show low CFTR mutation detection rates in the Illinois newborn screening program. J Genet Couns 2012;21(5):671–5.
13. Rosenfeld M, Davis R, FitzSimmons S, et al. Gender gap in cystic fibrosis mortality. Am J Epidemiol 1997;145(9):794–803.
14. Demko CA, Byard PJ, Davis PB. Gender differences in cystic fibrosis: Pseudomonas aeruginosa infection. J Clin Epidemiol 1995;48(8):1041–9.
15. Cooney AL, McCray PB Jr, Sinn PL. Cystic fibrosis gene therapy: looking back, looking forward. Genes (Basel) 2018;9(11).
16. Pittman JE, Ferkol TW. The evolution of cystic fibrosis care. Chest 2015;148(2):533–42.
17. Fuchs HJ, Borowitz DS, Christiansen DH, et al. Effect of aerosolized recombinant human DNase on exacerbations of respiratory symptoms and on pulmonary function in patients with cystic fibrosis. The Pulmozyme Study Group. N Engl J Med 1994;331(10):637–42.

18. Elkins MR, Robinson M, Rose BR, et al. A controlled trial of long-term inhaled hypertonic saline in patients with cystic fibrosis. N Engl J Med 2006;354(3):229–40.
19. Nixon GM, Armstrong DS, Carzino R, et al. Clinical outcome after early Pseudomonas aeruginosa infection in cystic fibrosis. J Pediatr 2001;138(5):699–704.
20. Ramsey BW, Pepe MS, Quan JM, et al. Intermittent administration of inhaled tobramycin in patients with cystic fibrosis. Cystic Fibrosis Inhaled Tobramycin Study Group. N Engl J Med 1999;340(1):23–30.
21. McCoy KS, Quittner AL, Oermann CM, et al. Inhaled aztreonam lysine for chronic airway Pseudomonas aeruginosa in cystic fibrosis. Am J Respir Crit Care Med 2008;178(9):921–8.
22. Saiman L, Marshall BC, Mayer-Hamblett N, et al. Azithromycin in patients with cystic fibrosis chronically infected with Pseudomonas aeruginosa: a randomized controlled trial. JAMA 2003;290(13):1749–56.
23. Konstan MW, Byard PJ, Hoppel CL, et al. Effect of high-dose ibuprofen in patients with cystic fibrosis. N Engl J Med 1995;332(13):848–54.
24. Ramsey BW, Davies J, McElvaney NG, et al. A CFTR potentiator in patients with cystic fibrosis and the G551D mutation. N Engl J Med 2011;365(18):1663–72.
25. Montemayor K, Lechtzin N. The PROSPECT Is Bright for CFTR Modulators. Ann Am Thorac Soc 2021;18(1):32–3.
26. Wainwright CE, Elborn JS, Ramsey BW, et al. Lumacaftor-Ivacaftor in Patients with Cystic Fibrosis Homozygous for Phe508del CFTR. N Engl J Med 2015;373(3):220–31.
27. Taylor-Cousar JL, Munck A, McKone EF, et al. Tezacaftor-ivacaftor in patients with cystic fibrosis homozygous for Phe508del. N Engl J Med 2017;377(21):2013–23.
28. Middleton PG, Mall MA, Drevinek P, et al. Elexacaftor-Tezacaftor-Ivacaftor for Cystic Fibrosis with a Single Phe508del Allele. N Engl J Med 2019;381(19):1809–19.
29. Heijerman HGM, McKone EF, Downey DG, et al. Efficacy and safety of the elexacaftor plus tezacaftor plus ivacaftor combination regimen in people with cystic fibrosis homozygous for the F508del mutation: a double-blind, randomised, phase 3 trial. Lancet 2019;394(10212):1940–8.
30. Stephenson AL, Tom M, Berthiaume Y, et al. A contemporary survival analysis of individuals with cystic fibrosis: a cohort study. Eur Respir J 2015;45(3):670–9.
31. Blanchard AC, Waters VJ. Microbiology of cystic fibrosis airway disease. Semin Respir Crit Care Med 2019;40(6):727–36.
32. Liou TG, Adler FR, Fitzsimmons SC, et al. Predictive 5-year survivorship model of cystic fibrosis. Am J Epidemiol 2001;153(4):345–52.
33. McGarry ME, Gibb ER, Oates GR, et al. Left behind: the potential impact of CFTR modulators on racial and ethnic disparities in cystic fibrosis. Paediatr Respir Rev 2021;42:35–42.
34. Buu MC, Sanders LM, Mayo JA, et al. Assessing differences in mortality rates and risk factors between hispanic and non-hispanic patients with cystic fibrosis in california. Chest 2016;149(2):380–9.
35. McGarry ME, McColley SA. Cystic fibrosis patients of minority race and ethnicity less likely eligible for CFTR modulators based on CFTR genotype. Pediatr Pulmonol 2021;56(6):1496–503.
36. Sawicki GS, Dasenbrook E, Fink AK, et al. Rate of Uptake of Ivacaftor Use after U.S. Food and Drug Administration Approval among Patients Enrolled in the U.S. Cystic Fibrosis Foundation Patient Registry. Ann Am Thorac Soc 2015;12(8):1146–52.

37. Carey MA, Card JW, Voltz JW, et al. It's all about sex: gender, lung development and lung disease. Trends Endocrinol Metab 2007;18(8):308–13.

38. Li Z, Kosorok MR, Farrell PM, et al. Longitudinal development of mucoid Pseudomonas aeruginosa infection and lung disease progression in children with cystic fibrosis. JAMA 2005;293(5):581–8.

39. Sanders DB, Hoffman LR, Emerson J, et al. Return of FEV1 after pulmonary exacerbation in children with cystic fibrosis. Pediatr Pulmonol 2010;45(2):127–34.

40. VanDevanter DR, Flume PA, Morris N, et al. Probability of IV antibiotic retreatment within thirty days is associated with duration and location of IV antibiotic treatment for pulmonary exacerbation in cystic fibrosis. J Cyst Fibros 2016;15(6):783–90.

41. Montemayor K, Psoter KJ, Lechtzin N, et al. Sex differences in treatment patterns in cystic fibrosis pulmonary exacerbations. J Cyst Fibros 2021;20(6):920–5.

42. Sutton S, Rosenbluth D, Raghavan D, et al. Effects of puberty on cystic fibrosis related pulmonary exacerbations in women versus men. Pediatr Pulmonol 2014;49(1):28–35.

43. Coakley RD, Sun H, Clunes LA, et al. 17beta-Estradiol inhibits Ca2+-dependent homeostasis of airway surface liquid volume in human cystic fibrosis airway epithelia. J Clin Invest 2008;118(12):4025–35.

44. Chotirmall SH, Smith SG, Gunaratnam C, et al. Effect of estrogen on pseudomonas mucoidy and exacerbations in cystic fibrosis. N Engl J Med 2012; 366(21):1978–86.

45. Holtrop M, Heltshe S, Shabanova V, et al. A Prospective Study of the Effects of Sex Hormones on Lung Function and Inflammation in Women with Cystic Fibrosis. Ann Am Thorac Soc 2021;18(7):1158–66.

46. Wang Y, Cela E, Gagnon S, et al. Estrogen aggravates inflammation in Pseudomonas aeruginosa pneumonia in cystic fibrosis mice. Respir Res 2010;11:166.

47. Abid S, Xie S, Bose M, et al. 17beta-Estradiol Dysregulates Innate Immune Responses to Pseudomonas aeruginosa Respiratory Infection and Is Modulated by Estrogen Receptor Antagonism. Infect Immun 2017;85(10):1–15.

48. Raghavan D, Gao A, Ahn C, et al. Lung transplantation and gender effects on survival of recipients with cystic fibrosis. J Heart Lung Transplant 2016;35(12): 1487–96.

49. Secunda KE, Guimbellot JS, Jovanovic B, et al. Females with cystic fibrosis demonstrate a differential response profile to Ivacaftor compared with males. Am J Respir Crit Care Med 2020;201(8):996–8.

50. Aalbers BL, Hofland RW, Bronsveld I, et al. Females with cystic fibrosis have a larger decrease in sweat chloride in response to lumacaftor/ivacaftor compared to males. J Cyst Fibros 2021;20(1):e7–11.

51. Zemanick ET, Konstan MW, VanDevanter DR, et al. Measuring the impact of CFTR modulation on sweat chloride in cystic fibrosis: Rationale and design of the CHEC-SC study. J Cyst Fibros 2021;20(6):965–71.

52. Flume PA, Liou TG, Borowitz DS, et al. Ivacaftor in subjects with cystic fibrosis who are homozygous for the F508del-CFTR mutation. Chest 2012;142(3):718–24.

Advances in Surgical and Mechanical Management of Chronic Obstructive Pulmonary Disease

Bilal H. Lashari, MD, MScPH[a],*, Gerard J. Criner, MD[b]

KEYWORDS

• COPD • Emphysema • BLVR • LVRS • Lung transplant

KEY POINTS

- Hyperinflation is a major cause of dyspnea in chronic obstructive pulmonary disease (COPD), especially in patients with an emphysematous phenotype.
- Lung volume reduction can be achieved bronchoscopically, as well as surgically.
- Bronchoscopic lung volume reduction using endobronchial valves achieves symptom and quality-of-life improvement that parallels surgical lung volume reduction.
- Surgical lung volume reduction has a mortality benefit in select patient populations.
- Lung transplantation is the ultimate treatment for COPD and is a highly selective process, which demands careful evaluation and early referral.

INTRODUCTION

Chronic obstructive pulmonary disease (COPD) is the third leading cause of mortality in the United States, behind cardiovascular and malignant disorders. It is also a common cause of significant morbidity and disability.

Initially thought of as only an airway disease, our understanding of COPD pathogenesis has evolved into a complex disorder of multiple interlocking pathways of repetitive inflammation, cellular injury, and aberrant repair that results in progressive lung damage to the parenchyma, airway, and vascular bed. This knowledge has been instrumental in developing numerous pharmaceutical targets and driving further research into drug development. However, the most successful current management targets lung hyperinflation. Dyspnea, exercise limitation, compromised cardiac function,

[a] Department of Thoracic Medicine and Surgery, Temple Lung Center, Temple University Hospital, 7 Parkinson Pavilion, 3401 North Broad Street, Philadelphia 19140, USA; [b] Department of Thoracic Medicine and Surgery, Lewis Katz School of Medicine at Temple University, Temple Lung Center, Temple University Hospital, 7 Parkinson Pavilion, 3401 North Broad Street, Philadelphia 19140, USA
* Corresponding author.
E-mail address: bilal.lashari@tuhs.temple.edu

Med Clin N Am 106 (2022) 1013–1025
https://doi.org/10.1016/j.mcna.2022.07.006
0025-7125/22/© 2022 Elsevier Inc. All rights reserved.

and increased mortality are all caused by hyperinflation. Most interventions aim to decrease or assist the patient to better tolerate hyperinflation. Although pharmacologic interventions can decrease hyperinflation, in those that are most severely hyperinflated (eg, due to emphysema), medical interventions alone are insufficient to reduce hyperinflation and beneficially alter the trajectory of the disease.

Herein, we provide an overview of the mechanical and surgical treatment of COPD and discuss nonsurgical or mechanical interventions, including bronchial occlusion therapies with endobronchial valves (EBVs), self-activating coils, foam sealants, thermal ablation, and airway bypass stenting, and then proceed to discuss surgical interventions, including lung volume reduction surgery (LVRS), bullectomy, and lung transplantation. Each section includes information on patient selection to assist clinicians in the timely identification and referral of patients who may benefit from these modalities.

RATIONALE FOR MECHANICAL OR SURGICAL INTERVENTION IN SEVERE CHRONIC OBSTRUCTIVE PULMONARY DISEASE

The 2022 Global Initiative for Chronic Obstructive Lung Disease report emphasizes patient symptoms and exacerbation history in the characterization of disease severity. It moves away from simple spirometric grading alone based on airflow limitation as measured by forced expiratory volume in 1 second (FEV_1). Patients with COPD form a heterogeneous group of individuals with a range of symptoms that require unique treatments despite having similar degrees of airflow obstruction. One of the most prevalent and important symptoms of COPD, especially emphysema, is dyspnea, with lung hyperinflation as the most important cause.

Lung hyperinflation results when there is an increase in the residual volume of the lung (RV). As the total lung capacity (TLC) is fixed, the volume available for tidal ventilation, also known as the inspiratory capacity, is reduced. This results in rapid shallow breathing to maintain adequate minute ventilation and contributes to a sensation of dyspnea. This problem is much more severe during exercise, as an increased respiratory demand requires a concomitant increase in minute ventilation. Additionally, because of airflow limitation, progressive dynamic hyperinflation results in further increases in RV with each successive breath. The dynamic reduction in inspiratory capacity further limits tidal volume, resulting in severe dyspnea and reduced exercise capacity (**Fig. 1**).[1]

Additionally, lung hyperinflation changes the anatomic configuration of the diaphragm to a mechanically disadvantageous one by causing it to foreshorten, decreasing its area of apposition to the rib cage and by increasing its radius of curvature. Hyperinflation also has direct and indirect effects on cardiac hemodynamics and may result in reduced cardiac output. It follows then that any intervention that successfully reduces RV size relative to the TLC would improve patient symptoms. This mechanical problem is the target for all current surgical interventions, with the aim being to reduce lung air trapping by removing diseased portions of the lung.

MECHANICAL MANAGEMENT OF CHRONIC OBSTRUCTIVE PULMONARY DISEASE
Mechanical Management of Emphysema

Reduction of total lung volume (TLV) can be achieved by either surgical removal of the most affected parts or through various means of bronchial occlusion, leading to atelectasis of the diseased segments and a functional reduction in lung volume achieved without surgical resection. As these interventions are usually performed via bronchoscopy, they are collectively termed bronchoscopic (BLVR) or endoscopic lung volume reduction. Several devices have been used to affect BLVR, including EBVs, metallic coils, foam sealants, and thermal vapor ablation. While many show promise, only

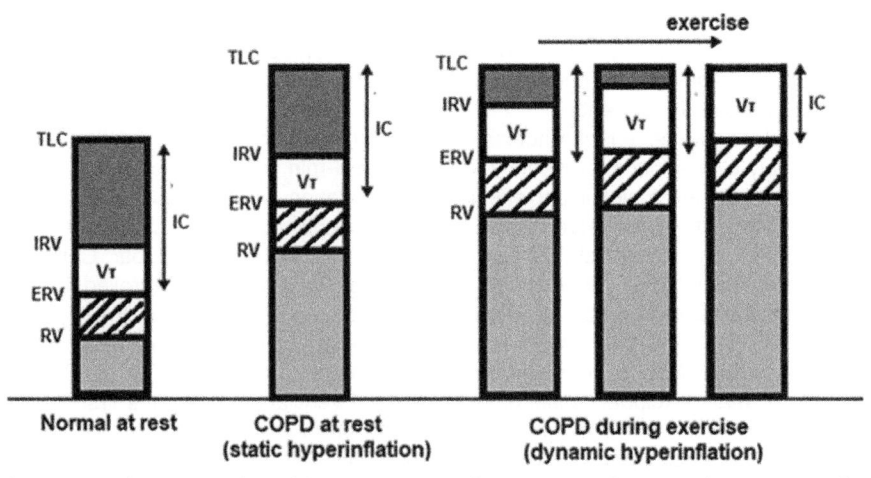

Fig. 1. Note the increased total lung capacity in the patient with COPD when compared to normal, even at rest. With sequential exercise, as tidal volume increases to meet metabolic demand, thr inspiratory reserve volume dimishes, this effect is augmented by dynamic increase in residual volume caused by inefficient exhalation, the net effect is the inability to increase tidal volume and progressive dyspnea.

EBVs are currently approved by the Food and Drug Administration (FDA) for use in COPD. We consider each of these following factors.

Endobronchial valves

Currently available EBVs include the Zephyr Endobronchial Valve (Pulmonx, Inc, Neuchatel, Switzerland) and the Spiration Valve System (Olympus, Tokyo, Japan). These are 1-way valves that, when deployed in the bronchial lumen, prevent air entry during inspiration while allowing air distal to the valve to slowly escape during expiration. This leads to the progressive collapse of distal alveoli and eventual atelectasis of the entire parenchyma distal to the deployed valve, reducing hyperinflation. This system assumes a closed airspace distal to the valve; efficacy is limited when collateral ventilation exists between airspaces. Collateral ventilation is an anatomic variation that exists when alveoli receive ventilation from 2 or more conducting airways. Collateral ventilation occurs through interalveolar communication called pores of Kohn, bronchiolar alveolar communications called channels of Lambert, or intrabronchial communications called channels of Martin. Regardless of the level of communication, the result is failure to achieve atelectasis with endobronchial occlusion if collateral ventilation exists. It is, therefore, a prerequisite that a closed system exists distal to the site chosen for occlusion. A specific marker for the presence of collateral ventilation is the presence of an incomplete lobar fissure on imaging. However, this finding is not sensitive and is limited by imaging and interpretation techniques. An incomplete fissure implies communication among lobes at a macroscopic level, and its presence immediately renders the success of the procedure doubtful. Evaluation of fissure integrity is followed by a physiologic assessment utilizing balloon occlusion of the airway of interest (Chartis, Pulmonx Inc, Neuchatel, Switzerland) and measuring airflow through it after complete lobar occlusion is achieved. Decremental airflow during exhalation, culminating in complete cessation of flow, is indicative of a closed system with no collateral ventilation. This method is superior to fissure integrity imaging evaluation.

While initial clinical trials evaluating the use of EBV were not consistently successful in improving FEV_1 or patient symptoms, significant improvement was apparent in the more selective trials later in its evolution. This evolution highlighted the importance of careful patient selection, operator expertise, foresight and aggressive management of complications, and continued follow-up at an experienced center in providing the best possible outcome for patients.

A decade ago, the endobronchial valve for emphysema palliation (VENT) trial[2] showed only a marginal improvement in FEV_1 and 6-min walk distance and was not able to demonstrate a significant effect on hyperinflation. This was perhaps the first study to demonstrate the importance of collateral ventilation, and subsequent trials, including the Endobronchial Valves for Emphysema without Interlobar Collateral Ventilation (STELVIO),[3] A Multi-center, Prospective, Randomized, Controlled Trial of Endobronchial Valve Therapy vs. Standard of Care in Heterogeneous Emphysema (TRANSFORM),[4] and Bronchoscopic lung volume reduction with endobronchial valves for patients with heterogeneous emphysema and intact interlobar fissures (BeLieVeR-HIFi study)[5] trials, excluded patients with collateral ventilation. While the first 2 trials showed a significant improvement in FEV_1, TLV, and 6-min walk distance, the results of the latter were less robust. STELVIO and TRANSFORM reported a mean decrease in TLV of more than 1000 mL, and this was reflected in an improvement in FEV_1 and patient symptoms.[3,4] The pivotal Lung Function Improvement After Bronchoscopic Lung Volume Reduction With Pulmonx Endobronchial Valves Used in Treatment of Emphysema (LIBERATE)[6] and A Prospective, Randomized, Controlled Multicenter Clinical Study to Evaluate the Safety and Effectiveness of the Spiration® Valve System for the Single Lobe Treatment of Severe Emphysema (EMPROVE)[7] trials established the role of EBV in the FDA-approved management of COPD. Similar to the TRANSFORM trial, these included only patients with a heterogeneous disease (defined as an absolute difference of 15 or greater in destruction scores between the targeted and ipsilateral lobes) with no collateral ventilation and were the most significant international multicenter trials to assess the intervention. Cumulative evidence now suggests that patients most likely to benefit from EBV are those with a heterogeneous disease and severe airflow limitation (FEV_1 <45%) but sufficient to undergo the procedure (FEV_1 >15%), with lung hyperinflation (defined as a TLC $\geq$ 100%) and no collateral ventilation. Patients with a homogeneous disease may also benefit from EBVs, and the most important limitation remains the presence of collateral ventilation. While no clinical trial has evaluated mortality as an endpoint in this context, patient-reported symptoms, 6-min walk distance, and airflow obstruction (FEV_1) have all shown improvement. A summary of criteria for referral to a BLVR program is provided in **Box 1**.

Pneumothorax, either from shear forces applied to the neighboring segments from lobar atelectasis or from compensatory hyperinflation of neighboring segments, remains the most common adverse event. Most clinical trials report a pneumothorax rate of 25% to 35%, with the majority occurring in the first few days after the procedure as

---

Box 1
Indications for EBVs

Limitation in exercise tolerance

TLC greater than 100%

FEV_1 less than 45%

Absence of collateral ventilation

Abbreviations: EBV, endobronchial valves; FEV_1, forced expiratory volume in 1 second; TLC, total lung capacity.

atelectasis of the target lobe ensues, and most require chest tube placement. Patients are therefore usually hospitalized for 3 to 4 days after the procedure.[8] When adequately managed, long-term outcomes are not adversely affected. Exacerbation of COPD along with non–life-threatening hemoptysis are other common complications of the procedure. Less common complications include migration of the EBV, pneumonia, and formation of granulation tissue. Despite the complications reported, BLVR provides benefits comparable to LVRS without the morbidity associated with major thoracic surgeries.

Areas for future study include the impact of BLVR on mortality and the role of EBV in patients with homogeneous emphysema.

Self-activating coils

Self-activating coils are nonocclusive devices. These are spring coils that are inserted into subsegmental airways bronchoscopically and are straight at the time of insertion. They recoil to their original configuration when released. These devices produce atelectasis by "pulling" the peribronchial parenchyma more centrally toward the hilum as they recoil. The major advantage of this approach is the independence from collateral ventilation as atelectasis is achieved by overcoming the distension pressure through the application of the coil. The procedure usually requires the placement of 10 coils in 2 sequential bronchoscopies.

The lung volume reduction coil treatment in patients with emphysema (RENEW) study[9] evaluated coils compared to medical therapy in 315 patients with severe homogeneous or heterogeneous emphysema with an $FEV_1 \leq 45\%$ and hyperinflation (TLC $\geq 100\%$). Investigators targeted the most affected lobes in patients with homogeneous emphysema and the upper lobes in patients with heterogeneous emphysema. Patients in the intervention arm showed a mean improvement of 10.3 m in the 6-minute walk distance at 12 months. Given the mean decline of 7.6 m in the control arm during the same period, the benefit of coils becomes apparent. The intervention group also had an improvement in FEV_1 of 12.3% and, more importantly, in patient-reported symptoms, as assessed by the St George's Respiratory Questionnaire (SGRQ), in 61.2% patients. Unfortunately, there were more in those treated. The intervention group had an increased incidence of lower respiratory tract infections (18.7% vs 4.5%) and pneumothorax (9.7% vs 0.6%). An interesting finding was that 35% of patients initially thought to have pneumonia were found to have a noninfectious cause of opacity; this was determined to be related to atelectasis and was called coil-related opacity. The presence of coil-related opacity was associated with better patient outcomes, indicating the success of the procedure.

A retrospective analysis of coils has unfortunately shown that the benefits are not long lasting, and benefit in the FEV_1 and symptoms were lost at 1 year.[10,11] These findings led to the development of the Randomized Controlled Study of the PneumRx Endobronchial Coil System versus Standard-of-Care Medical Management in the Treatment of Subjects with Severe Emphysema (ELEVATE) trial.[12] This trial was terminated early for financial reasons; however, it did show an improvement in FEV_1 and SGRQ scores in the intervention arm. There is a need for further study in this area, as coils are not FDA-approved for the treatment of COPD; however, these devices may return to the treatment landscape in the future.

Foam sealants

Foam sealants trigger an inflammatory response in the airway wall when deployed leading to fibrosis and subsequent airway occlusion. The AeriSeal (Aeris Therapeutics, Inc, Woburn, MA) is one such system. The sealant was evaluated compared to medical therapy in the ASPIRE study.[13] This study too was terminated early for business-related reasons; however, investigators were able to randomize 95 patients before termination. Patients in the intervention group had an 11.4% improvement in FEV_1, as well as improved SGRQ when compared to the control group at 6 months. Despite the overall improvement in respiratory status, patients in the intervention group had an unacceptable incidence of adverse events, with 2 deaths. Three patients developed severe respiratory failure requiring mechanical ventilation. Other adverse events included pneumonia, pneumothoraces, COPD exacerbation, and cavitary lung disease.[13] It is postulated that these adverse events are secondary to an intense inflammatory response to the sealant.

Because of the early termination of the trial and the burden of adverse events, sealants are not currently used in clinical practice.

Thermal vapor ablation

Vapor ablation uses water vapor to induce inflammation like that caused by sealants, albeit with thermal injury. The result is fibrosis and subsequent atelectasis, causing a decrease in lung volume. As with sealants, the advantage of this technique is that it does not require the absence of collateral ventilation, and smaller areas of the lung can be treated preserving healthy segments or subsegments even in diseased lobes by being selective in targeting airways. In the Sequential Segmental Treatment of Emphysema With Upper Lobe Predominance (STEP-UP) trial,[14] investigators randomized patients with upper-lobe-predominant emphysema with hyperinflation to treatment with thermal ablation and medical therapy and found an improvement in the FEV_1 of 14.7% as well as the SGRQ. However, there was no significant difference in the 6-minute walk distance. This modality too had an excess of adverse events, with up to one-fourth of the patients in the treatment group experiencing an exacerbation of COPD requiring hospitalization, and up to a fifth developing pneumonia. These limit the utility of thermal ablation now.

Airway bypass stents

Bypass stents are unique in that they are designed to be used in patients with homogeneous emphysema. These drug-eluting stents are placed bronchoscopically and create artificial airway connections between central airways and emphysematous lung parenchyma allowing escape of trapped gas. This reduces both static and dynamic hyperinflation. The Safety and Effectiveness of the Exhale® Drug-Eluting Stent in Homogeneous Emphysema Subjects With Severe Hyperinflation (EASE) trial[15] evaluated this technique in patients with severe emphysema and hyperinflation. The study was unable to show a difference in FEV_1 or dyspnea as reported by the modified Medical Research Council score (mMRC) between the intervention and control groups at 6 and 12 months. The authors postulate the lack of long-term benefit from (1) unstented pathways that initially improved air trapping but could not sustain this effect, (2) expectoration of stents leading to occlusion of the artificial communication, and (3) loss of stent patency from debris, granulation, and mucus.[15]

This technique is currently not employed in clinical practice. It remains to be seen whether further research and development will make this viable.

Mechanical Management in Chronic Bronchitis

We have considered the major target for mechanical intervention in COPD as hyperinflation, which is predominantly a feature of the emphysematous phenotype of COPD. However, chronic bronchitis can be extremely debilitating and is characterized by mucosal and goblet cell hyperplasia with excessive mucus secretion as an important feature. There has been interest in the mechanical disruption of mucus hypersecretion through 2 distinct mechanisms.

Targeted lung denervation

Targeted lung denervation aims to exploit the cholinergic innervation of airways which physiologically promotes bronchoconstriction and mucus secretion. Disruption of cholinergic signaling is the target for inhaled muscarinic antagonists which form a mainstay of pharmacologic therapy for COPD. Targeted lung denervation employs radiofrequency ablation to disrupt cholinergic nerves that accompany the mainstem bronchi. The radiofrequency catheter is encapsulated in a coolant-containing balloon which prevents epithelial damage as the thermal energy is directed to the deeper structures. Randomized Study to Optimize Dose Selection and Evaluate Safety After Treatment With the Holaira™ Lung Denervation System in Patients With Moderate to Severe COPD. (AIRFLOW-1)[16] and Randomized Study to Optimize Dose Selection and Evaluate Safety After Treatment With the Holaira™ Lung Denervation System in Patients With Moderate to Severe COPD. (AIRFLOW-2)[17] trials have evaluated lung denervation to establish safety. AIRFLOW-1 resulted in impaired gastric emptying from vagal nerve disruption in 5 of 13 patients, prompting the investigators to amend the protocol to include an esophageal balloon and measure the distance between the radiofrequency catheter and the distal esophagus. The AIRFLOW-2 study showed a lower risk of COPD exacerbation but no difference in patient-related symptoms in the intervention group. This has led to the currently on-going Study to Evaluate Safety and Efficacy After Treatment With the Nuvaira™ Lung Denervation System in Patients With COPD (AIRFLOW-3) study (NCT03639051) which is currently recruiting participants.

Bronchial cryospray

Bronchial cryospray aims to flash freeze and kill the bronchial epithelium including hyperplastic goblet cells, with the assumption that new epithelium will regrow with a normal phenotype without producing inflammation and scarring. This is done using a liquid nitrogen spray. The RejuvenAir (CSA Medical, Lexington, MA) system is currently being evaluated in clinical trials, and the Sham Controlled Prospective Randomized Clinical Trial of the RejuvenAir® System for the Treatment of Moderate to Severe Chronic Obstructive Pulmonary Disease With Chronic Bronchitis (SPRAY-CB) trial (NCT03893370) is currently enrolling patients. The primary endpoint is change in the SGRQ score at 12 months, whereas secondary endpoints include reduction of cough, sputum, and acute exacerbation rate.

Bronchial rheoplasty

Bronchial rheoplasty targets epithelium and goblet cells using short electrical bursts. Electrical energy is applied throughout the accessible airway. Similar to other modalities, it aims at destruction of diseased epithelium and replacement by healthy mucosa. The Evaluation of the Gala Airway Treatment System on Patients With Chronic Bronchitis (GALA) trial (NCT03107494) is an ongoing clinical trial evaluating the use of bronchial rheoplasty, and interim results have indicated that the procedure is safe, as there were no device-related adverse events and only 4 procedure-related events in the first 6 months. Significant changes in the SGRQ (mean decrease of 14.6 points) and COPD assessment test (mean decrease of 7.9 points) were observed in favor of the intervention.[18] These preliminary data suggest efficacy of the technique; trial completion is necessary for full evaluation.

SURGICAL TREATMENT FOR CHRONIC OBSTRUCTIVE PULMONARY DISEASE

Surgical management of COPD patients is limited to those with emphysema and includes bullectomy, LVRS, and lung transplantation.

Lung Volume Reduction Surgery

LVRS along with smoking cessation and oxygen supplementation in hypoxemic patients are the only interventions in COPD that have shown a decrease in mortality in selected individuals. LVRS is employed in symptomatic patients who have not had relief of symptoms despite other therapies. The evolution of this modality has not only informed treatment of COPD but have also led to important lessons in understanding the disease.

LVRS is performed via median sternotomy or video-assisted thoracoscopic surgery, removing the apical 20% to 30% of the parenchyma by wedge resection. As described previously, the major target of this intervention is hyperinflation and was first described in 1959 by Brantigan and colleagues[19] as a restoration of physiology rather than removal of pathology. However, it was not widely adopted until the 1990s, when Cooper and colleagues[20] reported the results from 20 consecutive cases showing a significant improvement in FEV_1 (of up to 1 L, 25%–38% predicted), a reduction in RV up to 1.7 L, a reduction in TLC up to 1.2 L, and improvement in symptoms and 6-minute walk distance.

In 2 randomized clinical trials, Criner and colleagues in 1999[21] and Geddes and colleagues in 2000,[22] patients were randomized to either LVRS or maximal medical therapy. These trials showed that LVRS improved FEV_1, TLC, RV, 6-minute walk distance, and quality of life. These findings helped in more widespread adoption of the procedure. Perhaps because of varied techniques and nonstandardized use of the procedure, 1-year mortality of 26% was reported by some authors.[23] The need for a prospective randomized clinical trial was recognized, which led to the National Emphysema Treatment Trial (NETT).[23] NETT is the pivotal trial that changed the landscape of COPD treatment. A total of 1218 patients from 17 centers were randomized to LVRS with maximal medical therapy versus maximal medical therapy alone. Patients underwent pulmonary function testing, lung perfusion, computed tomography imaging, and exercise testing. Additionally, patients were characterized as having upper-lobe-predominant emphysema (two-third patients) or non–upper-lobe-predominant emphysema (one-third of patients). Patients with FEV_1 less than 45%, TLC greater than 100%, and RV greater than 150% predicted were enrolled into the trial. The study showed that patients with upper-lobe-predominant emphysema and low exercise capacity (<40 W [W] in men and less than 25 W in women) had improved exercise capacity and mortality benefits with surgical intervention. Patients with upper-lobe emphysema but a high exercise capacity improved exercise capacity and symptoms but had no mortality benefit.[24] Long-term analysis showed that exercise capacity, symptoms, quality of life, and mortality benefits persisted in the upper-lobe-emphysema and low-exercise-tolerance groups at 4.3 years.[25] Importantly, the study showed that patients with non–upper-lobe-predominant emphysema had no improvement in symptoms, exercise capacity, or mortality, and those with a high exercise capacity within this group had worsened mortality. Additionally, patients with non–upper-lobe-predominant pattern of emphysema with either an FEV_1 less than 20% or diffusing capacity of lung for carbon monoxide (DLCO) less than 20% had increased mortality.[24] Post-hoc analysis of the NETT data also showed a decreased exacerbation rate for LVRS patients (~29% reduction)[26] and cardiovascular function and pulmonary mechanics.[27]

In addition to establishing the importance of LVRS in the management of emphysema, this trial clarified selection criteria. It cemented the role of careful patient selection in achieving the best results.

However, despite the evidence supporting its use, LVRS remains underutilized. This may be due to the significant morbidity associated with major thoracic surgery and the development of newer, less invasive techniques described previously. The most significant morbidity associated with the procedure is the development of an air leak in the

Box 2
Indications for LVRS
Limitation in exercise tolerance
Upper-lobe-predominant emphysema
TLC greater than 100% predicted
RV greater than 150% predicted
Abbreviation: RV, residual volume.

30-day postoperative period in 90% of the patients, with a median duration of 7 days. However, this can persist beyond 30 days in up to 12% of patients. The presence of an air leak does not affect mortality, and only about 4% of patients require reoperation.[28]

Current recommendations are to consider LVRS in patients with upper-lobe emphysema and low exercise capacity to improve mortality and in those with upper-lobe emphysema and high exercise tolerance to improve symptoms based on the benefits seen in NETT. Recommendations for referral to an LVRS program are listed in **Box 2**.

Bullectomy

Bullae are large airspaces in the lung with an internal diameter of greater than 1 cm, usually asymptomatic. Bullae large enough to occupy a significant portion of the hemithorax are rare and almost exclusively seen as a result of cigarette smoking but can also be associated with intravenous drug use and HIV infection. If a bulla occupies more than one-third of a hemithorax, it may cause ipsilateral lobar extrinsic compression. Surgical resection can be considered in patients in whom a bulla is contributing significantly to symptoms. Snider reported that bullectomy was successful in patients when a bulla occupied at least 30% of a hemithorax in patients with FEV_1 greater than 50% of predicted.[29] Long-term follow-up of patients undergoing bullectomy has shown improvements in FEV_1 and exercise capacity, and symptoms can persist at least 3 years after the procedure.[30] Similar to LVRS, smaller studies have shown that bullectomy has a favorable effect on cardiac function and lung and respiratory muscle mechanics.[31]

Bullectomy remains an attractive treatment option for patients with bullous emphysema, with hyperinflation and a giant bulla occupying a third of a hemithorax with symptoms despite maximal medical management. Indications for bullectomy are summarized in **Box 3**.

Lung Transplantation

Lung transplantation is the ultimate therapeutic intervention for patients with advanced COPD. COPD is the most common indication for transplant worldwide and is second only to idiopathic pulmonary fibrosis in the United States. Lung transplantation can

Box 3
Indications for bullectomy
Bulla occupying one-third of the hemithorax
FEV_1 greater than 50% predicted
Compressed adjacent lung parenchyma
Limitation in exercise tolerance

Box 4
Referral and listing criteria for lung transplantation in patients with advanced COPD[33]

Timing of referral for transplantation in patients with COPD
  BODE index of 5 to 6
  Frequent acute exacerbations
  Increase in BODE score greater than 1 over 24 months
  Pulmonary artery to aorta diameter greater than 1 on CT scan
  FEV_1 20% to 25%
  For a patient who is a candidate for BLVR or LVRS, simultaneous referral to lung reduction and transplant programs is appropriate.

Timing of listing for transplantation in patients with COPD
  BODE index score 7 to 10
  FEV_1 less than 20% predicted
  Presence of moderate to severe pulmonary hypertension
  History of severe exacerbations
  Chronic hypercapnia

Abbreviations: BLVR, bronchoscopic lung volume reduction; BODE, Body Mass Index, Airway Obstruction, Dyspnea, and Exercise tolerance; LVRS, lung volume reduction surgery.

---

improve patient mortality and dramatically improve quality of life in patients with end-stage COPD. It offers a posttransplant median survival of 5.6 years; however, it should be noted that there is considerable morbidity associated with this procedure, and careful patient selection is key to success.

Lung transplantation should be considered in any patient with COPD with (1) a Body Mass Index, Airway Obstruction, Dyspnea, and Exercise tolerance (BODE) index of 5 or

---

Box 5
Contraindications to lung transplantation[33]

- Lack of patient willingness
- Malignancy with high risk of recurrence or death related to cancer
- Acute renal failure with rising creatinine or on dialysis and low likelihood of recovery
- Glomerular filtration rate less than 40 mL/min unless being considered for multiorgan transplant
- Acute coronary syndrome or myocardial infarction within 30 days
- Stroke within 30 days
- Liver cirrhosis with portal hypertension or synthetic dysfunction
- Unless being considered for multiorgan transplant
- Acute hepatic failure
- Septic shock
- Active extrapulmonary or disseminated infection
- Active tuberculosis infection
- Limited functional status for posttransplant rehabilitation
- Progressive cognitive impairment
- Repeated episodes of nonadherence
- Active substance use or dependence including current tobacco use, marijuana smoking, or intravenous drug use
- Other severe uncontrolled medical conditions expected to limit survival after transplant

6, (2) FEV_1 less than 25% predicted, (3) ineligibility for LVRS, and (4) progressive respiratory failure as defined by a $Paco_2$ greater than 50 mm Hg or Pao_2 less than 60 mm Hg. Patients meeting these criteria should be referred to a lung transplant center for evaluation (**Box 4**). The BODE index is a multidimensional scoring system that outperforms FEV_1 alone when describing disease severity and predicting mortality. Decreasing FEV_1, distance ambulated during the 6-minute walk test, and body mass index are correlated with a higher score and increased mortality. An increasing mMRC dyspnea scale score is also correlated with a higher score and risk of all-cause mortality.[32]

Listing for transplant is indicated if the BODE index rises to ≥ 7 (which predicts an 80% 4-year mortality), the FEV_1 decreases to 15% to 20% of predicted, moderate or severe pulmonary hypertension is discovered on evaluation, and if the patient experiences ≥ 3 exacerbations in 1 year or 1 severe exacerbation with hypercapnic respiratory failure. Depending on the center and local experience, either a single or double lung transplant can be offered to the patient, which depends on many factors and is outside the scope of this discussion. It should be noted, however, that both methods offer acceptable survival benefit, with double lung transplant offering a slight advantage.

A particular problem to note is the choice between LVRS and lung transplantation. In patients with an FEV_1 of less than 25% but greater than 20% and a DLCO of greater than 20%, both interventions can be offered; however, lung transplantation is a highly morbid procedure and demands lifelong immune suppression and many changes to patient lifestyle which may not be palatable for some patients. It is also important to note that LVRS is not a contraindication to subsequent transplantation; however, for patients not in the small subset that will benefit from LVRS, lung transplantation may be offered as an alternative. Excluding immediate surgical complications, 5 years after the lung transplant, recipients are likely to suffer from hypertension (58.1%), renal dysfunction (27.2%), hyperlipidemia (26.6%), diabetes (22.8%), chronic lung allograft dysfunction (16.7%), and dialysis dependence (3.1%). A summary of contraindications for transplant is provided in **Box 5**.

SUMMARY

Modern management of COPD offers a variety of mechanical and surgical treatments for patients with advanced disease without significant benefits from maximal medical therapy. While some modalities are established and have proven physiologic and mortality benefits, others are under development or investigation. The landscape of COPD management promises to evolve as further options become available. It is important for clinicians to recognize patients that may benefit from these interventions and coordinate timely referral to maximize benefit.

CLINICS CARE POINTS

- Mechanical and surgical management of emphysema should be considered in patients who are symptomatic despite optimal medical management and referral to a specialized center should be made early.
- BLVR has comparable benefits to LVRS in select patients.
- LVRS offers improvement in symtoms and functional capacity and should be considered in patients with upper lobe predominant emphysema with hyperinflation.
- Lung transplantation may be the only treatment option in patients with advanced COPD who do not qualify for other treatment modalities, early referral to a transplant program should be considered.

DISCLOSURE

The authors have nothing to disclose.

REFERENCES

1. Kakavas S, Kotsiou OS, Perlikos F, et al. Pulmonary function testing in COPD: looking beyond the curtain of FEV1. Npj Prim Care Respir Med 2021;31(1):1–11.
2. Sciurba FC, Ernst A, Herth FJF, et al. A randomized study of endobronchial valves for advanced emphysema. N Engl J Med 2010;363(13):1233–44.
3. Klooster K, ten Hacken, Nick HT, et al. Endobronchial Valves for Emphysema without Interlobar Collateral Ventilation. N Engl J Med 2015;373(24):2325–35.
4. Kemp SV, Slebos D, Kirk A, et al. A Multicenter Randomized Controlled Trial of Zephyr Endobronchial Valve Treatment in Heterogeneous Emphysema (TRANS-FORM). Am J Respir Crit Care Med 2017;196(12):1535–43.
5. Davey C, Zoumot Z, Jordan S, et al. Bronchoscopic lung volume reduction with endobronchial valves for patients with heterogeneous emphysema and intact interlobar fissures (the BeLieVeR-HIFi study): a randomised controlled trial. Lancet 2015;386(9998):1066–73.
6. Criner GJ, Sue R, Wright S, et al. A Multicenter Randomized Controlled Trial of Zephyr Endobronchial Valve Treatment in Heterogeneous Emphysema (LIBERATE). Am J Respir Crit Care Med 2018;198(9):1151–64.
7. Criner GJ, Delage A, Voelker K, et al. Improving Lung Function in Severe Heterogenous Emphysema with the Spiration Valve System (EMPROVE). A Multicenter, Open-Label Randomized Controlled Clinical Trial. Am J Respir Crit Care Med 2019;200(11):1354–62.
8. Marchetti N, Duffy S, Criner GJ. Interventional Bronchoscopic Therapies for Chronic Obstructive Pulmonary Disease. Clin Chest Med 2020;41(3):547–57.
9. Sciurba FC, Criner GJ, Strange C, et al. Effect of Endobronchial Coils vs Usual Care on Exercise Tolerance in Patients With Severe Emphysema: The RENEW Randomized Clinical Trial. JAMA 2016;315(20):2178–89.
10. Kontogianni K, Gerovasili V, Gompelmann D, et al. Coil therapy for patients with severe emphysema and bilateral incomplete fissures - effectiveness and complications after 1-year follow-up: a single-center experience. Int J Chron Obstruct Pulmon Dis 2017;12:383–94.
11. Hartman JE, Klooster K, Gortzak K, et al. Long-term follow-up after bronchoscopic lung volume reduction treatment with coils in patients with severe emphysema. Respirology 2015;20(2):319–26.
12. Klooster K, Valipour A, Marquette C, et al. Endobronchial Coil System versus Standard-of-Care Medical Management in the Treatment of Subjects with Severe Emphysema. Respiration 2021;100(8):804–10.
13. Come CE, Kramer MR, Dransfield MT, et al. A randomised trial of lung sealant versus medical therapy for advanced emphysema. Eur Respir J 2015;46(3):651–62.
14. Herth FJF, Valipour A, Shah PL, et al. Segmental volume reduction using thermal vapour ablation in patients with severe emphysema: 6-month results of the multicentre, parallel-group, open-label, randomised controlled STEP-UP trial. Lancet Respir Med 2016;4(3):185–93.
15. Shah PL, Slebos D, Cardoso P, et al. Bronchoscopic lung-volume reduction with Exhale airway stents for emphysema (EASE trial): randomised, sham-controlled, multicentre trial. Lancet 2011;378(9795):997–1005.

16. Valipour A, Shah PL, Pison C, et al. Safety and Dose Study of Targeted Lung Denervation in Moderate/Severe COPD Patients. Respiration 2019;98(4):329–39.
17. Slebos D, Shah PL, Herth FJF, et al. Safety and Adverse Events after Targeted Lung Denervation for Symptomatic Moderate to Severe Chronic Obstructive Pulmonary Disease (AIRFLOW). A Multicenter Randomized Controlled Clinical Trial. Am J Respir Crit Care Med 2019;200(12):1477–86.
18. Valipour A, Fernandez-Bussy S, Ing AJ, et al. Bronchial Rheoplasty for Treatment of Chronic Bronchitis. Twelve-Month Results from a Multicenter Clinical Trial. Am J Respir Crit Care Med 2020;202(5):681–9.
19. Brantigan OC, Mueller E, Kress MB. A surgical approach to pulmonary emphysema. Am Rev Respir Dis 1959;80(1, Part 2):194–206.
20. Cooper JD, Trulock EP, Triantafillou AN, et al. Bilateral pneumectomy (volume reduction) for chronic obstructive pulmonary disease. J Thorac Cardiovasc Surg 1995;109(1):106–16.
21. Criner GJ, Cordova FC, Furukawa S, et al. Prospective randomized trial comparing bilateral lung volume reduction surgery to pulmonary rehabilitation in severe chronic obstructive pulmonary disease. Am J Respir Crit Care Med 1999;160(6):2018–27.
22. Geddes D, Davies M, Koyama H, et al. Effect of lung-volume-reduction surgery in patients with severe emphysema. N Engl J Med 2000;343(4):239–45.
23. Weinmann GG, Chiang Y, Sheingold S. The National Emphysema Treatment Trial (NETT): a study in agency collaboration. Proc Am Thorac Soc 2008;5(4):381–4.
24. Fishman A, Martinez F, Naunheim K, et al. A randomized trial comparing lung-volume-reduction surgery with medical therapy for severe emphysema. N Engl J Med 2003;348(21):2059–73.
25. Naunheim KS, Wood DE, Mohsenifar Z, et al. Long-term follow-up of patients receiving lung-volume-reduction surgery versus medical therapy for severe emphysema by the National Emphysema Treatment Trial Research Group. Ann Thorac Surg 2006;82(2):431–43.
26. Washko GR, Fan VS, Ramsey SD, et al. The effect of lung volume reduction surgery on chronic obstructive pulmonary disease exacerbations. Am J Respir Crit Care Med 2008;177(2):164–9.
27. Jörgensen K, Houltz E, Westfelt U, et al. Effects of lung volume reduction surgery on left ventricular diastolic filling and dimensions in patients with severe emphysema. Chest 2003;124(5):1863–70.
28. DeCamp MM, Blackstone EH, Naunheim KS, et al. Patient and surgical factors influencing air leak after lung volume reduction surgery: lessons learned from the National Emphysema Treatment Trial. Ann Thorac Surg 2006;82(1):197–207.
29. Snider GL. Health-care technology assessment of surgical procedures: the case of reduction pneumoplasty for emphysema. Am J Respir Crit Care Med 1996;153(4 Pt 1):1208–13.
30. Schipper PH, Meyers BF, Battafarano RJ, et al. Outcomes after resection of giant emphysematous bullae. Ann Thorac Surg 2004;78(3):976–82.
31. Travaline JM, Addonizio VP, Criner GJ. Effect of bullectomy on diaphragm strength. Am J Respir Crit Care Med 1995;152(5):1697–701.
32. Ko FWS, Tam W, Tung AHM, et al. A longitudinal study of serial BODE indices in predicting mortality and readmissions for COPD. Respir Med 2010;105(2):266–73.
33. Leard LE, Holm AM, Valapour M, et al. Consensus document for the selection of lung transplant candidates: An update from the International Society for Heart and Lung Transplantation. J Heart Lung Transplant 2021;40(11):1349–79.

Disparities in Disease Burden and Treatment of Patients Asthma and Chronic Obstructive Pulmonary Disease

Adam W. Gaffney, MD MPH

KEYWORDS

- Asthma • COPD • Disparities • Air pollution • Healthcare access
- Healthcare reform

KEY POINTS

- Low socioeconomic status individuals and people of color bear a disproportionate burden of lung disease in the US, including asthma and chronic obstructive pulmonary disease (COPD). Disparities in lung health, moreover, may be widening.
- Numerous adverse exposures, including air pollution, cigarette smoke, occupational hazards, household allergens, and respiratory viruses may help explain the connection between social class (and race/ethnicity) with respiratory illness.
- Disparities in the burden of lung disease are exacerbated by unequal access to medical care. Black, Hispanic, and low-income patients with asthma and COPD have inferior access to medical care in the US, which may undercut the management of their illnesses and lead to worse outcomes.
- Physicians can help patients with lung disease identify and potentially mitigate adverse pulmonary exposures, and ensure that disadvantaged patients obtain needed care, such as pulmonary rehabilitation for patients with COPD.
- However, to achieve equity in lung health, policy change is needed to ensure clean air, safe working conditions, good housing, and high-quality medical care to all.

INTRODUCTION

The lungs are an internal organ in direct and unique communication with the external environment. It is, therefore, unsurprising that they reflect the inequities of our surroundings and society. This reality was laid bare by SARS-CoV-2, a respiratory virus that continues to inflict disproportionate harm on the working class, Black, Hispanic, and indigenous communities. Yet disparities in the incidence of lung infections, in lung

Harvard Medical School, Cambridge Health Alliance, 1493 Cambridge Street, Cambridge, MA 02138, USA
E-mail address: agaffney@cha.harvard.edu

Med Clin N Am 106 (2022) 1027–1039
https://doi.org/10.1016/j.mcna.2022.08.005
0025-7125/22/© 2022 Elsevier Inc. All rights reserved.

function, and in morbidity and mortality from chronic respiratory disease are long-standing. These disparities in disease burden are, moreover, exacerbated by inequities in access to quality medical care for those who live with lung disease in the US.

A better understanding of such disparities is needed to address them, both among physicians and by society. In this review, I explore the myriad ways that social inequity is mirrored in the health or sickness of the lungs of Americans. I focus on two conditions commonly treated in general medical practice: asthma and chronic obstructive pulmonary disease (COPD). I examine social inequities in disease burden, but also in medical care faced by patients with each condition. I conclude with a discussion of reforms and strategies to mitigate these disparities, both at the level of the individual patient and on the national stage.

ASTHMA
Disparities in Disease Burden

The disparate impact of asthma is today widely recognized. However, socioeconomic and racial/ethnic disparities in asthma were not clearly appear until the 1980s, at the outset of what has been dubbed an "asthma epidemic" of unclear cause.[1] Colleagues and I examined long-term trends in socioeconomic disparities in asthma prevalence, from the 1960s – 2018, using the National Health and Nutrition Survey (NHANES).[2] As seen in **Fig. 1**, we found little evidence of socioeconomic (SES) disparities before the 1980s; subsequently, asthma prevalence increased among both children and adults of all income levels, but more sharply among poorer individuals, giving rise to a marked socioeconomic gap in recent years.[2] Whether this reflects lower rates of recognition of asthma among poorer individuals in earlier decades, a true widening in disparities during a period of rising economic inequality, or a combination of the 2, is unclear. However, other studies using other data sources have also identified rising pediatric asthma prevalence after 1980, with a disproportionate rise among Black, Puerto Rican, and lower income children giving rise to widening socioeconomic and racial/ethnic gaps.[3,4] Other data, meanwhile, have identified growing Black-White differences in adult asthma prevalence in the twenty-first century.[5]

Disparities are also present in morbidity and mortality from asthma. Black children have far higher rates of emergency room visits for asthma than white children.[6] The asthma hospitalization rate is 12.5 per 10,000 Black individuals and 5.6 per 10,000 Hispanic individuals — far higher than the rate among White people of 2.6 per 10,000.[7] And although asthma mortality fell overall from 1999 to 2015, it remained far higher among Black relative to White individuals, particularly among women.[8] Together, such statistics lay bare the extraordinarily disparate burden of asthma in the US.

A key question pertains to what underlies such disparities: to mitigate inequities it helps to understand mechanisms. Research in recent decades has identified multiple factors that contribute. First, disparities in exposure to outdoor air pollution play a role. Air pollution is associated both with incident asthma[9] and asthma exacerbations.[10] Black and Hispanic individuals, in turn, have higher exposure to particulate matter (PM) 2.5 components from a wide variety of sources.[11,12] People of low-socioeconomic status also have greater exposure to pollutants.[13] A notable recent analysis found that "redlined" census tracts in California — neighborhoods that received worse ratings by the Home Owners' Loan Corporation in the 1930s — today have higher proportions of Hispanic, Black, and low-income residents, higher diesel PM exposure, and higher rates of ER visits for asthma.[14] Hence, as a consequence of economic disadvantage, racist housing policy, and past and present segregation, disparities in air pollution exposure may contribute to contemporary asthma disparities.

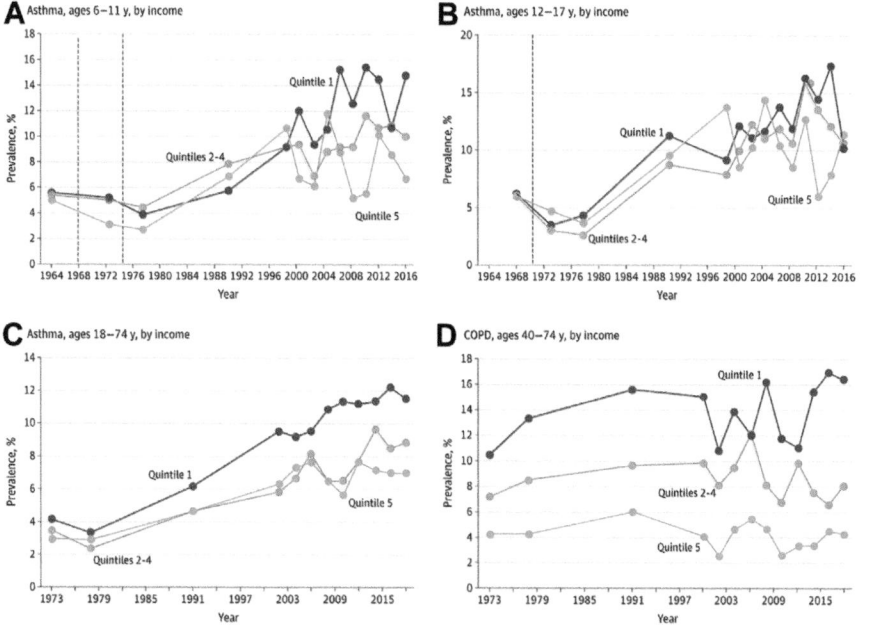

Fig. 1. Lung Disease Prevalence by Quintile of Family Income in the US, 1962 to 2018. Note: Dashed *lines* are used to indicate significant changes in question wording. Data are from the National Health Examination Survey (NHANES). See source for details on question wording, analysis, sample sizes, and other details. Panel A: Asthma, ages 6-11 years. Panel B: Asthma, ages 12-17 years. Panel C: Asthma, ages 18-74 years. Panel D: COPD, ages 40-74 years. (*From:* Gaffney AW, Himmelstein DU, Christiani DC, Woolhandler S. Socioeconomic Inequality in Respiratory Health in the US From 1959 to 2018. JAMA Intern Med 2021;181(7):968–76; with permission.)

Housing quality is another likely contributor to asthma disparities. Early life allergen exposure may result in allergen sensitization and consequently asthma.[15] The legacy of slavery and Jim Crow, exclusionary housing policies, and economic disadvantage has also produced disparities in housing quality that may lead to greater exposure to allergens for some, including dust mite mitogen, cockroach, rodent, and mold.[15] And, indeed, mitigation of such exposures through multi-pronged home repair program aimed at reducing allergen exposures[16] can improve asthma control.[15] However, evidence on the prevention of asthma itself via such interventions is still accumulating, and some randomized trials limited to house dust mite avoidance failed to show benefits on asthma outcomes.[17]

Another plausible factor that could drive asthma disparities, one that has garnered attention in the COVID-19 era, is the role of common circulating respiratory viruses. The disparate impact of COVID-19 is well described, yet a variety of investigations have also demonstrated inequities in the burden of respiratory syncytial virus (RSV) and influenza infections.[18,19] Notably, early in the COVID-19 pandemic, such viruses underwent an extraordinary decline in prevalence due to lockdowns and social distancing measures, asthma and COPD exacerbations fell sharply in multiple locales.[20] Although not confirmed, it is possible that this widespread decline in airway disease exacerbations had the effect of reducing disparities in asthma morbidity. Additionally, some have posited that early life respiratory tract infections could play a role in the pathogenesis of asthma itself.[21,22] Consequently, it is plausible, although unproven, that widespread disparies in exposure to respiratory viruses might contribute to disparities in asthma morbidity and potentially to incidence. The sources of disparities in respiratory viral exposure, in turn, are not obvious, although again there are lessons from COVID-19, with occupational exposures and household crowding 2 likely culprits. How to mitigate such exposures in the long-term, however, is less clear. The development of effective vaccines for common circulating respiratory viruses like RSV might make a difference.

Psychosocial strain, often downstream from economic deprivation and racism, is another commonly cited contributor to asthma disparities. A growing body of evidence has identified associations between exposures to violence, natural disasters, posttraumatic stress disorder, discrimination, and chronic stress with asthma incidence and morbidity.[23] The biological pathways connecting psychosocial strain with asthma are still unclear, however, but could involve upregulation of stress hormones, cytokines, and epigenetic change.[23] At the same time, disentangling psychosocial strain from the wide range of environmental exposures associated with adverse pulmonary effects can be challenging. Another complicating factor—with important clinical ramifications—is the potential role of dysfunctional breathing, which can coexist with asthma and exacerbate respiratory symptoms, and which is itself thought to be tied to psychosocial strain. One longitudinal study, for instance, found a link between sexual assault and dysfunctional breathing as well as (among women) asthma—yet not a correlation with lung function.[24]

Finally, growing data pointing to early life determinants of lung disease shed further light on how asthma disparities may emerge. For instance, multiple studies have found that such exposures as cigarette smoke, air pollution, and maternal hypertension can impair fetal lung structure and immunology either directly or indirectly (eg, via low birth weight or prematurity), with consequences for lung health later in life.[25] In the Tucson Children's Respiratory Study, lung function measured at only 2 months of age was associated with asthma in childhood and adulthood[26] and with lung function at age 22,[27] suggesting that asthma disparities may actually emerge in utero. If asthma indeed has fetal origins, efforts to mitigate disparities in asthma prevalence must go even further upstream—to the complex array of interconnected adverse exposures that affect pregnant people and newborns, and probably to inequality itself.

Disparities in Medical Care

Asthma is, fortunately, a treatable illness, which helps explain the reduction in morbidity and (likely) mortality from this illness in recent decades. However, the treatability of asthma also means that disparities in access to medical care exacerbate disparities in the burden of disease.

Disparities in access to, and quality of, medical care among individuals with asthma have long been observed.[28] From 1988 through 2008, although the use of preventive asthma medications among asthmatic children increased overall, there were significant disparities in the prescription of preventive asthma medications such as inhaled corticosteroids, with lower rates among Black and uninsured children.[29] Studies have similarly demonstrated Black-white disparities in long-term control medication use among adults.[30] Such disparities in the provision of this critical form of asthma therapy may have several underlying causes.

In a recent investigation, colleagues and I examined long-term trends in coverage and affordability of care for adults with asthma and COPD,[31] and observed stark disparities. **Fig. 2** provides data on trends in inadequate insurance—defined as those who are uninsured and those who are insured but go without needed care or

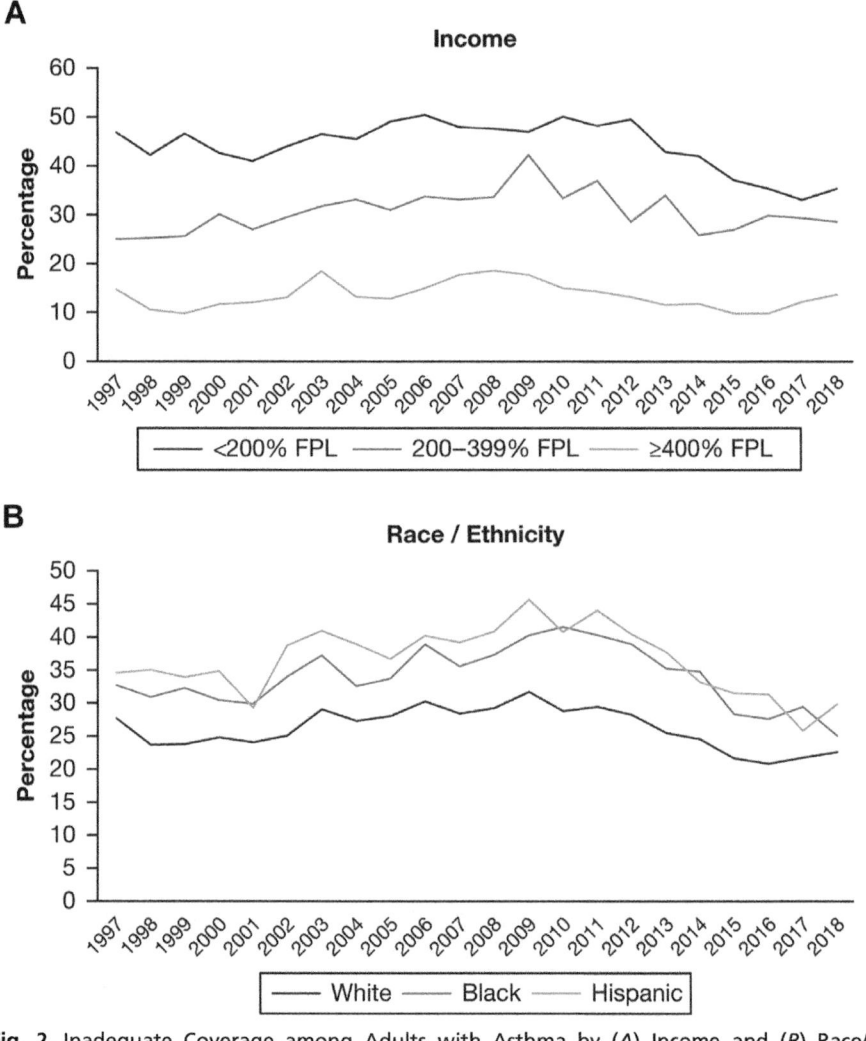

Fig. 2. Inadequate Coverage among Adults with Asthma by (*A*) Income and (*B*) Race/Ethnicity in the United States, 1997 to 2018. Note: Inadequate coverage defined as those (1) uninsured, (2) with delayed or foregone medical care because of costs, or (3) foregone prescription medications because of cost. Data are from the National Health Interview Survey (NHIS). (*From*: Gaffney AW, Hawks L, Bor D, White AC, Woolhandler S, McCormick D, et al. National trends and disparities in health care access and coverage among adults with asthma and COPD: 1997 - 2018. Chest. 2021 Jan 23; with permission.)

medications due to cost—among adults with asthma from 1997 to 2018. While the Affordable Care Act realized progress in reducing inadequate insurance among adults with asthma, large socioeconomic and racial/ethnic disparities in access to care persisted through the end of this period. Similar disparities have been identified among children with asthma by others: a recent investigation found that 10.6% of Black children with asthma with health insurance face cost barriers to seeing a doctor for asthma care, compared with only 2.9% of White children.[32]

Uninsurance and underinsurance no doubt contribute to disparities in care among individuals with asthma. Cost barriers can be onerous for patients with lung disease, and might deter the use of expensive medications such as inhalers, as well as other forms of care. One study examined data from the Kaiser Permanente health system, and found that 16% of families experienced financial stress stemming from the cost of care for children with asthma.[33] Another investigation found that, among lower-income families, those with higher cost-sharing for care had higher rates of delayed care or avoided physician and emergency department visits entirely.[33] Another study found that among US children with asthma over age 5, higher out-of-pocket cost exposure for asthma medications was associated with lower adherence to asthma medications and more hospitalizations.[34] An analysis conducted in Ontario similarly found that higher cost-sharing for medications was associated with lower use of controller medications.[35] Given the disparate impact of such cost-sharing for those with lower incomes, who are disproportionately members of racial/ethnic minorities, it is probable that financing features of US health care exacerbate underlying inequities in asthma prevalence and morbidity.

However, other factors—including geographic access to providers and mistrust provoked by longstanding racism in the medical care system—no doubt also contribute to disparities in care.

CHRONIC OBSTRUCTIVE PULMONARY DISEASE
Disparities in Impact

A discussion of the disparate impact of COPD must begin with the primary risk factor for this disease: cigarette smoking. In the 1970s, most American adults were current or former smokers, and there was little socioeconomic divide between those who smoked and who did not.[2] Over the next 5 decades, the creation of smoke-free workplaces, smoking bans in restaurants and bars, restrictions on marketing, educational campaigns, and other policies led to a major decline in smoking prevalence. However, over the same period, there was a widening in socioeconomic disparities in past or present exposure to tobacco smoke: in 2017-18, 34.2% of those in the highest income quintile were past or present smokers, compared with 57.9% among those in the lowest quintile.[2] It is unsurprisingly, then, that these decades also saw a widening socioeconomic divide in the prevalence of COPD. From 1971 to 2018, as seen in **Fig. 1**, the prevalence of self-reported COPD among those in the highest income quintile remained at 4%, while the prevalence among those in the lowest quintile increased from 10% to 16%.[2] This period also saw a widening in mortality from chronic lower respiratory disease overall among counties.[36]

However, disparities in the burden of COPD are incompletely explained by differences in smoking behavior. For instance, poverty and rural residence are both associated with COPD *independently* of smoking,[37] and individuals with COPD in rural areas have lower FEV1 and more respiratory symptoms compared with those in urban ones.[38] As demonstrated in **Fig. 3**, there is also a sharp rural/urban divide in mortality from COPD.[39] Such findings suggest that factors beyond smoking contribute to COPD disparities, including agricultural exposures, second-hand smoke, and deprivation itself. Worldwide, COPD among never-smokers is a major and increasingly recognized problem, and likely stems from a complex array of adverse exposures across the life course.[40] As a growing body of research demonstrates, some of the key factors in the pathogenesis of COPD occur early in life, well before the onset of cigarette smoking, as with asthma.

Traditionally, COPD was perceived as the consequence of an accelerated loss of lung function in adulthood caused by smoke exposure, as described in a famous

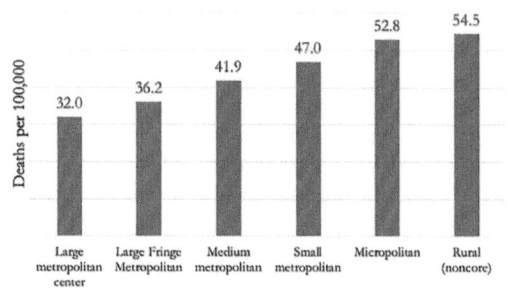

Fig. 3. Deaths from COPD across the urban – rural divide, 2015. (*Data from*: Croft JB. Urban-Rural County and State Differences in Chronic Obstructive Pulmonary Disease — United States, 2015. *MMWR Morb Mortal Wkly Rep.* 2018;67. https://doi.org/10.15585/mmwr.mm6707a1.)

article by Fletcher and Peto in 1977.[41] More recent research, however, has found that while accelerated loss of lung function explains the development of airway obstruction for some, others who go on to develop COPD have a normal rate of lung function decline in adulthood but failed to attain "normal" lung function in early adulthood.[42,43] A number of early life exposures associated with "childhood disadvantage" have been associated with subnormal maximal lung function in early adulthood, such as preterm birth, nutrition, childhood asthma, cigarette smoke exposure, pollution, and early life pneumonia.[43,44] Hence, some of the same early life exposures that may contribute to asthma early in life could also contribute to COPD later in life – and likely disparities in this illness.

In summary, disparities both in smoking and in the distribution of numerous other determinants of good pulmonary health contribute to inequities in COPD. A widening divide in smoking exposure will contribute to COPD disparities, but so too will broader social inequities that are persisting and possibly widening today.

Disparities in Medical Care

As with asthma, disparities in access to care among those with COPD exacerbate disparities in impact. Affordability of care is one major factor faced by disadvantaged individuals with COPD. While rates of uninsurance among the (nonelderly) with COPD fell after the 2014 implementation of the ACA, the proportion unable to afford care has changed little and the share unable to afford medications has actually risen.[31]

There are also rural/urban and racial/ethnic disparities in care access. Those with COPD living in rural areas have higher rates of underinsurance relative to those in urban areas.[45] Meanwhile, on both sides of the urban/rural divide, Black, American Indian, and Hispanic individuals with COPD are more likely to be underinsured relative to whites.[45] Underinsurance can be driven by high deductible health plans (HDHP), which impose steep out-of-pocket payments on individuals before insurance "kicks in." Our analysis of national survey data found high rates of foregone care among Americans with COPD, particularly among those with HDHPs. For instance, among individuals with COPD and an HDHP, 24.2% reported delaying care due to cost, 10.2% couldn't afford specialist care, 20.2% took less medicine to save money, 21.3% had in excess of $5000 in family out-of-pocket expenses, and 32.9% had problems paying medical bills.[46]

The high price of inhaled medications may impose a particularly heavy burden on such patients. For instance, a senior with COPD on triple inhaler therapy has estimated out-of-pocket inhaler costs of $2811 a year—a steep price particularly for patients on fixed incomes.[47] A large body of literature has found that such cost barriers tend to reduce health care utilization, regardless of whether the health care is "high" or "low" value. One study found a link between inhaler costs and medication nonadherence among those with COPD,[48] which could compromise disease control. A recent study found that COPD prescription "abandonment" rates increased with higher cost-sharing, from 10.1% for those with copays to 17.7% among those with deductibles.[49] High-deductibles were also associated with higher ER and hospital utilization among those with COPD in one cross-sectional national US-based study.[46] Another analysis similarly found an increase in admissions for airway disease after the introduction of higher drug cost-sharing in the province of British Columbia.[50] While these sorts of cost-barriers may serve to reduce care for patients with COPD in general, they could contribute to disparities in lung health for 2 reasons. First, they could disproportionately impact low-income individuals and members of racial/ethnic minorities, as these patients have fewer resources available to afford payments and hence may be more likely to forgo needed care. Second, they disproportionately impact patients with a greater burden of illness, who, again, are more likely to belong to disadvantaged groups.

Disparities in access to pulmonary rehabilitation care could also compound broader disparities in COPD burden. Pulmonary rehabilitation has been found to have a slew of benefits for patients with COPD, including improved quality of life and exercise tolerance, and is a critical part of treatment of these patients.[51] Yet pulmonary rehabilitation uptake remains suboptimal and inequitable. One analysis found that only 3.7% of COPD patients with Medicare had used pulmonary rehabilitation in 2020; among those of low SES, the rate was even lower (2.0%).[52] Another analysis using Medicare data found low rates of uptake of pulmonary rehabilitation following a COPD exacerbation, with significantly lower rates among Black and Hispanic individuals relative to whites.[53] Racial disparities in the uptake of pulmonary rehabilitation may not necessarily be driven by reduced geographic accessibility[54]; biases in referral patterns or cost-barriers are 2 alternative explanations. Another study, however, did find less geographic accessibility to pulmonary rehabilitation in rural counties relative to urban counties, where, as noted, the burden of COPD is higher.[55] Hence, again, disparities in burden are compounded by disparities in access to quality medical care.

SUMMARY

Social position distributes the means of good pulmonary health. Lower SES individuals and members of racial/ethnic minorities often experience more outdoor air pollution, occupational hazards, respiratory tract infections, tobacco smoke, adverse *in utero* exposures, and greater barriers to medical care. This, in turn, produces social and racial disparities in lung disease burden and treatment. Consequently, inequities in lung health can persist or increase even as overall adverse pulmonary exposures such as air quality improvement and smoking prevalence declines, and new useful therapies emerge.

For physicians, awareness of social inequities in lung health has important ramifications. Clinicians can elicit and potentially help their patients mitigate adverse household and occupational exposures. Awareness of the financial constraints of patients with lung disease is also important: prescriptions for inhalers that cannot be filled will not do very much good. Knowledge of disparities in the utilization of key forms of care such as pulmonary rehabilitation can also help lead to prompt referrals for disadvantaged patients with COPD who could benefit from this intervention. Although not explored in this review, there are also marked disparities in lung transplantation[56];

early referral of patients with advanced lung disease, and advocacy for greater equity in lung transplantation within institutions, is another way physicians can make a difference. Still, achieving equity in lung health and disease management clearly requires policy change.

Reducing disparities in pulmonary health necessitates the identification and mitigation of the numerous intermediate mechanisms that connect disadvantage with poor respiratory health, such as reducing indoor and outdoor air pollution, and improving working conditions and housing conditions for all. Rising inequality itself, however, is upstream of these exposures and must be addressed. Policy reform is also needed to achieve equity in medical care for patients with lung disease. Universal coverage would be an important first step: the 30 million who are uninsured in the US, including many with lung disease, often go without even basic medical care. To achieve equity, health care reform must go further, because many with health insurance still cannot access or afford needed care due to high copays, deductibles, narrow provider networks, or geographic disparities in access to care. National health insurance with first dollar coverage could go some way in realizing more equitable care for all with lung disease.[57–59]

The COVID-19 pandemic demonstrated how an ostensibly color-blind, class-blind respiratory virus can inflict such disproportionate harm on working-class people and members of racial and ethnic minorities. As we have seen in this review, however, pulmonary inequity is a far broader problem. Both in their clinical practice and in their engagement in the public sphere, physicians can be a force of change for the better for their patients with lung disease.

CLINICS CARE POINTS

- Physicians caring for patients with asthma and COPD should be cognizant of large gaps in lung health, access to care, and affordability of medicines faced by members of racial/ethnic minority and low socioeconomic groups.

- Exposures throughout the lifespan — ranging from pollution to respiratory infections and tobacco smoke — may contribute to disparities in lung disease incidence and disease control. An awareness of relevant exposures, such as home allergens or unhealthy workplaces, may help physicians to identify and potentially help mitigate them.

- Patients with COPD and asthma may be unable to afford care that physicians prescribe, such as increasingly expensive inhaled therapies. While it is important for physicians to be aware of these barriers, addressing them requires policy reform. National health insurance without cost barriers, for instance, would help ensure care is received based on need and not ability to pay.

- Pulmonary rehabilitation is a helpful but underused therapy for patients with COPD, and disadvantaged patients are even less likely to undergo it. Clinicians caring for such patients may be able to address such disparities with proactive and early referral when indicated, although disparities in travel time or affordability may also be a barrier.

- There are substantial equity gaps in pulmonary transplantation among patients with advanced lung disease. While again, early referral to pulmonologists or pulmonary transplant referrals for patients with advanced lung disease may help, institutional and societal reforms are needed to close such gaps.

DISCLOSURE

A.W. Gaffney is on the board of directors of Physicians for a National Health Program (PNHP), a nonprofit organization that favors coverage expansion through a single-payer program; however, he has not received compensation from that group, although some of his travel on behalf of the organization was previously reimbursed by it. The spouse of A.W. Gaffney is an employee of Treatment Action Group (TAG), a nonprofit research and policy think tank focused on HIV, TB, and Hepatitis C treatment.

REFERENCES

1. Eder W, Ege MJ, von Mutius E. The Asthma Epidemic. N Engl J Med 2006; 355(21):2226–35.
2. Gaffney AW, Himmelstein DU, Christiani DC, et al. Socioeconomic Inequality in Respiratory Health in the US From 1959 to 2018. JAMA Intern Med 2021.
3. Akinbami LJ, Moorman JE, Garbe PL, et al. Status of childhood asthma in the United States, 1980-2007. Pediatrics 2009;123(Suppl 3):S131–45.
4. Akinbami LJ, Simon AE, Rossen LM. Changing trends in asthma prevalence among children. Pediatrics 2016;137(1). https://doi.org/10.1542/peds.2015-2354.
5. Bhan N, Kawachi I, Glymour MM, et al. Time trends in racial and ethnic disparities in asthma prevalence in the United States from the Behavioral Risk Factor Surveillance System (BRFSS) study (1999–2011). Am J Public Health 2015;105(6): 1269–75.
6. Urquhart A, Clarke P. US racial/ethnic disparities in childhood asthma emergent health care use: National Health Interview Survey, 2013-2015. J Asthma 2020; 57(5):510–20.
7. Centers for Disease Control adn Prevention. Asthma Data Visualizations. 2021. Available at: https://www.cdc.gov/asthma/data-visualizations/default.htm. Accessed July 21, 2022.
8. Pennington E, Yaqoob ZJ, Al-kindi SG, et al. Trends in asthma mortality in the United States: 1999 to 2015. Am J Respir Crit Care Med 2019;199(12):1575–7.
9. Garcia E, Berhane KT, Islam T, et al. Association of Changes in Air Quality With Incident Asthma in Children in California, 1993-2014. JAMA 2019;321(19): 1906–15.
10. Orellano P, Quaranta N, Reynoso J, et al. Effect of outdoor air pollution on asthma exacerbations in children and adults: Systematic review and multilevel meta-analysis. PLoS One 2017;12(3):e0174050.
11. Bell Michelle L, Ebisu Keita. Environmental inequality in exposures to airborne particulate matter components in the United States. Environ Health Perspect 2012;120(12):1699–704.
12. Tessum CW, Paolella DA, Chambliss SE, et al. PM2.5 polluters disproportionately and systemically affect people of color in the United States. Sci Adv 2021;7(18): eabf4491.
13. Hajat A, Hsia C, O'Neill MS. Socioeconomic Disparities and Air Pollution Exposure: a Global Review. Curr Environ Health Rep 2015;2(4):440–50.
14. Nardone A, Casey JA, Morello-Frosch R, et al. Associations between historical residential redlining and current age-adjusted rates of emergency department visits due to asthma across eight cities in California: an ecological study. Lancet Planet Health 2020;4(1):e24–31.
15. Bryant-Stephens TC, Strane D, Robinson EK, et al. Housing and asthma disparities. J Allergy Clin Immunol 2021;148(5):1121–9.
16. Wilson J, Dixon SL, Breysse P, et al. Housing and allergens: A pooled analysis of nine US studies. Environ Res 2010;110(2):189–98.

17. Beasley R, Semprini A, Mitchell EA. Risk factors for asthma: is prevention possible? Lancet 2015;386(9998):1075–85.
18. Chandrasekhar R, Sloan C, Mitchel E, et al. Social determinants of influenza hospitalization in the United States. Influenza Other Respir Viruses 2017;11(6): 479–88.
19. Hutchins SS, Fiscella K, Levine RS, et al. Protection of Racial/Ethnic Minority Populations During an Influenza Pandemic. Am J Public Health 2009;99(Suppl 2): S261–70.
20. Cookson W, Moffatt M, Rapeport G, et al. A Pandemic Lesson for Global Lung Diseases: Exacerbations Are Preventable. Am J Respir Crit Care Med 2022; 205(11):1271–80.
21. Wang G, Kull I, Bergström A, et al. Early-life risk factors for reversible and irreversible airflow limitation in young adults: findings from the BAMSE birth cohort. Thorax 2021;76(5):503–7.
22. Martinez FD. The Origins of Asthma and Chronic Obstructive Pulmonary Disease in Early Life. Proc Am Thorac Soc 2009;6(3):272–7.
23. Landeo-Gutierrez J, Forno E, Miller GE, et al. Exposure to Violence, Psychosocial Stress, and Asthma. Am J Respir Crit Care Med 2020;201(8):917–22.
24. Hancox RJ, Morgan J, Dickson N, et al. Rape, asthma and dysfunctional breathing. Eur Respir J 2020;55(6).
25. Bush A. Lung Development and Aging. Ann ATS 2016;13(Supplement_5): S438–46.
26. Guerra S, Lombardi E, Stern DA, et al. Fetal Origins of Asthma: A Longitudinal Study from Birth to Age 36 Years. Am J Respir Crit Care Med 2020;202(12): 1646–55.
27. Stern DA, Morgan WJ, Wright AL, et al. Poor airway function in early infancy and lung function by age 22 years: a non-selective longitudinal cohort study. Lancet 2007;370(9589):758–64.
28. Cabana MD, Lara M, Shannon J. Racial and Ethnic Disparities in the Quality of Asthma Care. Chest 2007;132(5, Supplement):810S–7S.
29. Kit BK, Simon AE, Ogden CL, et al. Trends in Preventive Asthma Medication Use Among Children and Adolescents, 1988–2008. Pediatrics 2012;129(1):62–9.
30. Oraka E, Iqbal S, Flanders WD, et al. Racial and Ethnic Disparities in Current Asthma and Emergency Department Visits: Findings from the National Health Interview Survey, 2001–2010. J Asthma 2013;50(5):488–96.
31. Gaffney AW, Hawks L, Bor D, et al. National trends and disparities in healthcare access and coverage among adults with asthma and COPD: 1997 - 2018. Chest 2021. https://doi.org/10.1016/j.chest.2021.01.035.
32. Pate CA, Qin X, Bailey CM, et al. Cost barriers to asthma care by health insurance type among children with asthma. J Asthma 2020;57(10):1103–9.
33. Fung V, Graetz I, Galbraith A, et al. Financial barriers to care among low-income children with asthma: health care reform implications. JAMA Pediatr 2014;168(7): 649–56.
34. Karaca-Mandic P, Jena AB, Joyce GF, et al. Out-of-pocket medication costs and use of medications and health care services among children with asthma. JAMA : J Am Med Assoc 2012;307(12):1284–91.
35. Ungar WJ, Kozyrskyj A, Paterson M, et al. Effect of cost-sharing on use of asthma medication in children. Arch Pediatr Adolesc Med 2008;162(2):104–10.
36. Dwyer-Lindgren L, Bertozzi-Villa A, Stubbs RW, et al. Trends and Patterns of Differences in Chronic Respiratory Disease Mortality Among US Counties, 1980-2014. JAMA 2017;318(12):1136–49.

37. Raju S, Keet CA, Paulin LM, et al. Rural Residence and Poverty are Independent Risk Factors for COPD in the United States. Am J Respir Crit Care Med 2018. https://doi.org/10.1164/rccm.201807-1374OC.

38. Raju S, Brigham EP, Paulin LM, et al. The Burden of Rural COPD: Analyses from the National Health and Nutrition Examination Survey (NHANES). Am J Respir Crit Care Med 2019. https://doi.org/10.1164/rccm.201906-1128LE.

39. Croft JB. Urban-Rural County and State Differences in Chronic Obstructive Pulmonary Disease — United States, 2015. MMWR Morb Mortal Wkly Rep 2018; 67. https://doi.org/10.15585/mmwr.mm6707a1.

40. Yang IA, Jenkins CR, Salvi SS. Chronic obstructive pulmonary disease in never-smokers: risk factors, pathogenesis, and implications for prevention and treatment. Lancet Respir Med 2022;0(0). https://doi.org/10.1016/S2213-2600(21)00506-3.

41. Fletcher C, Peto R. The natural history of chronic airflow obstruction. Br Med J 1977;1(6077):1645–8.

42. Marott JL, Ingebrigtsen TS, Çolak Y, et al. Lung Function Trajectories Leading to Chronic Obstructive Pulmonary Disease as Predictors of Exacerbations and Mortality. Am J Respir Crit Care Med 2020;202(2):210–8.

43. Martinez FD. Early-Life Origins of Chronic Obstructive Pulmonary Disease. N Engl J Med 2016;375(9):871–8.

44. Svanes C, Sunyer J, Plana E, et al. Early life origins of chronic obstructive pulmonary disease. Thorax 2010;65(1):14–20.

45. Gaffney AW, Hawks L, White AC, et al. Health Care Disparities Across the Urban-Rural Divide: A National Study of Individuals with COPD. J Rural Health 2022. https://doi.org/10.1111/jrh.12525.

46. Gaffney A, White A, Hawks L, et al. High Deductible Health Plans and Healthcare Access, Use, and Financial Strain in Those with COPD. Ann ATS 2019. https://doi.org/10.1513/AnnalsATS.201905-400OC.

47. Tseng CW, Yazdany J, Dudley RA, et al. Medicare Part D Plans' Coverage and Cost-Sharing for Acute Rescue and Preventive Inhalers for Chronic Obstructive Pulmonary Disease. JAMA Intern Med 2017;177(4):585–8.

48. Castaldi PJ, Rogers WH, Safran DG, et al. Inhaler Costs and Medication Nonadherence Among Seniors With Chronic Pulmonary Disease. Chest 2010;138(3):614–20.

49. Patel B, Mayne P, Patri T, et al. Out-of-Pocket Costs and Prescription Filling Behavior of Commercially Insured Individuals With Chronic Obstructive Pulmonary Disease. JAMA Health Forum 2022;3(5):e221167.

50. Dormuth CR, Maclure M, Glynn RJ, et al. Emergency hospital admissions after income-based deductibles and prescription copayments in older users of inhaled medications. Clin Ther 2008;30:1038–50. Part 1(0).

51. Spruit MA, Singh SJ, Garvey C, et al. An Official American Thoracic Society/European Respiratory Society Statement: Key Concepts and Advances in Pulmonary Rehabilitation. Am J Respir Crit Care Med 2013;188(8):e13–64.

52. Nishi SPE, Zhang W, Kuo YF, et al. Pulmonary Rehabilitation Utilization in Older Adults With Chronic Obstructive Pulmonary Disease, 2003 to 2012. J Cardiopulm Rehabil Prev 2016;36(5):375–82.

53. Spitzer KA, Stefan MS, Priya A, et al. Participation in Pulmonary Rehabilitation after Hospitalization for Chronic Obstructive Pulmonary Disease among Medicare Beneficiaries. Ann ATS 2018;16(1):99–106.

54. Spitzer KA, Stefan MS, Priya A, et al. A Geographic Analysis of Racial Disparities in Use of Pulmonary Rehabilitation After Hospitalization for COPD Exacerbation. Chest 2020;157(5):1130–7.
55. Moscovice IS, Casey MM, Wu Z. Disparities in Geographic Access to Hospital Outpatient Pulmonary Rehabilitation Programs in the United States. Chest 2019;156(2):308–15.
56. Gaffney AW. Lung Transplantation Disparities among Patients with IPF: Recognition and Remedy. Ann ATS 2022;19(6):899–901.
57. Gaffney AW. ICU Equity and Regionalization in the COVID-19 Era. Ann ATS 2022. https://doi.org/10.1513/AnnalsATS.202110-1200VP.
58. Gaffney AW. Full Coverage of COVID-19-Related Care Was Necessary. But Do Other Pulmonary Patients Deserve Any Less? Ann ATS 2021. https://doi.org/10.1513/AnnalsATS.202106-683VP.
59. Gaffney AW, Verhoef PA, Hall JB. POINT: Should Pulmonary/ICU Physicians Support Single-payer Health-care Reform? Yes. Chest. 2016;150(1):9–11. https://doi.org/10.1016/j.chest.2016.02.660.

Lung Cancer Screening

Humberto K. Choi, MD, FCCP*, Peter J. Mazzone, MD, MPH, FCCP

KEYWORDS

- Lung cancer • Screening • Computed tomography

KEY POINTS

- Lung cancer screening with low-radiation dose chest computed tomography scans reduces lung cancer deaths.
- Screening involves optimizing the balance of mortality reduction and the potential harms related to the evaluation of false-positive results, overdiagnosis, invasive procedures, and radiation exposure.
- Components of a high-quality screening program include the identification of eligible individuals, shared decision-making, performing a low-dose computed tomography and reporting the results, management of screen-detected findings, smoking cessation, ensuring adherence, data collection, and quality improvement.

INTRODUCTION

Lung cancer screening (LCS) with low-dose computed tomography (LDCT) reduces lung cancer deaths by early detection.[1,2] LCS is a program that includes offering LDCT to individuals who are at high risk of developing lung cancer to detect the disease at an early stage when curative intent treatment is more likely to be successful.

The aim of an LCS program is to find a balance between maximizing mortality reduction and avoiding potential harms. It is a complex task, and a multidisciplinary team is necessary to build a high-quality program. Screening programs can be structured in different ways, but each program should include the following processes: identifying eligible individuals; shared decision-making (SDM); performing the LDCT and structured reporting of LDCT results; a strategy to manage lung nodule and non-lung nodule findings; smoking cessation support for individuals who smoke; and quality improvement processes (**Box 1**).

EVIDENCE BASE FOR LUNG CANCER SCREENING

Chest radiographs (CXR) and sputum cytology have been evaluated as screening tests in early screening trials. Despite finding improved survival for those with screen-detected lung cancer, the trials failed to demonstrate a reduction in lung-cancer-specific

Respiratory Institute, Cleveland Clinic, 9500 Euclid Avenue Mail Code A90, Cleveland, OH 44195, USA
* Corresponding author.
E-mail address: choih@ccf.org

Med Clin N Am 106 (2022) 1041–1053
https://doi.org/10.1016/j.mcna.2022.07.007
0025-7125/22/© 2022 Elsevier Inc. All rights reserved.

Box 1
Components of a high-quality LCS program

Components of a lung cancer screening program
- Criteria for lung cancer screening (LCS) eligibility
  Current policy includes age of 50 to 80 years, at least 20 pack-year smoking history and current smoking or quit within the past 15 years from the US Preventive Services Task Force and Centers for Medicare and Medicaid Services. Include asymptomatic and healthy enough to benefit from screening.
- Criteria for the frequency and duration of screening
  In keeping with best evidence and current policy. Current policy is annual screening until no longer eligible.
- Performance of the low-dose computed tomography (LDCT)
  Following American College of Radiology-Society of Thoracic Radiology technical specifications[61];
- Structured reporting of LDCT results
  Reporting of lung nodule findings based on current guidance (eg, Lung-RADS), with recommendations for follow-up and reporting of significant non-nodule findings.
- Criteria for lung nodule size that is labeled as a test positive
  In keeping with best evidence and current recommendations (eg, Lung-RADS—6 mm or larger if a solid nodule on the prevalence screen).
- Lung nodule management algorithms and team
  Algorithms for small solid, large solid, and subsolid lung nodules based on best evidence and current guidelines, connection to a multidisciplinary team with lung nodule management expertise.
- Smoking-cessation expertise
  Either part of the screening program or as a connection to a smoking-cessation program.
- A means to promote patient and provider education.
- A patient navigation and scheduling system
  To promote outreach to eligible patients and ensure compliance with testing and annual screening recommendations.
- Data collection
  To assist with patient tracking and management as well as to drive quality improvement initiatives.

---

mortality.[3–5] Therefore, CXR or sputum cytology should not be used as lung-cancer-screening tests.

The chase to find an effective screening test shifted to LDCT due to its increased sensitivity in detecting small lung cancers. Several randomized controlled trials evaluating LDCT screening provided insight about the effectiveness of the test as a screening method and about the natural course of the disease.[1,2,6,7,8,9,10,11,12] The National Lung Screening Trial (NLST) and the Nederlands-Leuvens Longkanker Screening Onderzoek (NELSON) screening trial are the only 2 trials that were powered to demonstrate lung-cancer-specific mortality reduction with LDCT screening.

The NLST enrolled 53,456 individuals between the ages of 55 and 74 years between 2002 and 2009. Participants had a history of smoking of at least 30 pack-years and were either current smokers or former smokers who had quit within the past 15 years. The trial randomized individuals to either LDCT or CXR screening with a baseline scan followed by 2 annual rounds with 6 to 7 years of follow-up. In the LDCT arm, there were 354 deaths from lung cancer, compared with 442 in the CXR arm. Three rounds of LDCT resulted in a 16% to 20% of relative reduction in lung cancer deaths. Based on these results, 320 subjects would need to undergo LDCT screening to avert 1 death due to lung cancer using the NLST protocol.

The NELSON trial had a smaller sample size of mostly male participants than NLST, longer follow-up (10 years), no scheduled screening in the control arm, screening rounds with different intervals, and used nodule volume and volume doubling time to identify potential cases of early lung cancer.[6] The trial confirmed the lung cancer mortality reduction with LDCT screening seen in the NLST. Lung cancer mortality was lower in the screening group by 24%.[2] The effect was more pronounced in women than in men. LDCT screening decreased mortality by 26% in men and 33% (not statistically significant) in women over a 10-year period.[2] However, the study was not powered to detect a significant difference in women due to the lower representation of women (only 16%).

There are potential harms from LDCT screening including physical harms related to the evaluation of screen-detected findings, psychological distress associated with knowledge of the results, overdiagnosis and overtreatment, and the risks related to radiation exposure.

The NLST used a lung nodule size threshold of 4 mm for positive results. In the LDCT group, 96% of all positive scans were not cancer.[1] Approximately 20% of all surgical resections were performed in patients with screen-detected benign nodules. The frequency of major complications occurring during a diagnostic evaluation of a detected finding was 33 per 10,000 individuals screened by LDCT and 10 per 10,000 individuals screened by CXR. The rates of complications after invasive diagnostic procedures are higher in the community setting.[13] Screen-detected findings also have the potential to cause short-term psychological distress; however, adverse effects do not appear to persist in long term (>6 months).[14]

Overdiagnosis in LCS refers to the detection of lung cancers that may be indolent enough that they do not progress to cause symptoms or be a cause of death. Individuals eligible for LCS may also have severe comorbidities that cause some of those individuals to die of other causes before lung cancer would have impacted their lives.

In the NLST, it is estimated that 18.5% of the lung cancers diagnosed were overdiagnosed cancer. The probability was higher if the histology was a noninvasive adenocarcinoma (79%).[15] The number of cases of overdiagnosis found among the 320 participants who would need to be screened in the NLST to prevent 1 death from lung cancer was 1.38.[15] These overdiagnosed cancers may cause anxiety, and their treatment could lead to morbidity.

The risks related to radiation exposure are more challenging to estimate. One study estimated that 1 in 2500 patients screened may die of radiation-related malignancy from the cumulative radiation received from screening.[16]

PROGRAM STRUCTURE

LCS programs can be structured using different models:

- *Centralized*: In this model, the program assumes the responsibility of most of the LCS processes. The program receives referrals from providers outside the program or actively identifies screen-eligible individuals. A dedicated team performs SDM visits and orders and schedules LDCT scans. The program is responsible for interpreting the LDCT scans, communicating results with patients and ordering providers, managing screen-detected findings, and tracking patients to ensure adherence with follow-up recommendations and annual screening.
- *Decentralized*: This model relies mostly on primary care providers (PCPs) who are generally responsible for identifying screen-eligible individuals, ordering LDCT scans, performing SDM, communicating results, managing screen-detected findings, and providing smoking cessation counseling. The program generally just performs and provides interpretation of LDCT scans. This model requires

PCPs to have the time and interest necessary to take ownership of most screening processes.

- *Hybrid*: This model incorporates elements of both centralized and decentralized approaches. Definitions of hybrid programs can vary. A hybrid program may have a centralized resource support (eg, program navigator) that manages certain screening processes for the referring providers who otherwise own the patients care. Another definition of a hybrid program is one that has one site performing screening with a centralized approach, whereas peripheral sites screen with a decentralized approach.

An LCS program can be successful in any setting with the appropriate support to provide all the components of high-quality screening (see **Box 1**). However, centralized and hybrid models are preferred to a fully decentralized program given the multiple demands put on PCPs. LCS programs using a centralized approached are more likely to include individuals who appropriately meet eligibility criteria and more likely to have screening participants adhere to annual screening than a decentralized program.[17] In locations where a fully centralized approach is not possible, a centralized team can assist with LCS processes such as scheduling individuals, assessing eligibility for screening, standardizing lung nodule management, providing smoking cessation counseling, tracking and ensuring adherence, maintaining a registry, and population management.

The coordinator or navigator is an important team member in centralized and hybrid models. The staffing and responsibilities of a coordinator varies among programs. Coordinators ensure that high-quality processes are present and performed.[18] In a study conducted at a large, academic center with a centralized LCS program, the hiring of a full-time coordinator improved participants' adherence to annual screening from 22% to 66%.[19]

WHO TO SCREEN

In 2013, the US Preventive Services Task Force (USPSTF) recommended annual LDCT screening for individuals between 55 and 80 years of age who have at least a 30 pack-year smoking history and who currently smoke or who have quit within the last 15 years in large part because of the results of the NLST.[20] These criteria were expanded in lieu of the more recent NELSON trial results that confirmed lung cancer mortality reduction with LDCT in a population with lower overall risk and from insight obtained by sophisticated modeling studies.[2] The current USPSTF recommendation for lung cancer screening is for adults aged 50 to 80 years who have at least a 20 pack-year smoking history and are currently smoking or have quit within the past 15 years.[21] In 2022, the Centers for Medicare and Medicaid Services (CMS) evaluated the evidence for coverage of lung cancer screening in the Medicare population, establishing similar eligibility criteria (upper age limit 77 years instead of 80).[22]

The current criteria not only expanded eligibility and access to LCS compared to the 2013 criteria but also are estimated to improve population-level health outcomes. Modeling analyses suggested that annually screening persons meeting the new USPSTF criteria would be associated with lung cancer mortality reduction of 13.0%, avoiding 503 lung cancer deaths and 6918 life-years gained per 100,000 persons in the population aged 45 to 90 years over a lifetime of screening.[23,24] In comparison, the 2013 USPSTF-recommended criteria were estimated to be associated with lung cancer mortality reduction of 9.8%, avoiding 381 lung cancer deaths, and 4882 life-years gained per 100,000 persons in the same population.[23,24]

A more complex approach to identify individuals who could benefit from screening is to estimate their risk of developing or dying from lung cancer or the potential of gaining life-years from screening by using validated prediction models.[25–33] These models are more cumbersome and challenging to implement, but they could lead to greater equity across gender and race in eligibility for LCS. The American College of Chest Physicians recommended the use of risk predictors and life-gained calculators to identify screen-eligible individuals who otherwise do not meet USPSTF criteria. However, it is important to note that health insurance providers may not pay for screening LDCT for those who do not meet the USPSTF criteria.[34]

LCS should be performed annually until individuals do not meet criteria anymore. It is recommended that screening should be discontinued once an individual develops a health problem that significantly limits life expectancy or the ability or willingness to have curative-intent treatment.[20]

SHARED DECISION-MAKING

Individual decisions about participation in LCS can be complex. SDM is a mandated component of LCS with the purpose of providing patients with the information and support they need to make value-based individualized decisions about whether to be screened. SDM allows individuals to learn about their risk of developing lung cancer and the benefits and potential harms of screening. Decision-aids and risk-prediction tools are effective ways to communicate complex topics to patients. They have been shown to improve knowledge and improve the comfort with decision-making by reducing decisional conflict.[35,36]

Components of counseling and SDM that should be performed and documented in the medical record include determination of LCS eligibility; the use of a decision aid; counseling on the importance of adherence to annual screening; the impact of comorbidities and the ability or willingness to undergo diagnosis and treatment; preparation for the likely findings of the LDCT; and counseling on the importance of maintaining cigarette smoking abstinence if a former smoker or of smoking cessation if a current smoker.[22]

In the community setting, the eligible population for LCS based on the USPSTF criteria is older, has a higher proportion of individuals who smoke, and has more comorbidities than in the screening trials.[37] In general, older patients with more comorbidities have lower life expectancies and are at higher risk of potential harms, especially complications related to invasive procedures, thus a lower net benefit from screening.[38] SDM is the opportunity to identify and discuss the factors that might affect someone's decision to participate in screening. A successful SDM means that the decision made was in line with the individual's values, preferences, and goals of care.

PERFORMING AND REPORTING LOW-DOSE COMPUTED TOMOGRAPHY

Screening LDCT should be performed with a volumetric computed tomography (CT) dose index of ≤ 3 mGy for a standard-size individual (height 5′ 7, weight 155 lbs).[22] The dose may need to be modified for smaller and larger individuals. The LDCT scans need to be interpreted by board-certified radiologists and use a standardized lung nodule identification, classification, and reporting system.[22] Data about the LDCT findings and participant characteristics should be collected for quality improvement purposes. Submission of data to a national registry is recommended but no longer mandated. The American College of Radiology developed a reporting system called the Lung CT Screening Reporting and Data System (Lung-RADS).[39,40] Lung-RADS standardizes screening LDCT reporting and provides management recommendations for screen-detected lung nodules (**Table 1**). This standardization facilitates result interpretation and outcome monitoring.

Table 1
Lung-RADS categories and management recommendations[39]

Lung-RADS Category and Score		Findings	Example	Management Recommendation
Incomplete	0	Prior chest CT examination(s) being located for comparison. Part or all of lungs cannot be evaluated.		Additional lung cancer screening CT images and/or comparison to prior chest CT examinations is needed
Negative	1	No lung nodules. Nodule(s) with specific calcifications: complete, central, popcorn, concentric rings and fat containing nodules.	Calcified nodule in the left lower lobe	
Benign appearance of behavior	2	Perifissural nodule(s) < 10 mm (524 mm³) Solid nodule(s): <6 mm (<113 mm³), new < 4 mm (<34 mm³) Part solid nodule(s): <6 mm total diameter (<113 mm³) on baseline screening Nonsolid nodule(s) (GGN): <30 mm (<14137 mm³) or ≥30 mm (≥14,137 m³) and unchanged or slowing growing. Category 3 or 4 nodules unchanged for ≥3 mo	Right lower lobe 1.2-cm ground glass nodule	Continue annual screening with LDCT in 12 mo

Probably benign	3	Solid nodule(s): ≥6 to <8 mm (≥113 to <268 mm³) at baseline or new **4 mm to <6 mm** (34 to < 113 mm³) Part solid nodule(s): ≥6 mm total diameter (≥113 mm³) with solid component < 6 mm (<113 mm³) or new < 6 mm total diameter (<113 mm³) Nonsolid nodule(s) (GGN): ≥30 mm (≥14,137 mm³) on baseline CT or new	New left lower lobe 4.2-mm nodule	6-mo LDCT
Suspicious	4A	Solid nodule(s): ≥8 to <15 mm (≥268 to <1767 mm³) at baseline or growing <8 mm (<268 mm³) or new 6 to <8 mm (113 to <268 mm³) Part solid nodule(s): ≥6 mm (≥113 mm³) with solid component ≥6 mm to <8 mm (≥113 to < 268 mm³) or with a new or growing Endobronchial nodule	New right upper lobe 7-mm nodule	3 mo LDCT; PET/CT may be used when there is a ≥8-mm (≥268 mm³) solid component
Very suspicious	4B	Solid nodule(s): ≥15 mm (≥1767 mm) or new or growing, and ≥8 mm (≥268 mm³) Part solid nodule(s): With a solid component ≥8 mm (≥268 mm³) or a new or growing ≥4 mm (≥34 mm³) solid component	Left upper lobe 21-mm nodule	Chest CT with or without contrast, PET/CT and/or tissue sampling depending on the probability of malignancy and comorbidities. PET/CT may be used when there is a ≥8 mm (≥268 mm³) solid component. For new large nodules that develop on an annual repeat screening CT, a 1-mo LDCT may be recommended to address potentially infectious or inflammatory conditions
	4X	Category 3 or 4 nodules with additional features or imaging findings that increases the suspicion of malignancy	Right perihilar 4 cm mass associated with right paratracheal adenopathy	

Table from American College of Radiology Committee on Lung-RADS. Lung-RADS Assessment Categories version 1.1. https://www.acr.org/-/media/ACR/Files/RADS/Lung-RADS/LungRADSAssessmentCategoriesv1-1.pdf. (Excluding images).

MANAGEMENT OF SCREEN-DETECTED LUNG NODULES

The NLST used a lung nodule size threshold of 4 mm for positive results. The overall positive rate of the baseline LDCT was 27.3% using this size threshold in this trial. Small nodules in the size range of 4-6 mm accounted for over half of all positive screens across all 3 screening time points. These nodules were found to be malignant less than 1% of the time.[1] Micronodules (less than 4 mm) are also common. In the NLST, 42% of participants had at least 1 micronodule.[41] However, micronodules that developed into a lung cancer represented only 1.2% of the lung cancers diagnosed in the LDCT arm and 0.11% of the total micronodule cases.[41]

Lung-RADS increased the size threshold for a positive result from a 4-mm to a 6-mm transverse average. The increase in the size threshold reduces the false-positive rate at the expense of a small compromise of test sensitivity. In a study where Lung-RADS was applied to the NLST group at baseline, the false-positive rate decreased from 26.6% to 12.8%, and baseline sensitivity fell from 93.5% to 84.9%.[42]

Screen-detected nodules can be challenging to evaluate and can lead to invasive procedures. There are several validated risk-prediction models to assist in malignancy risk estimation.[43] The Brock model is likely the best fit as it was derived from an LCS population.[44] The integration of clinical, blood, and imaging biomarkers has been shown to improve noninvasive diagnosis of indeterminate nodules.[45] Further research is still needed, but this combined biomarker model could potentially reduce the rate of unnecessary invasive procedures while shortening the time to diagnosis.

NON-LUNG NODULE FINDINGS

Non-lung nodule findings are common on screening LDCT.[46] The prevalence depends on how these findings are defined and each program's threshold to report them. In the authors' program, 94% of the individuals screened had incidental non-nodule findings.[46] Most incidental non-nodule findings are not actionable.[47] The most common incidental findings are non-nodule pulmonary abnormalities and coronary calcifications.[46,48]

LCS programs should incorporate a discussion of nonlung nodule findings into SDM and develop management strategies for the most common findings.[49] Although most non-nodule findings do not require additional evaluation, serious diagnoses can be found including extrapulmonary malignancies and severe coronary artery disease (**Fig. 1**).[46] The evaluation of incidental findings can significantly impact reimbursement generated by an LCS program. We estimated Medicare reimbursement to be approximately $817 per patient in our LCS program.[46] Fourteen percent of patients required referral to specialists, and 12% required additional testing. Of the total reimbursement, 46.2% was related to the evaluation of non-nodule findings.

INTEGRATION OF SMOKING-CESSATION INTERVENTIONS

LCS is a "teachable moment" for smoking cessation. However, undergoing screening alone is not enough to modify smoking behavior.[50,51] CMS and the USPSTF recommend that smoking-cessation interventions are integrated into LCS programs.[21] It has been demonstrated that the combination of LCS with smoking cessation improved the cost-effectiveness of screening while maximizing its clinical benefits.[52,53]

Integrating a smoking-cessation intervention into an LCS program is strongly recommended; however, studies have not shown any specific intervention to increase cessation rates within the LCS setting.[54,55]

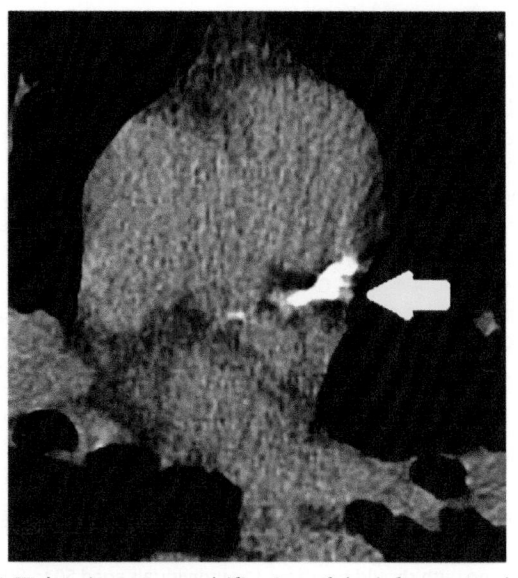

Fig. 1. Screening LDCT showing severe calcification of the left anterior descendant coronary artery that required further evaluation with cardiac stress test and cardiac catheterization.

Although the best approaches and interventions for smoking cessation have not been determined in the LCS setting, LCS programs should continue to offer tobacco treatment for individuals who smoke. Smoking cessation has several clinical benefits including reducing the risk of developing cancer.[56] There are several smoking-cessation resources that can assist in building a standardized approach.[57–60] It is important for LCS programs to develop their own smoking-cessation interventions or establish relationships with tobacco treatment programs.

CLEVELAND CLINIC LUNG CANCER SCREENING PROGRAM

At Cleveland Clinic, our LCS program has adopted a centralized approach. We have a multidisciplinary central leadership with pulmonologists and thoracic radiologists. The team also comprises regional physician champions, primary care partnerships, advanced practice providers (APPs), nonclinical coordinators, schedulers, a program manager, and IT support. Any provider in our health system can make a referral to the program. Our team reviews eligibility criteria and places the LDCT order. We have established eligibility criteria in keeping with USPSTF recommendations. We actively remind providers of eligible individuals with best practice alerts on the electronic medical records. Provider and patient access to self-scheduling complements our scheduling resources.

SDM is performed by our APP team at our main campus hospital and in the regional hospitals and health centers. The visit begins with a review of patient eligibility for screening and assessment of general health. A 6-minute narrated video developed by our program explains the benefits, potential harms, and other components of screening. We use an online decision aid to review the individual risk of developing lung cancer (www.shouldiscreen.com) and the net benefit of screening. We discuss possible screen-detected findings, stress importance of annual screening, and decide on how to communicate results. We incorporate smoking-cessation counseling and connect individuals who smoke to local resources.

Lung-RADS is used for reporting results and management recommendations. Our team is responsible for communicating and managing screen-detected findings. Participants receive written and/or verbal communication of LDCT results. Cases of individuals who had LDCT that received Lung-RADS category 4 A/B/X or cases with potentially significant non-nodule findings (eg, mediastinal adenopathy) are reviewed weekly at a conference similar to a tumor board. Decisions about continuing surveillance or performing invasive procedure are made in collaboration with expert pulmonologists, thoracic radiologists, and the APP team. Care paths have been developed for common non-nodule findings (eg, thyroid nodules, coronary calcifications) in collaboration with our subspecialty colleagues.

We use electronic medical records and a templated note with extractable data elements. We use a commercially available patient-management platform for data collection and reporting. These data are reviewed regularly, guiding quality-improvement efforts.

CLINICS CARE POINTS

- Lung cancer screening with low-radiation dose chest computed tomography scans reduces lung cancer deaths.
- Lung cancer screening with should be offered to individuals aged 50 to 80 years who have at least a 20 pack-year smoking history and are currently smoking or have quit within the past 15 years.
- A high-quality screening program has processes implemented for appropriate patient selection, shared-deicsion making, balancing benefits and potential harms, and management of screen-detected findings.

DISCLOSURE

The authors have nothing to disclose.

REFERENCES

1. National Lung Screening Trial Research T, Aberle DR, Adams AM, et al. Reduced lung-cancer mortality with low-dose computed tomographic screening. N Engl J Med 2011;365(5):395–409.
2. de Koning HJ, van der Aalst CM, de Jong PA, et al. Reduced Lung-Cancer Mortality with Volume CT Screening in a Randomized Trial. N Engl J Med 2020;382(6): 503–13.
3. Brett GZ. The value of lung cancer detection by six-monthly chest radiographs. Thorax 1968;23(4):414–20.
4. Fontana RS, Sanderson DR, Taylor WF, et al. Early lung cancer detection: results of the initial (prevalence) radiologic and cytologic screening in the Mayo Clinic study. Am Rev Respir Dis 1984;130(4):561–5.
5. Melamed MR, Flehinger BJ, Zaman MB, et al. Screening for early lung cancer. Results of the Memorial Sloan-Kettering study in New York. Chest 1984;86(1): 44–53.
6. van Klaveren RJ, Oudkerk M, Prokop M, et al. Management of lung nodules detected by volume CT scanning. N Engl J Med 2009;361(23):2221–9.
7. Sverzellati N, Silva M, Calareso G, et al. Low-dose computed tomography for lung cancer screening: comparison of performance between annual and biennial screen. Eur Radiol 2016;26(11):3821–9.

8. Paci E, Puliti D, Lopes Pegna A, et al. Mortality, survival and incidence rates in the ITALUNG randomised lung cancer screening trial. Thorax 2017;72(9):825–31.
9. Infante M, Cavuto S, Lutman FR, et al. Long-Term Follow-up Results of the DANTE Trial, a Randomized Study of Lung Cancer Screening with Spiral Computed Tomography. Am J Respir Crit Care Med 2015;191(10):1166–75.
10. Wille MM, Dirksen A, Ashraf H, et al. Results of the Randomized Danish Lung Cancer Screening Trial with Focus on High-Risk Profiling. Am J Respir Crit Care Med 2016;193(5):542–51.
11. Becker N, Motsch E, Gross ML, et al. Randomized Study on Early Detection of Lung Cancer with MSCT in Germany: Results of the First 3 Years of Follow-up After Randomization. J Thorac Oncol 2015;10(6):890–6.
12. Field JK, Duffy SW, Baldwin DR, et al. The UK Lung Cancer Screening Trial: a pilot randomised controlled trial of low-dose computed tomography screening for the early detection of lung cancer. Health Technol Assess 2016;20(40):1–146.
13. Huo J, Xu Y, Sheu T, et al. Complication Rates and Downstream Medical Costs Associated With Invasive Diagnostic Procedures for Lung Abnormalities in the Community Setting. JAMA Intern Med 2019;179(3):324–32.
14. Wu GX, Raz DJ, Brown L, et al. Psychological Burden Associated With Lung Cancer Screening: A Systematic Review. Clin Lung Cancer 2016;17(5):315–24.
15. Patz EF Jr, Pinsky P, Gatsonis C, et al. Overdiagnosis in low-dose computed tomography screening for lung cancer. JAMA Intern Med 2014;174(2):269–74.
16. Bach PB, Mirkin JN, Oliver TK, et al. Benefits and harms of CT screening for lung cancer: a systematic review. JAMA 2012;307(22):2418–29.
17. Smith HB, Ward R, Frazier C, et al. Guideline-Recommended Lung Cancer Screening Adherence Is Superior With a Centralized Approach. Chest 2022;161(3):818–25.
18. Tanner NT, Brasher PB, Wojciechowski B, et al. Screening Adherence in the Veterans Administration Lung Cancer Screening Demonstration Project. Chest 2020;158(4):1742–52.
19. Spalluto LB, Lewis JA, LaBaze S, et al. Association of a Lung Screening Program Coordinator With Adherence to Annual CT Lung Screening at a Large Academic Institution. J Am Coll Radiol 2020;17(2):208–15.
20. Moyer VA, USPST Force. Screening for lung cancer: U.S. Preventive Services Task Force recommendation statement. Ann Intern Med 2014;160(5):330–8.
21. US Preventive Services Task Force Final Recommendation Statement. Lung cancer: screening. Available at: https://www.uspreventiveservicestaskforce.org/uspstf/recommendation/lung-cancer-screening. Accessed February 1, 2022.
22. National Coverage Analysis. Decision memo. Screening for lung cancer with low dose computed tomography. Available at: https://www.cms.gov/medicare-coverage-database/view/ncacal-decision-memo.aspx?proposed=N&NCAId=274. Accessed May 11, 2022.
23. Oken MM, Hocking WG, Kvale PA, et al. Screening by chest radiograph and lung cancer mortality: the Prostate, Lung, Colorectal, and Ovarian (PLCO) randomized trial. JAMA 2011;306(17):1865–73.
24. Meza R, Jeon J, Toumazis I, et al. Evaluation of the Benefits and Harms of Lung Cancer Screening With Low-Dose Computed Tomography: Modeling Study for the US Preventive Services Task Force. JAMA 2021;325(10):988–97.
25. Bach PB, Kattan MW, Thornquist MD, et al. Variations in lung cancer risk among smokers. J Natl Cancer Inst 2003;95(6):470–8.
26. Spitz MR, Hong WK, Amos CI, et al. A risk model for prediction of lung cancer. J Natl Cancer Inst 2007;99(9):715–26.

27. Cassidy A, Myles JP, van Tongeren M, et al. The LLP risk model: an individual risk prediction model for lung cancer. Br J Cancer 2008;98(2):270–6.

28. Hoggart C, Brennan P, Tjonneland A, et al. A risk model for lung cancer incidence. Cancer Prev Res (Phila) 2012;5(6):834–46.

29. Marcus MW, Chen Y, Raji OY, et al. LLPi: Liverpool Lung Project Risk Prediction Model for Lung Cancer Incidence. Cancer Prev Res (Phila) 2015;8(6):570–5.

30. Wilson DO, Weissfeld J. A simple model for predicting lung cancer occurrence in a lung cancer screening program: The Pittsburgh Predictor. Lung Cancer 2015; 89(1):31–7.

31. Kovalchik SA, Tammemagi M, Berg CD, et al. Targeting of low-dose CT screening according to the risk of lung-cancer death. N Engl J Med 2013;369(3):245–54.

32. Katki HA, Kovalchik SA, Berg CD, et al. Development and Validation of Risk Models to Select Ever-Smokers for CT Lung Cancer Screening. JAMA 2016; 315(21):2300–11.

33. Cheung LC, Berg CD, Castle PE, et al. Life-Gained-Based Versus Risk-Based Selection of Smokers for Lung Cancer Screening. Ann Intern Med 2019;171(9): 623–32.

34. Mazzone PJ, White CS, Kazerooni EA, et al. Proposed Quality Metrics for Lung Cancer Screening Programs: A National Lung Cancer Roundtable Project. Chest 2021;160(1):368–78.

35. Wiener RS, Gould MK, Arenberg DA, et al. An official American Thoracic Society/ American College of Chest Physicians policy statement: implementation of low-dose computed tomography lung cancer screening programs in clinical practice. Am J Respir Crit Care Med 2015;192(7):881–91.

36. Fukunaga MI, Halligan K, Kodela J, et al. Tools to Promote Shared Decision-Making in Lung Cancer Screening Using Low-Dose CT Scanning: A Systematic Review. Chest 2020;158(6):2646–57.

37. Ma J, Ward EM, Smith R, et al. Annual number of lung cancer deaths potentially avertable by screening in the United States. Cancer 2013;119(7):1381–5.

38. Howard DH, Richards TB, Bach PB, et al. Comorbidities, smoking status, and life expectancy among individuals eligible for lung cancer screening. Cancer 2015; 121(24):4341–7.

39. American College of Radiology Committee on Lung-RADS. Lung-RADS Assessment Categories version 1.1. https://www.acr.org/-/media/ACR/Files/RADS/Lung-RADS/LungRADSAssessmentCategoriesv1-1.pdf. Accessed May 11, 2022.

40. D'Orsi CJ, Kopans DB. Mammography interpretation: the BI-RADS method. Am Fam Physician 1997;55(5):1548–50, 1552.

41. Munden RF, Chiles C, Boiselle PM, et al. Micronodules Detected on Computed Tomography During the National Lung Screening Trial: Prevalence and Relation to Positive Studies and Lung Cancer. J Thorac Oncol 2019;14(9):1538–46.

42. Pinsky PF, Gierada DS, Black W, et al. Performance of Lung-RADS in the National Lung Screening Trial: a retrospective assessment. Ann Intern Med 2015;162(7): 485–91.

43. Choi HK, Ghobrial M, Mazzone PJ. Models to Estimate the Probability of Malignancy in Patients with Pulmonary Nodules. Ann Am Thorac Soc 2018;15(10): 1117–26.

44. McWilliams A, Tammemagi MC, Mayo JR, et al. Probability of cancer in pulmonary nodules detected on first screening CT. N Engl J Med 2013;369(10):910–9.

45. Kammer MN, Lakhani DA, Balar AB, et al. Integrated Biomarkers for the Management of Indeterminate Pulmonary Nodules. Am J Respir Crit Care Med 2021; 204(11):1306–16.

46. Morgan L, Choi H, Reid M, et al. Frequency of Incidental Findings and Subsequent Evaluation in Low-Dose Computed Tomographic Scans for Lung Cancer Screening. Ann Am Thorac Soc 2017;14(9):1450–6.
47. Kucharczyk MJ, Menezes RJ, McGregor A, et al. Assessing the impact of incidental findings in a lung cancer screening study by using low-dose computed tomography. Can Assoc Radiol J 2011;62(2):141–5.
48. Janssen K, Schertz K, Rubin N, et al. Incidental Findings in a Decentralized Lung Cancer Screening Program. Ann Am Thorac Soc 2019;16(9):1198–201.
49. Tanoue L, Sather P, Cortopassi I, et al. Standardizing the Reporting of Incidental, Non-Lung Cancer (Category S) Findings Identified on Lung Cancer Screening Low-Dose CT Imaging. Chest 2022.
50. Slatore CG, Baumann C, Pappas M, et al. Smoking behaviors among patients receiving computed tomography for lung cancer screening. Systematic review in support of the U.S. preventive services task force. Ann Am Thorac Soc 2014;11(4):619–27.
51. Tammemagi MC, Berg CD, Riley TL, et al. Impact of lung cancer screening results on smoking cessation. J Natl Cancer Inst 2014;106(6):dju084.
52. Villanti AC, Jiang Y, Abrams DB, et al. A cost-utility analysis of lung cancer screening and the additional benefits of incorporating smoking cessation interventions. PLoS One 2013;8(8):e71379.
53. Tanner NT, Kanodra NM, Gebregziabher M, et al. The Association between Smoking Abstinence and Mortality in the National Lung Screening Trial. Am J Respir Crit Care Med 2016;193(5):534–41.
54. Iaccarino JM, Duran C, Slatore CG, et al. Combining smoking cessation interventions with LDCT lung cancer screening: A systematic review. Prev Med 2019;121: 24–32.
55. Tremblay A, Taghizadeh N, Huang J, et al. A Randomized Controlled Study of Integrated Smoking Cessation in a Lung Cancer Screening Program. J Thorac Oncol 2019;14(9):1528–37.
56. Samet JM. Health benefits of smoking cessation. Clin Chest Med 1991;12(4): 669–79.
57. A clinical practice guideline for treating tobacco use and dependence: 2008 update. A U.S. Public Health Service report. Am J Prev Med 2008;35(2):158–76.
58. Barua RS, Rigotti NA, Benowitz NL, et al. ACC Expert Consensus Decision Pathway on Tobacco Cessation Treatment: A Report of the American College of Cardiology Task Force on Clinical Expert Consensus Documents. J Am Coll Cardiol 2018;72(25):3332–65.
59. Centers for Disease Control and Preventtion. Smoking and Tobacco Use. Available at: https://www.cdc.gov/tobacco. Accessed March 1st, 2022.
60. Amercian Lung Association. Quit Smoking. Available at: https://www.lung.org/quit-smoking. Accessed March 1st, 2022.
61. American College of Radiology. ACR–SCBT-MR–SPR Practice Parameters for the Performance of Thoracic Computed Tomography (CT). Available at: https://www.acr.org/-/media/ACR/Files/Practice-Parameters/CT-Thoracic.pdf. Accessed March 12, 2022.

Hypersensitivity Pneumonitis

An Updated Diagnostic Guide for Internists

Megan A. Koster, MD, PharmD

KEYWORDS

- Hypersensitivity pneumonitis • Interstitial lung disease • Pulmonary fibrosis

KEY POINTS

- Hypersensitivity pneumonitis (HP) is an immune-mediated interstitial lung disease characterized by inflammatory and/or fibrotic destruction of the lung parenchyma and small airways in a susceptible individual exposed to an inhaled antigen.
- A new classification system categorizes HP into fibrotic and nonfibrotic subtypes based on the presence or absence of radiographic or histopathologic fibrosis. These subtypes replace prior categories of subacute, acute, or chronic HP.
- Radiographic findings of nonfibrotic HP include ground-glass opacities, centrilobular nodules, air trapping, or mosaic attenuation. Radiographic findings in fibrotic HP include lung fibrosis with centrilobular nodules, air trapping, mosaic attenuation or a new radiographic term entitled the three-density pattern.
- Formal exposure questionnaires, serum IgG testing, or bronchoalveolar lavage lymphocytosis can be used to provide additional data to support the diagnosis of HP in the appropriate context. In isolation, these tests are insufficient to rule in or exclude HP.
- Multidisciplinary discussion may suggest tissue sampling for histopathologic analysis in cases where improved diagnostic confidence will yield changes to treatment strategy.

INTRODUCTION

Hypersensitivity pneumonitis (HP) is an uncommon interstitial lung disease, which manifests with symptoms of dyspnea and cough following exposure to an inhaled antigen.[1] The pathophysiology of HP is best characterized by an inflammatory and/or fibrotic destruction of the lung parenchyma and small airways.[2] HP remains a diagnostic and therapeutic challenge to the practicing clinician due to the heterogeneity of disease presentation, ubiquity of potential inciting agents, variation in diagnostic criteria, and the lack of a standardized diagnostic approach. Despite international

Division of Pulmonary and Critical Care, Department of Medicine, Mount Auburn Hospital, Harvard Medical School, 300 Mount Auburn Street, # 419, Cambridge, MA 02138, USA
E-mail address: megan.koster@mah.org

Med Clin N Am 106 (2022) 1055–1065
https://doi.org/10.1016/j.mcna.2022.08.007
medical.theclinics.com

collaboration, these factors have also affected research efforts in HP, perpetuating uncertainty regarding optimal diagnosis and clinical management.[3–5]

Now, two recent clinical practice guidelines have proposed a consensus definition of HP and new classification systems with structured radiographic and pathologic criteria for diagnosis.[6,7] Each proposed diagnostic algorithm highlights the importance of a thorough exposure history to identify the inciting antigen. Internists are uniquely poised to identify potential cases of HP given their insight into the social, environmental, vocational, and occupational facets of their patients' lives. The aim of this summary is to equip internists with an updated understanding of HP manifestations, recommended diagnostic steps, and strategies for referral.

DEFINITIONS AND TERMINOLOGY

HP is an immune-mediated interstitial lung disease affecting the lung parenchyma and small airways.[6,7] The definition has several key components:

- Inflammatory and/or fibrotic destruction of the lung parenchyma and small airways,
- Mediated by dysregulated immune response to an inhaled antigen, and
- Occurring in a genetically susceptible, sensitized individual.

HP has been previously described as "extrinsic allergic alveolitis," which is considered historic terminology that is no longer used.[8] In addition, the literature is full of case reports of specific instances of HP named according to the cause of the exposure. Examples range from the traditional "farmer's lung," which implicates thermophilic actinomycetes or Aspergillus from contaminated plant materials to "bird fancier's disease" caused by avian feathers and droppings to the esoteric "hair-remover lung," which impugns the chemical hydrofluorocarbon-134a found in the coolant fluid of laser hair-removal devices.[9–12] Use of these named entities, although memorable, is discouraged in favor of the umbrella term of "hypersensitivity pneumonitis" itself.

CLASSIFICATION

Clinicians familiar with HP will recall categorization of HP as subacute, acute, and chronic, based on the duration of symptoms at the time of presentation.[4] However, this approach has several flaws. First, distinctions between these time intervals are arbitrary, vague, or variably defined in the HP literature. Second, these categories do not reliably correlate with prognosis.[1,13] Although it is tempting to conceptualize "acute" HP as benign or reversible and "chronic" HP as the opposite, patients with HP can recover with avoidance of the offending antigen or progress to respiratory failure regardless of categorization as subacute, acute, or chronic.[6,14]

In addition to identification and elimination of the inciting antigen, the factor most reliably correlated with patient outcomes is the presence or absence of fibrosis, either on high-resolution computed tomography (HRCT) or on histopathology.[15–20] Based on this emerging data, with the goal of achieving greater clinical, prognostic, and research utility, clinical practice guidelines now recommend classification of HP into 2 distinct subtypes:[6,7,21,22]

- Nonfibrotic HP.
- Fibrotic HP.

Fibrotic HP may include a purely fibrotic phenotype or a mixed phenotype with elements of inflammation and fibrosis, as long as fibrosis is the predominant feature of disease.[6]

CLINICAL PRESENTATION

The presentation of HP is heterogenous. Patients with both nonfibrotic and fibrotic HP can present with the following symptoms:[1]

- Most common: dyspnea, cough
- Less common: low-grade fever, chills, chest tightness, weight loss, body aches, wheezing

Symptoms may develop suddenly, over hours to days to weeks, or insidiously, over months to years, and may be episodic or relapsing/remitting, in concert with antigen exposure.[1,5]

On physical examination, patients may present with the following signs:[1,5]

- Most common: inspiratory crackles;
- Less common: wheezing, cyanosis; and
- Characteristic if present: inspiratory squeaks.

EPIDEMIOLOGY

Determining the epidemiology of HP is challenging due to regional differences in climate, antigens, and activities that predispose to exposure. Estimates of incidence are generally about 0.9 per 100,000 persons, although rates are higher among specific at-risk groups, for example, up to 4.95 per 100,000 among bird-breeders.[23–26] In the United States, an insurance claims analysis identified a 1-year prevalence from 1.67 to 2.61 per 100,000 persons from 2004 to 2013.[25] Rates varied substantially by state and were highest among individuals aged 65 years and older. Mortality rates were higher for men, individuals aged $\geq$65 years and individuals with fibrotic HP. The following factors have been associated with a poorer prognosis:[14–20,25,27]

- Demographic: male gender, aged 65 years and older;
- Clinical presentation: fibrotic HP, reduced baseline pulmonary function tests (PFTs); and
- Exposure: cigarette smoking, persistent exposure to the inciting antigen, inability to identify the inciting antigen.

PATHOPHYSIOLOGY

HP emerges in susceptible individuals following serial exposure to a wide array of inciting antigens. Lists of antigens known to induce HP and the sources by which patients encounter them are vast and ever-expanding, with geographic variation.[6,8] There is no clearly defined frequency, concentration, or duration of exposure that correlates with clinical phenotype. The most common route of exposure is via inhalation.[28] Although not exhaustive, general categories of implicated antigens include the following:[6]

- Organic material:
  - Microbes: fungi, molds, yeasts, bacteria;
  - Animal proteins: fur, feathers, droppings, and milk; and
  - Plant proteins: flour, dusts, powders, and wood fibers.
- Inorganic material:
  - Chemical: foam, sprays, paints, pharmaceuticals, metal liquids, or fumes.

Despite a thorough history of occupational, recreational, or household exposures, the inciting antigen is not identified in up to 60% of confirmed cases of HP.[13,14] Given the prognostic implications of identification and elimination of the inciting antigen, some guidelines recommend the use of a questionnaire tailored to geographic region and/or site visits from an occupational medicine or environmental hygiene specialist to help identify the inciting antigen in suspected cases.[7]

Following exposure, a dysregulated immune response incorporating both humoral (ie, antigen-specific IgG antibodies) and cellular (ie, T-helper cell type 1) components mediates lymphocytic inflammation and granuloma formation.[28] This inflammation of the lung parenchyma and small airways characterizes HP and may be followed by fibroblast accumulation and lung fibrosis.[28]

RADIOGRAPHIC PRESENTATION
Imaging Test of Choice

The preferred imaging test for the diagnosis of HP is a HRCT of the chest. Plain radiographs lack the required sensitivity and may seem normal.[1,3] Crucial elements of the HRCT include:[6]

- Two distinct series of images: one at deep *inspiration*, one after prolonged *exhalation*,
- Without contrast enhancement,
- Without prone images, and
- With reconstruction of thin-section CT images 1.5 mm or lesser.

Obtaining the additional series of images after prolonged exhalation is necessary because 'air-trapping', a key radiographic feature in HP, is only apparent on exhalation.[29]

Understanding Key Terms

Several terms may be used to describe the radiographic appearance of HP (**Table 1**). Ground-glass opacities (GGOs) and mosaic attenuation are the radiologic correlates of inflammatory lung infiltration.[6] Small airways disease or obstruction is manifest by centrilobular nodules and air trapping.[7] The three-density pattern is a new term to replace the "headcheese sign" and is considered highly specific for fibrotic HP.[6,30] Lung fibrosis is suggested by the presence of coarse reticulation associated with the following:[29]

- Architectural distortion: displacement of lung structures, eg, bronchi, fissures, or septa,
- Traction bronchiectasis: irregular bronchial dilation caused by retraction of adjacent lung parenchyma, and
- Honeycombing: cystic airspaces with thickened, fibrous walls.

Radiographic Findings According to Hypersensitivity Pneumonitis Subtype

The new classification system categorizing HP into nonfibrotic and fibrotic subtypes has specific radiographic criteria for each subtype (**Table 2**).[6] Findings considered "typical" are highly suggestive of HP. Findings that are less common or nonspecific but still consistent with HP are listed as "compatible." For fibrotic HP, there is an additional category of findings "indeterminate" for HP, which is neither suggestive nor compatible with HP. In these cases, histopathology would be required for confident diagnosis.

Nonfibrotic hypersensitivity pneumonitis

Typical nonfibrotic HP requires evidence of inflammatory lung infiltration (GGOs or mosaic attenuation) plus evidence of small airways disease (centrilobular nodules or air trapping). The findings are diffusely distributed to all lung fields but may spare the bases. Lung cysts,

Table 1
Radiographic terms on high-resolution computed tomography used in the diagnosis of hypersensitivity pneumonitis[6,7,29]

Term	View	Description
Centrilobular nodules	Inhalation	Typically small ($\leq$3 mm), profuse, and ill-defined
Ground-glass opacity	Inhalation	Hazy increased opacification of the lung, which is less opaque than a consolidation
Mosaic attenuation	Inhalation	Patchwork of regions with different attenuation, which, in HP, represents either: • Region with inflammatory lung infiltration/GGO (increased attenuation) adjacent to normal lung OR • Normal lung adjacent to region with small airway obstruction (decreased attenuation)
Three-density pattern	Inhalation	New term referring to three different attenuations above seen adjacent to one another • Increased attenuation: GGO • Normal lung • Decreased attenuation: small airway obstruction and/or decreased vascularity
Air-trapping	Exhalation	Regions of decreased attenuation corresponding to retained air in lung tissue distal to an obstruction Seen on expiratory images as a lack of the normal increased attenuation that occurs with exhalation
Fibrosis	Inhalation	Reticulation or GGO with architectural distortion, traction bronchiectasis, or honeycombing

Key terms used to describe radiographic findings of HP.

airspace consolidations, or GGOs in a uniform and subtle distribution are nonspecific but compatible with nonfibrotic HP diagnosis in the right clinical context.[6,7]

Fibrotic hypersensitivity pneumonitis

Typical fibrotic HP requires lung fibrosis with evidence of airway obstruction that may include centrilobular nodules, air trapping, mosaic attenuation, or the three-density pattern. Lung fibrosis may be distributed randomly, midlung predominant, or in a manner sparing the bases. Less commonly, lung fibrosis may present with extensive GGO, with a usual interstitial pneumonia (UIP) pattern, or with a peribronchovascular or upper-lobe predominant distribution.[31] These variants are considered compatible with fibrotic HP if they are associated with evidence of airway obstruction.[6] Fibrosis alone, of any variant, including fibrotic nonspecific interstitial pneumonia (NSIP) or organizing pneumonia-like patterns, without evidence of airway obstruction, would be indeterminate for fibrotic HP.

ADJUNCTIVE TESTING

Beyond a thorough exposure history and HRCT, several other tests have been investigated as potential sources of support for an HP diagnosis. In isolation, no single diagnostic element is sufficient to confirm a diagnosis of HP.

Antigen-specific antibody testing

Measurement of serum IgG specific to antigens known to cause HP has been suggested in numerous proposed diagnostic algorithms for HP.[1,4,5,21] Testing is commonly performed with a panel of potentially causative antigens, either via

Table 2
Radiographic findings on resolution computed tomography according to hypersensitivity pneumonitis subtype[6,7]

Subtype	Findings	
Nonfibrotic	Typical	GGO or mosaic attenuation, plus either centrilobular nodules or air-trapping
	Compatible	Uniform and subtle GGO, airspace consolidation, or lung cysts
Fibrotic	Typical	Lung fibrosis plus either centrilobular nodules, air-trapping, mosaic attenuation, or the three-density pattern
	Compatible	Lung fibrosis with a variant pattern (extensive GGO or UIP) or distribution (peribronchovascular or upper-lobe) plus either centrilobular nodules, air-trapping, mosaic attenuation, or the three-density pattern
	Indeterminate	UIP, fibrotic-NSIP or organizing pneumonia-like pattern alone[a]

Findings are defined in **Table 1** unless otherwise specified.
[a] UIP, fibrotic-NSIP and organizing pneumonia-like patterns are described elsewhere.[29,31]

precipitins or, increasingly, ELISA. Technique and panel of antigens vary across laboratories and institutions. There is no standardized list of antigens to include.[6]

Serum IgG testing has demonstrated an ability to distinguish patients with known HP from controls.[1,32] However, test characteristics (sensitivity, specificity) are poorer when serum IgG testing was used to distinguish HP from other ILDs.[32]

Current clinical practice guidelines disagree regarding the role of serum IgG testing in the diagnostic evaluation of HP.[6,7] There is consensus that serum IgG testing is convenient and noninvasive, and may support a diagnosis of HP, but alone is inadequate to confidently rule in or exclude the diagnosis. In addition, a positive serum IgG test indicates the patient was exposed to a particular antigen but it does not necessarily imply causation for the patient's lung disease.

Bronchoalveolar lavage lymphocytosis

Bronchoscopy with bronchoalveolar lavage (BAL) is used to provide diagnostic information for patients with suspected ILD in conjunction with clinical and imaging data. Analysis of BAL fluid in ILD is useful to rule out infection and to identify findings that suggest alternative diagnoses, such as eosinophilia and alveolar hemorrhage.[33]

In HP, the production of lymphocytic inflammation in response to an inciting antigen is considered a key element of pathophysiology.[28] Systematic reviews and meta-analyses indicate that lymphocyte count in BAL fluid is elevated in patients with HP compared with patients with sarcoidosis or idiopathic pulmonary fibrosis (IPF).[34,35] However, results from the literature are conflicting, and there is no clearly proven threshold for what lymphocyte percentage to use as a cutoff. Test characteristics for BAL lymphocytosis of 20%, 30%, and 40% indicate that higher thresholds have poorer sensitivity but better specificity for HP.[6,34]

Current clinical guidelines suggest BAL lymphocytosis can increase diagnostic confidence in distinguishing nonfibrotic HP from sarcoidosis and potentially to distinguish fibrotic HP from sarcoidosis and IPF.[6,7] In nonfibrotic HP, BAL may additionally be useful to rule out infection. In the absence of clear data, a threshold lymphocyte count of 30% has been suggested.[6]

Pulmonary function testing

PFTs have not been shown to be helpful in establishing the diagnosis of HP. There is no characteristic pattern or deficit in PFTs that is unique to HP in comparison to other lung diseases.[1,3] As such, PFTs were not included in two recently published algorithms for the diagnosis of HP.[6,7] Once a diagnosis of HP has been established, PFTs can be used to assess the degree of respiratory system impairment, response to treatment, or indicate prognosis, particularly in fibrotic HP.[36]

HISTOPATHOLOGY

If a confident diagnosis of HP cannot be made from evidence of exposure, imaging, or multidisciplinary discussion (MDD), obtaining a tissue sample may be required, particularly if confirmation would result in a change in management. Specimens may be obtained from transbronchial biopsy, transbronchial lung cryobiopsy, or surgical lung biopsy. Tissue sampling may be combined with BAL for lymphocyte count if not already obtained.

Histopathologic Findings Inconsistent with Hypersensitivity Pneumonitis

The following findings suggest an alternative diagnosis that is *not* HP:[6]

- More plasma cells present than lymphocytes,
- Extensive lymphoid hyperplasia,
- Extensive, well-formed sarcoidal or necrotizing granulomas, and
- Aspirated particles.

Histopathologic Findings in Nonfibrotic Hypersensitivity Pneumonitis

Presence of the following findings in one specimen is highly suggestive of nonfibrotic HP:[6,7]

- Airway-centered (bronchiolocentric) cellular interstitial pneumonia,
- Cellular bronchiolitis with or without foamy macrophages,
- Lymphocyte-predominant inflammation in each of the above, and
- Small, poorly formed, nonnecrotizing granulomas ± multinucleated giant cells.

Histopathologic Findings in Fibrotic Hypersensitivity Pneumonitis

In fibrotic HP, cellular interstitial pneumonia and bronchiolitis has given way to fibrosis. The findings may be patchy, interspersed with regions typical for nonfibrotic HP, and may require sampling of more than one biopsy site, similar to IPF.[6,37,38] Presence of the following is highly suggestive of fibrotic HP:[6,7]

- Chronic fibrosing interstitial pneumonia with architectural distortion, fibroblast foci, and/or subpleural honeycombing, which may be in a UIP or fibrotic NSIP pattern,[31]
- Airway-centered fibrosis with or without peribronchiolar metaplasia, and
- Small, poorly formed, nonnecrotizing granulomas.

DIAGNOSTIC STEPS

Internists who encounter patients with a clinical presentation suggestive of HP are faced with the dilemma of integrating a complex array of historical, radiographic, laboratory, and pathologic data to make the diagnosis. Numerous attempts to codify a diagnostic algorithm for HP have all been hindered by the lack of clear diagnostic criteria. Now, new, detailed algorithms are available, which incorporate the updated diagnostic criteria and classification system of HP into nonfibrotic and fibrotic subtypes.[6,7]

Both algorithms stress the importance of MDD in assessing diagnostic confidence based on evidence for exposure, HRCT findings, BAL lymphocytosis, and

Compile Evidence of Exposure	Obtain High-Resolution CT Chest	Referral for Multidisciplinary Discussion	Consider Utility & Necessity of Invasive Procedures
• Thorough history of potential vocational, occupational, or household exposures • Questionnaire if locally available • Serum IgG testing	• Include inspiratory & expiratory views • Without contrast • Without prone images	• Include individuals with expertise in pulmonology, radiology and pathology	• Bronchoscopy for BAL lymphocytosis and/or • Tissue sampling for histopathologic assessment

Fig. 1. Diagnostic approach for the internist in cases of suspected HP. **Fig. 1** Diagnostic elements in the leftmost columns, including exposure evidence and HRCT, are available in the general internal medicine setting and helpful to obtain before specialty referral. Diagnostic elements in the rightmost column may be recommended following multidisciplinary discussion.

histopathology. MDD has been studied favorably in ILD and IPF, and although data supporting the benefits of MDD in HP is less robust, this is thought to reflect the previous lack of consensus diagnostic criteria.[39–41]

Yet, there is disagreement, even between algorithms incorporating the latest data, classification system, and diagnostic criteria. Each algorithm is complex and includes elements not widely available to the internist, such as bronchoscopy and tissue sampling. There is no consensus on when internists should refer patients for specialty care and no roadmap for what data would be helpful to obtain before referral. In light of this need, **Fig. 1** synthesizes the available recommendations and outlines a reasonable diagnostic approach for the internist with a suspected case of HP.

SUMMARY

HP is a complex immune-mediated interstitial lung disease, which manifests in lymphocytic inflammation of the lung parenchyma and small airways. Classification according to fibrotic or nonfibrotic subtypes based on the presence or absence of fibrosis offers an objective categorization with specific radiographic and histopathologic criteria, which may be better aligned with patient prognosis. The internist is well positioned to elicit history of potential exposures and obtain clinical data relevant to an HP diagnosis before referral for specialty care. Hopefully, future studies will apply new diagnostic algorithms to the identification of treatment standards by HP subtype.

CLINICS CARE POINTS

- Hypersensitivity pneumonitis (HP) is characterized by inflammatory and/or fibrotic destruction of the lung parenchyma and small airways due to a dysregulated immune response to an inhaled antigen in a susceptible, sensitized individual.

- Patients with HP present with dyspnea, cough, and inspiratory crackles. Less common presentations include low-grade fever, chills, wheezing, and cyanosis. Inspiratory squeaks are characteristic if present.

- A new classification system categorizes HP into fibrotic and nonfibrotic subtypes based on the presence or absence of radiographic or histopathologic fibrosis. These subtypes replace prior categories of subacute, acute, or chronic HP.

- Inciting antigens may include microorganisms, animal and plant proteins (such as feathers, fur, droppings, and dust), or chemical sprays or fumes encountered from a variety of sources. In many cases of HP, the exposure is not identified despite a thorough history. Tools such as questionnaires and serum IgG testing may provide supportive evidence for an exposure in the right clinical context and geographic region.

- Radiographic findings of nonfibrotic HP include ground-glass opacities, centrilobular nodules, air trapping, or mosaic attenuation. Radiographic findings in fibrotic HP include lung fibrosis with centrilobular nodules, air trapping, mosaic attenuation, or a new radiographic term entitled the three-density pattern.

- Histopathologic findings of HP include evidence of lymphocytic, airway-centered interstitial pneumonia and bronchiolitis with poorly formed nonnecrotizing granulomas, with or without associated lung fibrosis.

- New diagnostic algorithms highlight the role of multidisciplinary discussion in making a confident diagnosis of HP.

DISCLOSURE

The author has nothing to disclose.

REFERENCES

1. Lacasse Y, Selman M, Costabel U, et al, HP Study Group. Clinical diagnosis of hypersensitivity pneumonitis. Am J Respir Crit Care Med 2003;168:952–8.
2. Koster MA, Thomson CC, Collins BF, et al. Diagnosis of hypersensitivity pneumonitis in adults, 2020 clinical practice guideline: summary for clinicians. Ann Am Thorac Soc 2021;18(4):559–66.
3. Fink JN, Ortega HG, Reynolds HY, et al. Needs and opportunities for research in hypersensitivity pneumonitis. Am J Respir Crit Care Med 2005;171:792–8.
4. Richerson HB, Bernstein IL, Fink JN, et al. Guidelines for the clinical evaluation of hypersensitivity pneumonitis: report of the Subcommittee on Hypersensitivity Pneumonitis. J Allergy Clin Immunol 1989;84:839–44.
5. Morisset J, Johannson KA, Jones KD, et al, HP Delphi Collaborators. Identification of diagnostic criteria for chronic hypersensitivity pneumonitis: an international modified Delphi survey. Am J Respir Crit Care Med 2018;197:1036–44.
6. Raghu G, Remy-Jardin M, Ryerson CJ, et al. Diagnosis of hypersensitivity pneumonitis in adults: an official ATS/JRS/ALAT clinical practice guideline. Am J Respir Crit Care Med 2020;202:e36–69.
7. Fernández Pérez ER, Travis WD, Lynch DA, et al. Diagnosis and evaluation of hypersensitivity pneumonitis: CHEST guideline and expert panel report. Chest 2021;160(2):e97–156.
8. Barnes H, Jones K, Blanc P. The hidden history of hypersensitivity pneumonitis. Eur Respir J 2022;59(1):2100252.
9. Ramazzini B. De morbis artificium diatribe. Modena (Italy): Antonio Capponi; 1700.
10. Zergham AS, Heller D. Farmers lung. In: StatPearls. StatPearls Publishing; 2022.
11. Sullivan A, Shrestha P, Lanham T, et al. Bird fancier's lung: an underdiagnosed etiology of dyspnea. Respir Med Case Rep 2020;31:101288.
12. Ishiguro T, Yasui M, Nakade Y, et al. Extrinsic allergic alveolitis with eosinophil infiltration induced by 1,1,1,2-tetrafluoroethane (HFC-134a): a case report. Intern Med 2007;46(17):1455–7.
13. Hanak V, Golbin JM, Ryu JH. Causes and presenting features in 85 consecutive patients with hypersensitivity pneumonitis. Mayo Clin Proc 2007;82:812–6.

14. Fernández Pérez ER, Swigris JJ, Forssén AV, et al. Identifying an inciting antigen is associated with improved survival in patients with chronic hypersensitivity pneumonitis. Chest 2013;144(5):1644–51.
15. De Sadeleer LJ, Hermans F, De Dycker E, et al. Effects of corticosteroid treatment and antigen avoidance in a large hypersensitivity pneumonitis cohort: a single-centre cohort study. J Clin Med 2018;8(1):14.
16. Hanak V, Golbin JM, Hartman TE, et al. High-resolution CT findings of paren-chymal fibrosis correlate with prognosis in hypersensitivity pneumonitis. Chest 2008;134(1):133–8.
17. Mooney JJ, Elicker BM, Urbania TH, et al. Radiographic fibrosis score predicts survival in hypersensitivity pneumonitis. Chest 2013;144(2):586–92.
18. Salisbury ML, Gu T, Murray S, et al. Hypersensitivity pneumonitis: radiographic phenotypes are associated with distinct survival time and pulmonary function tra-jectory. Chest 2019;155:699–711.
19. Chiba S, Tsuchiya K, Akashi T, et al. Chronic hypersensitivity pneumonitis with a usual interstitial pneumonia-like pattern: correlation between histopathologic and clinical findings. Chest 2016;149(6):1473–81.
20. Lima MS, Coletta ENAM, Ferreira RG, et al. Subacute and chronic hypersensitiv-ity pneumonitis: histopathological patterns and survival. Respir Med 2009;103(4):508–15.
21. Vasakova M, Morell F, Walsh S, et al. Hypersensitivity pneumonitis: perspectives in diagnosis and management. Am J Respir Crit Care Med 2017;196:680–9.
22. Salisbury ML, Myers JL, Belloli EA, et al. Diagnosis and treatment of fibrotic hy-persensitivity pneumonia: where we stand and where we need to go. Am J Respir Crit Care Med 2017;196:690–9.
23. Solaymani-Dodaran M, West J, Smith C, et al. Extrinsic allergic alveolitis: inci-dence and mortality in the general population. QJM 2007;100(4):233–7.
24. Yoshida K, Suga M, Nishiura Y, et al. Occupational hypersensitivity pneumonitis in Japan: data on a nationwide epidemiological study. Occup Environ Med 1995;52(9):570–4.
25. Fernández Pérez ER, Kong AM, Raimundo K, et al. Epidemiology of hypersensi-tivity pneumonitis among an insured population in the United States: a claims-based cohort analysis. Ann Am Thorac Soc 2018;15(4):460–9.
26. Morell F, Villar A, Ojanguren I, et al. Hypersensitivity pneumonitis and (idiopathic) pulmonary fibrosis due to feather duvets and pillows. Arch Bronconeumol (Engl Ed 2021;57(2):87–93.
27. Ohtsuka Y, Munakata M, Tanimura K, et al. Smoking promotes insidious and chronic farmer's lung disease and deteriorates the clinical outcome. Intern Med 1995;34:966–71.
28. Vasakova M, Selman M, Morell F, et al. Hypersensitivity pneumonitis: current con-cepts of pathogenesis and potential targets for treatment. Am J Respir Crit Care Med 2019;200:301–8.
29. Hansell DM, Bankier AA, MacMahon H, et al. Fleischner Society: glossary of terms for thoracic imaging. Radiology 2008;246(3):697–722.
30. Barnett J, Molyneaux PL, Rawal B, et al. Variable utility of mosaic attenuation to distinguish fibrotic hypersensitivity pneumonitis from idiopathic pulmonary fibrosis. Eur Respir J 2019;54:1900531.
31. Raghu G, Remy-Jardin M, Myers JL, et al. American Thoracic Society; European Respiratory Society; Japanese Respiratory Society; Latin American Thoracic So-ciety. Diagnosis of idiopathic pulmonary fibrosis: an official ATS/ERS/JRS/ALAT clinical practice guideline. Am J Respir Crit Care Med 2018;198:e44–68.

32. Jenkins AR, Chua A, Chami H, et al. Questionnaires or serum IgG testing in the diagnosis of hypersensitivity pneumonitis among patients with interstitial lung disease. Ann Am Thorac Soc 2021;18(1):130–47.

33. Meyer KC, Raghu G, Baughman RP, et al. An official American Thoracic Society clinical practice guideline: the clinical utility of bronchoalveolar lavage cellular analysis in interstitial lung disease. Am J Respir Crit Care Med 2012;185(9): 1004–14.

34. Patolia S, Tamae Kakazu M, Chami HA, et al. Bronchoalveolar lavage lymphocytes in the diagnosis of hypersensitivity pneumonitis among patients with interstitial lung disease. Ann Am Thorac Soc 2020;17(11):1455–67.

35. Adderley N, Humphreys CJ, Barnes H, et al. Bronchoalveolar lavage fluid lymphocytosis in chronic hypersensitivity pneumonitis: a systematic review and meta-analysis. Eur Respir J 2020;56(2):200026.

36. Macaluso C, Boccabella C, Kokosi M, et al. Short-term lung function changes predict mortality in patients with fibrotic hypersensitivity pneumonitis. Respirology 2022;27(3):202–8.

37. Flaherty KR, Travis WD, Colby TV, et al. Histopathologic variability in usual and nonspecific interstitial pneumonias. Am J Respir Crit Care Med 2001;164(9): 1722–7.

38. Akashi T, Takemura T, Ando N, et al. Histopathologic analysis of sixteen autopsy cases of chronic hypersensitivity pneumonitis and comparison with idiopathic pulmonary fibrosis/usual interstitial pneumonia. Am J Clin Pathol 2009;131: 405–15.

39. De Sadeleer LJ, Meert C, Yserbyt J, et al. Diagnostic ability of a dynamic multidisciplinary discussion in interstitial lung diseases: a retrospective observational study of 938 cases. Chest 2018;153(6):1416–23.

40. Walsh SLF, Wells AU, Desai SR, et al. Multicentre evaluation of multidisciplinary team meeting agreement on diagnosis in diffuse parenchymal lung disease: a case-cohort study. Lancet Respir Med 2016;4(7):557–65.

41. Dodia N, Amariei D, Kenaa B, et al. A comprehensive assessment of environmental exposures and the medical history guides multidisciplinary discussion in interstitial lung disease. Respir Med 2021;179:106333.

Initiating Pharmacologic Treatment in Tobacco-Dependent Adults

Alejandra Ellison-Barnes, MD, MPH[a,b],
Panagis Galiatsatos, MD, MHS[a,c],*

KEYWORDS

- Tobacco dependence • Nicotine addiction • Pharmacotherapy • Smoking cessation

KEY POINTS

- Nicotine addiction is complex and warrants insight into the patient's behavior and tobacco dependence.
- Pharmacotherapy can assist in the ability to manage a patient's nicotine addiction, with the goal becoming tobacco independent.
- There are several medications to select from for tobacco dependence management, and insight into their mechanisms and side-effects will allow for more precise clinical care.

INTRODUCTION

French diplomat Jean Nicot de Villemain introduced tobacco to France at a time the nation was exerting its cultural influence throughout the world.[1] The tobacco plant *Nicotiana tabacum* and its addictive chemical, nicotine—both named after Nicot de Villemain—were praised and promoted for their potential use in medicine and health.[1] The purported medical and health benefits continued to be touted centuries later, when Army surgeons in World War I praised tobacco in the form of cigarettes for aiding wounded military personnel in relaxation and pain mitigation.[2] However, the medical perspective on tobacco, especially cigarette consumption, pivoted in the 1950s and 1960s when it was linked to irreversible pulmonary pathologic conditions, from chronic bronchitis to lung cancer.[3] Since then, the aim of assisting the population in becoming tobacco-independent has been a priority of health care and medicine, as tobacco

Funding: This research received no external funding.
[a] The Tobacco Treatment and Cancer Screening Clinic, The Johns Hopkins Health System, Baltimore, MD, USA; [b] Division of General Internal Medicine, The Johns Hopkins School of Medicine, Baltimore, MD, USA; [c] Division of Pulmonary and Critical Care Medicine, The Johns Hopkins School of Medicine, Baltimore, MD, USA
* Corresponding author. 4940 Eastern Avenue, 4th Floor, Asthma and Allergy Building, Baltimore, MD 21224.
E-mail address: panagis@jhmi.edu

smoking is the leading cause of preventable morbidity and mortality.[4] Although counseling and behavior change remain at the forefront of addressing tobacco dependence,[5] pharmacotherapy has a vital role in curbing tobacco cravings and assisting in smoking cessation overall. In this review, the authors discuss the pharmacotherapies currently used as frontline agents for tobacco dependence as well as their benefit in diverse populations.

THE BIOLOGY OF NICOTINE ADDICTION

In 1988, the US Surgeon General's report declared that nicotine is the chemical in tobacco that results in addiction.[6] Nicotine's addictive properties have much to do with where it binds in the central nervous system and the resulting behaviors that reinforce the addiction. Nicotine, a volatile alkaloid, binds to acetylcholine receptors (AChR), a class of ligand-gated ion channels that open and allow the flow of positive ions, such as potassium and sodium.[7] AChR have a significant role in cellular excitability and neuronal integration, as well as in releasing various neurotransmitters throughout the brain.[8] With nicotine binding to AChR—converting them into nicotine AChR (nAChR)—nicotine is able to influence various parts of the brain as it acts on the most abundant nAChR, $\alpha_4\beta_2$ nAChR, in mammalian brains.[9] In particular, nicotine is able to activate the mesocorticolimbic dopamine system, a portion of the brain that is capable of inducing emotions of reward, survival, and aversion.[8,10] This activation and resulting arborization within the mesocorticolimbic dopamine system result in much of the behavior of addiction for the patients.

The mesocorticolimbic anatomic portion of the brain is vital to nicotine's addictive properties. The mesocorticolimbic system is anchored by the midbrain area known as the ventral tegmental area (VTA). The VTA has an abundance of nAChR, which when activated, transmit dopamine to the cortical area and limbic area of the brain. Specifically, dopamine is transmitted to the prefrontal cortex and the nucleus accumbens (NAc).[5] The associated reward sensation within the brain owing to the release of dopamine within this mesolimbic portion of the brain is the underlying, crucial mechanism for the development of nicotine addiction and subsequent strong physical dependence on tobacco.[11,12] This pathway of dopamine release and dopamine-related action is central to smoking cessation pharmacotherapy targets.

The chronicity of behavioral adaptations and abnormalities that characterize nicotine addiction warrants attention. Their persistence is due in part to the neural gene expressions activated by nicotine and its resulting in addiction.[13] As in earlier discussion, nicotine promotes the release of dopamine in the VTA through nAChR-mediated mechanisms, with further activation of specific subsets of nAChR on dopamine cell bodies, increasing their excitability and reinforcing nicotine-related influences.[13] The dopamine release and resulting transmission in the NAc results in the accumulation of a key molecule: ΔFosB, a transcription factor and member of the Fos family with extraordinary stability.[14] The NAc is one of the vital brain regions responsible for the compulsive behaviors and motivations of addiction. With repeated exposure to nicotine, ΔFosB accumulates in the NAc and persists in its neurons for significantly long periods of time, in some cases permanently.[15] ΔFosB in the NAc represents one of the vital molecular mechanisms that sustain gene expressions long after nicotine exposure and cessation.[13,15] ΔFosB functions as a type of "molecule switch" that converts the immediate nicotine-related behavior into persistent adaptations, contributing to the long-term neural and behavioral plasticity of nicotine addiction.[13] Such persistent adaptations lead to habits and compulsions that may become conditioned, potentially permanently, for the person with nicotine addiction, leading to tobacco dependence.

Understanding of the biology of nicotine addiction and, specifically, that it occurs in the mesocorticolimbic dopamine neural circuitry system of the brain—the brain's reward circuitry—also gives insight into the behaviors that occur in persons with nicotine addiction and tobacco dependence. The brain reward circuitry has diverse nAChR subtypes and receives afferent cholinergic innervation from nearby structures.[16] Nicotine acts directly on the reward circuitry as a type of reward-related sensory input, resulting in dopamine neuronal phasic bursts and inducing dopamine release.[17] These reward circuits that experience significant neuroplasticity related to nicotine manifest clinically in patients with nicotine addiction as conditional responses. Learned responses become conditional responses for persons with nicotine addiction, resulting in cigarette cravings when prompted by external and/or internal cues.[17] This results in persons with nicotine addiction attaching meaning to their smoking, creating a complex, multidimensional and developmental nature of tobacco dependence.[18] These attachments are diverse, from social to pleasure to emotional functions of nicotine addiction that may translate into tobacco dependence that is sociopsychologic as well as physical.[18] Therefore, when aiming to manage tobacco dependence's nicotine addiction with the use of pharmacotherapy, understanding the aforementioned mesocorticolimbic dopamine system (the brain reward circuitry) is key to a clinical understanding of what current medications are intended to do for the patient.

PHARMACOTHERAPY FOR NICOTINE ADDICTION AND TOBACCO DEPENDENCE

In assisting patients to manage their tobacco dependence, clinicians should recognize that such management warrants sustained, longitudinal care and strategies that take into account the biology of nicotine addiction and its resulting compulsion toward smoking. In essence, a chronic care model is needed to effectively manage a patient's tobacco dependence,[19] with treatments that may include counseling and pharmacotherapy. Such an emphasis on nicotine's addictive element has been established since the US Surgeon General's 1988 report, updated in 2008, linking tobacco use as the principal sign of nicotine addiction.[6,20] Additional guidelines around nicotine addiction have also been released, emphasizing pharmacotherapy especially as key to the management and treatment of tobacco dependence.[21,22] Given that smoking cessation has well-established health benefits, as the act of smoking greatly influences many diseases and their respective disease management, the management of tobacco dependence should be a priority for all clinicians and their patients. The current evidence base that has accumulated over the last 4 decades supports the inclusion of pharmacotherapy in the clinical workflow for effective management of tobacco dependence.

Moving forward, this article explores how pharmacotherapies currently approved by the Food and Drug Administration (FDA) assist in the management of tobacco dependence through their actions on nicotine addiction. Specifically, the authors focus on first-line pharmacotherapies that include nicotine replacement therapy (NRT), varenicline, and bupropion, exploring the biological basis of these medications and their respective pharmacology, and understanding how they attenuate the influence of nicotine addiction.[5,22,23] Furthermore, the authors explore tobacco dependence management in special populations, such as persons who are pregnant and persons with significant mental health morbidities, in an effort to understand potential challenges and confounders to effective tobacco dependence management with pharmacotherapy. Finally, they explore the future directions of potential pharmacotherapies currently under investigation.

Nicotine Replacement Therapy

NRTs were the first effective pharmacotherapies for the treatment of nicotine addiction, with nicotine gum having been approved by the FDA in 1984.[24] The administration of nicotine through NRTs has been shown to assist in the cravings experienced by persons who smoke, even weeks after smoking cessation, as well as to assist with nicotine withdrawal.[25] NRTs come in various forms, including transdermal patches, gum, lozenges, nasal sprays, and inhalers. The multiple formulations of NRT products should be considered by clinicians and patients in an effort to identify preferred route of administration and appropriate timing of the products (eg, use daily, use as needed, or both), to assist in making the management of nicotine addiction comfortable, and reducing dependence on tobacco products.

As previously mentioned, nicotine is the primary alkaloid and principal chemical driving the psychopharmacologic addiction to tobacco products. However, how NRTs are formulated and administered warrants attention, as nicotine from these products does not reproduce similar feelings and sensations on par with nicotine delivered by cigarettes.[26] First, the belief that NRT products trade 1 addiction for another is unwarranted, as the overall incidence of dependence on NRT products is low.[26,27] This is due in part to the low amount of nicotine in NRT products and that NRT-specific nicotine takes longer to reach the brain given its route of administration. This greatly attenuates nicotine's addictive potential, which is in part dependent on high concentrations rapidly reaching the brain. Second, clinicians should be prepared to discuss the various routes of administration and their impact on the patient's desire to smoke. NRT transdermal patches offer a slower and more sustained delivery of nicotine throughout the day to provide a general control over cravings through buildup of plasma nicotine levels, thereby acting as a type of "controller medication." In contrast, formulations such as gum, lozenges, inhalers, sublingual tablets, and nasal spray are all acute-dosing nicotine delivery products. This self-dosing mechanism provides patients control over the timing of nicotine delivery, allowing these NRT products to be used at times when immediate cravings are particularly problematic.[28] In this regard, acute-dosing nicotine delivery products should be thought of as a type of "rescue medication" in the patient's tobacco dependence treatment. Note that tolerance may build over time with the nontransdermal NRT products. Clinicians should be prepared to mitigate concerns over forming dependence on NRTs and to discuss how to appropriately use controller versus rescue medications in the management of nicotine addiction.

The efficacy of NRTs for the management of nicotine addiction has been reaffirmed over the years, and as a result, these pharmacotherapies are still considered first-line agents for tobacco dependence. In a 2018 review of all NRT products, Hartmann-Boyce and colleagues[29] found 133 trials using NRTs, totaling 64,640 participants, and concluded that all forms of NRT medications (transdermal patch, gum, lozenge, nasal spray, inhaler) increase the probability of smoking cessation versus the studies' control groups, finding the relative risk (RR) for cessation of all NRT formulations was 1.55 (95% confidence interval [CI], 1.49–1.61). The NRT transdermal patch had an RR of smoking cessation of 1.64 (95% CI, 1.53–1.75; 25,754 participants) as compared with the control group.[29] As for pharmacotherapy formulations for the acute delivery of nicotine, NRT gum was found to have an RR of cessation of 1.49 (95% CI, 1.40–1.60; 22,581 participants).[29]

Although the success of NRTs assures their current place within the arsenal of tools for clinicians to use for patients attempting to quit smoking, a few side effects should be emphasized to patients. First, all NRT products can cause local irritation of skin, buccal mucosa, nasal passages, or airways, depending on route of administration. It is recommended that the transdermal patch be rotated to different places of the patient's body to reduce skin irritation. Second, NRT transdermal patches may cause nightmares or sleeping interruptions if worn for 24 hours; for such patients, discussion of using the patch during the day with removal at night may be needed.[30] Chest discomfort and heart palpitations have also been reported, warranting discussions of dosing changes and/or further cardiac evaluation.[31] Finally, other common symptoms include dizziness and nausea. Preparing patients for the side effects will assure they can tolerate the medications in an effort to achieve their ultimate goal: quitting smoking and becoming tobacco independent.

Bupropion

Bupropion was the first non-NRT medication approved by the FDA for use as pharmacotherapy for smoking cessation. Developed for the treatment of major depressive disorder (MDD), bupropion was introduced in 1989 as a short-acting, immediate release medication.[32] Bupropion blocks the reuptake of neurotransmitters norepinephrine and dopamine, with resulting efficacy as an antidepressant comparable to other antidepressants, such as selective serotonin reuptake inhibitors.[32] Almost a decade after its introduction of MDD, bupropion's potential as a smoking cessation pharmacotherapy began to receive attention.[33] This smoking cessation property is due to bupropion's inhibition of dopamine reuptake, specifically in the mesolimbic region, given that dopamine release is a consequence of nAChR stimulation by nicotine and reinforces nicotine's addiction.[33,34] In addition to bupropion's intervention on neural pathways that aids in smoking cessation, given bupropion's antidepressant properties, it may also assist with nicotine withdrawal-related depressive symptoms. A sustained release formulation was introduced in 1996 and is often the formulation used for bupropion and nicotine addiction. Bupropion is now considered a first-line agent in the United States for the treatment of tobacco dependence.

Bupropion's role as effective pharmacotherapy for smoking cessation has been reaffirmed over the decades in many clinical trials. In a recent meta-analysis, Howes and colleagues[35] found in 45 studies (17,866 participants) that the RR of bupropion leading to long-term smoking cessation was statistically significant and clinically superior to that of a placebo (RR, 1.64; 95% CI, 1.52–1.77). Because bupropion works on a different neurologic pathway than NRTs, they may be combined, which may result in greater smoking cessation rates compared with a placebo or an NRT alone.[36,37] Furthermore, bupropion, alone or in combination with NRTs, may be more advantageous in specific patient populations, such as those with mental health issues such as depression.[37]

The clinical side effects of bupropion warrant consideration to either prepare patients for these adverse effects or determine that the medication may not be appropriate for certain patients. For instance, bupropion can result in weight loss, usually within 8 weeks of initiation of the medication.[38] Therefore, if an adult patient with tobacco dependence is underweight (body mass index <18.5 kg/m^2), the patient may not be a suitable candidate for bupropion treatment. In addition, bupropion lowers the seizure threshold and is contraindicated in patients with established seizure disorders, in patients with active heavy alcohol intake,[39] and in patients who have sustained a recent head injury.[34] Finally, bupropion can lead to adverse psychiatric effects, resulting in intolerance of the medication.[35] Each patient's mental health, including mood, affect, and suicidal ideation, should be monitored after initiation of bupropion, especially for patients with established psychiatric morbidities.

Varenicline

Varenicline is a α4β2 nAChR partial agonist that was approved by the FDA as a pharmacotherapy for smoking cessation in 2006.[40] A partial agonist against α4β2 nAChR has several key advantages for persons with tobacco dependence. First, it leads to a sustained increase of dopamine in the mesolimbic region.[41] This sustained level of dopamine attenuates the cravings, and potentially the withdrawal effects, of nicotine in persons with tobacco dependence. Second, the partial agonist effect on the nAChR may also prevent nicotine-induced increases in dopamine levels, resulting in a gradual lack of reward from tobacco for the person who smokes, assisting in both cessation and potential future relapse.[40,41] Finally, in recent guidelines, varenicline was evaluated against the NRT transdermal patch and bupropion and was found to be superior, likely owing to the aforementioned pharmacokinetics.[22] Of note, the development of varenicline was inspired by cytisine, a natural alkaloid and known partial agonist of nAChR.[42] However, cytisine has failed to show efficacy similar to varenicline for patients with tobacco dependence.[43]

Varenicline is offered in 2 doses, 0.5 mg and 1.0 mg, and for new users to the medication, a 7-day lead-in week is provided, ultimately to be titrated to 1.0 mg twice a day.[25] Adjustments to dosing should be considered for patients receiving hemodialysis. Medication duration is often up to 6 months. However, for certain patients struggling to quit smoking, it may be reasonable to discuss extending the medication beyond 6 months.[22] Varenicline is safe overall, with phase 2 and phase 3 placebo-controlled trials showing discontinuation rates (12%) comparable to placebo (10%).[44,45] However, with regard to common side effects that may impact tolerability of varenicline, the adverse effects that occurred at higher rates in trials include nausea, headache, insomnia, and abnormal dreams.[40] Of note, some of these side effects may occur at higher rates when using varenicline with NRT products. Although the combination of the two has been shown to be more efficacious than varenicline alone,[21,22] side effects were more common when compared with varenicline alone.[22]

Clinicians should also be aware of the history of varenicline's black box warnings. A black box warning by the FDA is the strongest warning the administration can place on a pharmacotherapy, and one placed on the medication due to its potential for serious adverse or life-threatening side effects. For Chantix, a black box warning was issued in 2009, 3 years after approval, owing to concerns over serious neuropsychiatric side effects, such as suicidal ideation.[46] However, a later randomized trial demonstrated that such risks were significantly lower than first reported, and in 2016, the FDA removed varenicline's black box warnings.[47] The safety has been reaffirmed in recent meta-analyses and guidelines.[22,48]

Given varenicline's efficacy profile and overall safety, clinicians should consider varenicline as a first-line agent for all eligible patients, either alone or in combination with the NRT products[21] or bupropion.[49]

CONSIDERATIONS IN SPECIFIC POPULATIONS
Pregnancy

Tobacco is associated with numerous adverse outcomes with respect to reproductive health. Although causality is not proven for all of these, associations include infertility, miscarriage, preterm delivery, low birthweight, and stillbirth, among others.[50] Approximately 7.2% of people who become pregnant smoke at some point during the pregnancy.[51] Rates are higher among younger people (ages 15–29), those of American Indian/Alaska Native or white race, and those with limited education (high school diploma or less).[51] It is recommended that current tobacco use be assessed for all pregnant people. It is important to assess not only cigarette use but also use of other forms of tobacco, such as e-cigarettes, hookah, and smokeless tobacco.[52]

Pregnant women should be advised to cease the use of tobacco products in any form and should be offered supportive interventions to achieve this.[52] The evidence for treatment of tobacco cessation in pregnancy is overall limited. The first-line intervention for cessation during pregnancy is typically behavioral or psychosocial interventions, which may include counseling, motivational interviewing, or financial incentives. These are associated with higher cessation rates later in pregnancy, whereas health education alone is not.[53]

The use of medication to facilitate cessation during pregnancy is also an option and should be considered through shared decision making following a discussion of risks and benefits. An individual's breastfeeding plans should also be taken into account, as this may affect which medications can be continued long term. It has been shown that NRT is likely beneficial, although data are not conclusive.[54] Increased metabolism of nicotine during pregnancy and poor adherence to NRT (studies report adherence rates as low as <10%) may explain the inconsistent efficacy.[54,55]

Currently, there is minimal evidence to demonstrate the efficacy of bupropion or varenicline for cessation during pregnancy. Pregnancy does not significantly alter the pharmacokinetics of bupropion or its metabolites during pregnancy; however, existing randomized controlled trials have not demonstrated increased cessation rates at the end of pregnancy.[56–58] No randomized trials exist for varenicline during pregnancy, but an observational study suggests it may be more effective than nicotine patches.[59] Importantly, no significant adverse birth outcomes have been identified with either bupropion or varenicline.[60,61] Additional randomized studies of the use of these medications during pregnancy are needed.

Although the greatest benefits are seen with cessation before 15 weeks' gestational age, cessation should be encouraged at any stage of pregnancy.[52] Notably, of those who do quit, approximately 50% to 60% will restart following delivery, so it is important to continue assessment and treatment in the postpartum period as well.[62]

Mental Health Disorders

More than one-fifth of adults in the United States have a mental health disorder.[63] Those with a diagnosis of a mental health disorder, including mood disorders, anxiety disorders, substance use disorder, and psychoses, are more likely to use tobacco than those without a diagnosis of mental health disorder. In 2019, 27.2% of those with any mental health disorder smoked cigarettes in the past month, whereas only 15.8% of those without mental illness reported tobacco use.[63] Certain psychiatric disorders are associated with even higher rates of tobacco use, with rates exceeding 70% in those with schizophrenia.[64] Tobacco use has been associated with poorer clinical outcomes in psychosis, with more missed antipsychotic doses and lower quality of life.[65]

Historically, tobacco cessation among those with mental health disorders has not always been a focus for their treating physicians.[66] However, smoking cessation has been associated with a reduction in depression and anxiety and improvement in both stress and quality of life, in both those with and those without formal psychiatric disorders and thus should be a priority.[67] Tobacco cessation treatments, including NRT, bupropion, and varenicline, have been shown to be safe and effective, even among those with serious mental illness, as long as there is adequate clinical monitoring.[68–70] Particular considerations for tobacco cessation treatments in patients with mental health disorders include medication effects (smoking can influence levels of psychotropic medications) and untreated nicotine withdrawal mimicking symptoms of psychiatric disorders.[71] Developing collaborations between tobacco control programs and mental health services may be particularly important.[72]

Race/Ethnicity

There are several salient differences in tobacco use and cessation patterns by race/ethnicity that are worth considering when approaching cessation. Bear in mind that there are wide variations in rates of tobacco use by racial subgroups/ethnicity that are often obscured by aggregated categories.[73]

Non-Hispanic black individuals who smoke tend to start smoking later and use fewer cigarettes per day.[74,75] They declare intention to quit within both 1-month and 6-month timeframes at higher rates than non-Hispanic whites and also have higher rates of past-year quit attempts than non-Hispanic whites.[76,77] Nevertheless, non-Hispanic blacks ultimately have more difficulty in quitting than non-Hispanic whites.[78] Of note, non-Hispanic blacks are more likely to smoke menthol cigarettes, which are associated with greater dependence and decreased cessation success.[79,80]

Similarly, Hispanics/Latinos are more likely to be light smokers yet do not have higher rates of success with cessation attempts.[78] Meanwhile, American Indian/Alaska Natives have the highest rates of tobacco use and the lowest quit ratio, which measures the population-level proportion of ever-smokers aged 25 or older who currently do not smoke.[73,81]

Possible reasons for these patterns include differences in health care utilization as well as access to and use of cessation treatments among racial/ethnic minorities than non-Hispanic whites.[78] Based on self-reported data, there do not seem to be major differences between racial/ethnic groups in terms of behavioral factors influencing intention to quit, such as duration of prior quit attempts or frequency of smoking, but it has been shown that receipt of cessation advice from a doctor may be particularly influential for non-Hispanic black as compared to non-Hispanic white individuals who smoke.[76] For all races/ethnicities, receipt of advice to quit is associated with higher odds of intending to quit, so ensuring universal screening, advising, and cessation support is crucial.[76] Preferences for counseling style should also be assessed to ensure an appropriate match.[82]

FUTURE DIRECTIONS
Nicotine Vaccines

One novel proposed cessation tool is immunization against nicotine. Antibodies against nicotine capture it in the bloodstream and reduce the amount of nicotine that is able to reach the brain when an individual uses a tobacco product. Immunization can be achieved through active immunization, in which exposure to an immunogen causes vaccine recipients to develop nicotine-specific antibodies, or through passive immunization, in which antibodies are produced in a laboratory setting and transferred to recipients.[83] Passive immunization strategies have so far been investigated only in animal models.[84]

Unfortunately, attempts to induce active immunization through a nicotine vaccine have not yet been successful. To date, no randomized controlled nicotine vaccine trial has demonstrated a statistically significant difference in long-term (12 months) cessation among those receiving vaccine versus placebo, although subgroup analyses conducted in 2 studies showed that those with high antibody levels sustained higher abstinence rates for longer periods of time.[85–87] There have been few serious adverse events, and no evidence of compensatory smoking, which is promising for future efforts in this field.[85]

Generating an adequate immune response is a clear challenge, and some candidate vaccines that have been studied required 5 or more doses to achieve an adequate response, which may limit utility in the clinical setting.[84] Future directions that may lead to improved, less heterogenous immune response include changes in adjuvants, the use of nanoparticle carriers, or alternate routes of administration.[84,88]

Psilocybin

Psychedelics have been proposed as another possible tobacco-cessation tool. Psilocybin is a naturally occurring 5-hydroxytryptamine (serotonin) 2A receptor agonist derived from fungi. It is a classic psychedelic with low physiologic toxicity that has shown promise as a treatment for mood disorders, including anxiety and depression as well as alcohol and tobacco dependence.[89] Typical exclusions in the limited studies to date include those with psychotic disorders or significant risk for psychotic disorders, who are thought to be at higher risk for prolonged reactions to psychedelics, and individuals with an elevated cardiovascular risk, because psilocybin increases blood pressure.[89] Psilocybin can cause anxiety or fear during administration with associated harmful behaviors, so participants must be prepared for and monitored during administration.

One small study of 15 participants administered 2 to 3 sessions of psilocybin with concomitant cognitive behavioral therapy.[90] This study found that at 12-month follow-up, 67% were biologically confirmed to be smoking abstinent. Long-term follow-up at an average of 30 months demonstrated that 60% of the original cohort remained abstinent. This long-term success with cessation after psychedelic use has been noted in naturalistic settings as well.[91]

SUMMARY

There is a strong evidence base for the use of existing pharmacotherapies to support tobacco cessation, alone or in combination, ideally with concurrent behavioral interventions. Future pharmacotherapies under development may assist in the most refractory cases. Incorporating current and future therapies into a longitudinal chronic care model for tobacco dependence will help a diverse range of patients achieve independence from nicotine addiction.

CLINICS CARE POINTS

- Pharmacotherapy for tobacco dependence is intended to assist in the management of the nicotine addiction, without challenging cravings or withdrawal symptoms that often result in relapse.

- Each available pharmacotherapy for tobacco dependence is able to achieve smoking cessation and should be tailored to the patient's co-morbidities and tolerance of the medication.

REFERENCES

1. Vigié M, Vigié M. Célébrations nationales 2004: Jean Nicot, sieur de Villemain. 2004. Available at: http://www2.culture.gouv.fr/culture/actualites/celebrations 2004/villemain.htm. Accessed 27 April 2022.
2. Smith EA, Malone RE. "Everywhere the soldier will be": wartime tobacco promotion in the US military. Am J Public Health 2009;99(9):1595–602.

3. Parascandola M. Cigarettes and the US Public Health Service in the 1950s. Am J Public Health 2001;91(2):196–205.

4. Samet JM. Tobacco smoking: the leading cause of preventable disease worldwide. Thorac Surg Clin 2013;23(2):103–12.

5. U.S. Department of Health and Human Services. Smoking Cessation, A Report of the Surgeon General. Atlanta, GA: U.S. Department of Health and Human Services, Centers for Disease Control and Prevention, National Center for Chronic Disease Prevention and Health Promotion, Office on Smoking and Health; 2020.

6. Services UDoHaH. Nicotine addiction: A report of the Surgeon General. DHHS Publication Number (CDC). 1988:88–8406.

7. Institute of Medicine (US) Committee to Assess the Science Base for Tobacco Harm Reduction; Stratton K, Shetty P, Wallace R, et al., editors. Clearing the Smoke: Assessing the Science Base for Tobacco Harm Reduction, Washington, DC, National Academies Press, US, 2001. Available at: https://www.ncbi.nlm.nih.gov/books/NBK222375/

8. D'Hoedt D, Bertrand D. Nicotinic acetylcholine receptors: an overview on drug discovery. Expert Opin Ther Targets 2009;13(4):395–411.

9. Maskos U, Molles BE, Pons S, et al. Nicotine reinforcement and cognition restored by targeted expression of nicotinic receptors. Nature 2005;436(7047): 103–7.

10. Picciotto MR, Zoli M, Rimondini R, et al. Acetylcholine receptors containing the beta2 subunit are involved in the reinforcing properties of nicotine. Nature 1998;391(6663):173–7.

11. Picciotto MR, Mineur YS. Molecules and circuits involved in nicotine addiction: The many faces of smoking. Neuropharmacology 2014;76 Pt B:545–53.

12. Picciotto MR, Addy NA, Mineur YS, et al. It is not "either/or": activation and desensitization of nicotinic acetylcholine receptors both contribute to behaviors related to nicotine addiction and mood. Prog Neurobiol 2008;84(4):329–42.

13. Centers for Disease Control and Prevention (US); National Center for Chronic Disease Prevention and Health Promotion (US); Office on Smoking and Health (US). How Tobacco Smoke Causes Disease: The Biology and Behavioral Basis for Smoking-Attributable Disease: A Report of the Surgeon General. Atlanta (GA): Centers for Disease Control and Prevention (US); 2010. Available at: https://www.ncbi.nlm.nih.gov/books/NBK53017/

14. Okuno H. Regulation and function of immediate-early genes in the brain: beyond neuronal activity markers. Neurosci Res 2011;69(3):175–86.

15. Nestler EJ, Barrot M, Self DW. DeltaFosB: a sustained molecular switch for addiction. Proc Natl Acad Sci U S A 2001;98(20):11042–6.

16. Omelchenko N, Sesack SR. Laterodorsal tegmental projections to identified cell populations in the rat ventral tegmental area. J Comp Neurol 2005;483(2):217–35.

17. De Biasi M, Dani JA. Reward, addiction, withdrawal to nicotine. Annu Rev Neurosci 2011;34:105–30.

18. Amos A, Wiltshire S, Haw S, et al. Ambivalence and uncertainty: experiences of and attitudes towards addiction and smoking cessation in the mid-to-late teens. Health Educ Res 2006;21(2):181–91.

19. Davy C, Bleasel J, Liu H, et al. Effectiveness of chronic care models: opportunities for improving healthcare practice and health outcomes: a systematic review. BMC Health Serv Res 2015;15:194.

20. Fiore M, United States. Tobacco Use and Dependence Guideline Panel. Treating tobacco use and dependence: 2008 update. 2008 update ed. Rockville, Md.: U.S. Dept. of Health and Human Services, Public Health Service; 2008.

21. Galiatsatos P, Garfield J, Melzer AC, et al. Summary for Clinicians: An ATS Clinical Practice Guideline for Initiating Pharmacologic Treatment in Tobacco-Dependent Adults. Ann Am Thorac Soc 2021;18(2):187–90.

22. Leone FT, Zhang Y, Evers-Casey S, et al. Initiating Pharmacologic Treatment in Tobacco-Dependent Adults. An Official American Thoracic Society Clinical Practice Guideline. Am J Respir Crit Care Med 2020;202(2):e5–31.

23. Barua RS, Rigotti NA, Benowitz NL, et al. 2018 ACC Expert Consensus Decision Pathway on Tobacco Cessation Treatment: A Report of the American College of Cardiology Task Force on Clinical Expert Consensus Documents. J Am Coll Cardiol 2018;72(25):3332–65.

24. Edens E, Massa A, Petrakis I. Novel pharmacological approaches to drug abuse treatment. Curr Top Behav Neurosci 2010;3:343–86.

25. Aubin HJ, Luquiens A, Berlin I. Pharmacotherapy for smoking cessation: pharmacological principles and clinical practice. Br J Clin Pharmacol 2014;77(2):324–36.

26. Carpenter MJ, Ford ME, Cartmell K, et al. Misperceptions of nicotine replacement therapy within racially and ethnically diverse smokers. J Natl Med Assoc 2011; 103(9–10):885–94.

27. Hughes JR, Pillitteri JL, Callas PW, et al. Misuse of and dependence on over-the-counter nicotine gum in a volunteer sample. Nicotine Tob Res 2004;6(1):79–84.

28. Wadgave U, Nagesh L. Nicotine Replacement Therapy: An Overview. Int J Health Sci (Qassim) 2016;10(3):425–35.

29. Hartmann-Boyce J, Chepkin SC, Ye W, et al. Nicotine replacement therapy versus control for smoking cessation. Cochrane Database Syst Rev 2018;5:CD000146.

30. Colrain IM, Trinder J, Swan GE. The impact of smoking cessation on objective and subjective markers of sleep: review, synthesis, and recommendations. Nicotine Tob Res 2004;6(6):913–25.

31. Mills EJ, Wu P, Lockhart I, et al. Adverse events associated with nicotine replacement therapy (NRT) for smoking cessation. A systematic review and meta-analysis of one hundred and twenty studies involving 177,390 individuals. Tob Induc Dis 2010;8:8.

32. Fava M, Rush AJ, Thase ME, et al. 15 years of clinical experience with bupropion HCl: from bupropion to bupropion SR to bupropion XL. Prim Care Companion J Clin Psychiatry 2005;7(3):106–13.

33. Tong EK, Carmody TP, Simon JA. Bupropion for smoking cessation: a review. Compr Ther 2006;32(1):26–33.

34. Wilkes S. The use of bupropion SR in cigarette smoking cessation. Int J Chron Obstruct Pulmon Dis 2008;3(1):45–53.

35. Howes S, Hartmann-Boyce J, Livingstone-Banks J, et al. Antidepressants for smoking cessation. Cochrane Database Syst Rev 2020;4:CD000031.

36. Jorenby DE, Leischow SJ, Nides MA, et al. A controlled trial of sustained-release bupropion, a nicotine patch, or both for smoking cessation. N Engl J Med 1999; 340(9):685–91.

37. Stapleton J, West R, Hajek P, et al. Randomized trial of nicotine replacement therapy (NRT), bupropion and NRT plus bupropion for smoking cessation: effectiveness in clinical practice. Addiction 2013;108(12):2193–201.

38. Jain AK, Kaplan RA, Gadde KM, et al. Bupropion SR vs. placebo for weight loss in obese patients with depressive symptoms. Obes Res 2002;10(10):1049–56.

39. Overview of Alcohol Consumption, National Institute on Alcohol Abuse and Alcoholism (NIAAA), Available from: https://www.niaaa.nih.gov/alcohols-effects-health/overview-alcohol-consumption.

40. Mohanasundaram UM, Chitkara R, Krishna G. Smoking cessation therapy with varenicline. Int J Chron Obstruct Pulmon Dis 2008;3(2):239–51.

41. Tonstad S, Arons C, Rollema H, et al. Varenicline: mode of action, efficacy, safety and accumulated experience salient for clinical populations. Curr Med Res Opin 2020;36(5):713–30.

42. Papke RL, Heinemann SF. Partial agonist properties of cytisine on neuronal nicotinic receptors containing the beta 2 subunit. Mol Pharmacol 1994;45(1):142–9.

43. Courtney RJ, McRobbie H, Tutka P, et al. Effect of Cytisine vs Varenicline on Smoking Cessation: A Randomized Clinical Trial. JAMA 2021;326(1):56–64.

44. Leas EC, Pierce JP, Benmarhnia T, et al, Effectiveness of Pharmaceutical Smoking Cessation Aids in a Nationally Representative Cohort of American Smokers. J Natl Cancer Inst 2018;110(6):581–7.

45. Nollen NL, Mayo MS, Sanderson Cox L, et al. Factors That Explain Differences in Abstinence Between Black and White Smokers: A Prospective Intervention Study. J Natl Cancer Inst 2019;111(10):1078–87.

46. Davies NM, Thomas KH. The Food and Drug Administration and varenicline: should risk communication be improved? Addiction 2017;112(4):555–8.

47. Lawler EC, Skira MM. Information shocks and pharmaceutical firms' marketing efforts: Evidence from the Chantix black box warning removal. J Health Econ 2022; 81:102557.

48. Anthenelli RM, Benowitz NL, West R, et al. Neuropsychiatric safety and efficacy of varenicline, bupropion, and nicotine patch in smokers with and without psychiatric disorders (EAGLES): a double-blind, randomised, placebo-controlled clinical trial. Lancet 2016;387(10037):2507–20.

49. Ebbert JO, Croghan IT, Sood A, et al. Varenicline and bupropion sustained-release combination therapy for smoking cessation. Nicotine Tob Res 2009; 11(3):234–9.

50. United States. Public Health Service. Office of the Surgeon General. How tobacco smoke causes disease: the biology and behavioral basis for smoking-attributable disease : a report of the Surgeon General. Washington, (DC): U.S. Dept. of Health and Human Services, Public Health Service.

51. Drake P, Driscoll AK, Mathews TJ. Cigarette Smoking During Pregnancy: United States, 2016. NCHS Data Brief 2018;(305):1–8.

52. Tobacco and Nicotine Cessation During Pregnancy: ACOG Committee Opinion, Number 807. Obstet Gynecol 2020;135(5):e221–9, https://pubmed.ncbi.nlm.nih.gov/32332417/.

53. Chamberlain C, O'Mara-Eves A, Porter J, et al. Psychosocial interventions for supporting women to stop smoking in pregnancy. Cochrane Database Syst Rev 2017;2:CD001055.

54. Claire R, Chamberlain C, Davey MA, et al. Pharmacological interventions for promoting smoking cessation during pregnancy. Cochrane Database Syst Rev 2020; 3:CD010078.

55. Bowker K, Lewis S, Coleman T, et al. Changes in the rate of nicotine metabolism across pregnancy: a longitudinal study. Addiction 2015;110(11):1827–32.

56. Fay EE, Czuba LC, Sager JE, et al. Pregnancy Has No Clinically Significant Effect on the Pharmacokinetics of Bupropion or Its Metabolites. Ther Drug Monit 2021; 43(6):780–8.

57. Nanovskaya TN, Oncken C, Fokina VM, et al. Bupropion sustained release for pregnant smokers: a randomized, placebo-controlled trial. Am J Obstet Gynecol 2017;216(4):420, e421-420 e429.

58. Kranzler HR, Washio Y, Zindel LR, et al. Placebo-controlled trial of bupropion for smoking cessation in pregnant women. Am J Obstet Gynecol MFM 2021;3(6): 100315.

59. Choi SKY, Tran DT, Kemp-Casey A, et al, The Comparative Effectiveness of Varenicline and Nicotine Patches for Smoking Abstinence During Pregnancy: Evidence From a Population-based Cohort Study. Nicotine Tob Res 2021;23(10): 1664–72.

60. Turner E, Jones M, Vaz LR, et al. Systematic Review and Meta-Analysis to Assess the Safety of Bupropion and Varenicline in Pregnancy. Nicotine Tob Res 2019; 21(8):1001–10.

61. Tran DT, Preen DB, Einarsdottir K, et al. Use of smoking cessation pharmacotherapies during pregnancy is not associated with increased risk of adverse pregnancy outcomes: a population-based cohort study. BMC Med 2020;18(1):15.

62. Colman GJ, Joyce T. Trends in smoking before, during, and after pregnancy in ten states. Am J Prev Med 2003;24(1):29–35.

63. 2019 National Survey on Drug Use and health: Detailed Tables. Rockville, MD: Substance Abuse and Mental Health Services Administration; 2020.

64. Kopczynska M, Zelek W, Touchard S, et al. Complement system biomarkers in first episode psychosis. Schizophr Res 2019;204:16–22.

65. Oluwoye O, Monroe-DeVita M, Burduli E, et al. Impact of tobacco, alcohol and cannabis use on treatment outcomes among patients experiencing first episode psychosis: data from the national RAISE-ETP study. Early Interv Psychiatry 2019; 13(1):142–6.

66. Physician behavior and practice patterns related to smoking cessation. Washington DC: Association of American Medical Colleges; 2007.

67. Taylor GM, Lindson N, Farley A, et al. Smoking cessation for improving mental health. Cochrane Database Syst Rev 2021;3:CD013522.

68. Tidey JW, Miller ME. Smoking cessation and reduction in people with chronic mental illness. BMJ 2015;351:h4065.

69. Shawen AE, Drayton SJ. Review of pharmacotherapy for smoking cessation in patients with schizophrenia. Ment Health Clin 2018;8(2):78–85.

70. Ahmed S, Virani S, Kotapati VP, et al. Efficacy and Safety of Varenicline for Smoking Cessation in Schizophrenia: A Meta-Analysis. Front Psychiatry 2018;9:428.

71. Das S, Prochaska JJ. Innovative approaches to support smoking cessation for individuals with mental illness and co-occurring substance use disorders. Expert Rev Respir Med 2017;11(10):841–50.

72. Williams JM, Willett JG, Miller G. Partnership between tobacco control programs and offices of mental health needed to reduce smoking rates in the United States. JAMA Psychiatry. 2013;70(12):1261–2.

73. United States. Department of Health and Human Services, National Center for Chronic Disease Prevention and Health Promotion (U.S.). Office on Smoking and Health. Tobacco use among U.S. racial/ethnic minority groups. Atlanta, Ga.: Dept. of Health and Human Services, Center for Disease Control and Prevention, National Center for Chronic Disease Prevention and Health Promotion For sale by the Supt. of Docs., U.S. G.P.O.; 1998.

74. Cantrell J, Bennett M, Mowery P, et al. Patterns in first and daily cigarette initiation among youth and young adults from 2002 to 2015. PLoS One 2018;13(8): e0200827.

75. Roberts ME, Colby SM, Lu B, et al. Understanding Tobacco Use Onset Among African Americans. Nicotine Tob Res 2016;18(Suppl 1):S49–56.

76. Soulakova JN, Li J, Crockett LJ. Race/ethnicity and intention to quit cigarette smoking. Prev Med Rep 2017;5:160–5.

77. Babb S, Malarcher A, Schauer G, et al. Quitting Smoking Among Adults - United States, 2000-2015. MMWR Morb Mortal Wkly Rep 2017;65(52):1457–64.

78. Trinidad DR, Perez-Stable EJ, White MM, et al. A nationwide analysis of US racial/ethnic disparities in smoking behaviors, smoking cessation, and cessation-related factors. Am J Public Health 2011;101(4):699–706.

79. Giovino GA, Villanti AC, Mowery PD, et al. Differential trends in cigarette smoking in the USA: is menthol slowing progress? Tob Control 2015;24(1):28–37.

80. Villanti AC, Collins LK, Niaura RS, et al. Menthol cigarettes and the public health standard: a systematic review. BMC Public Health 2017;17(1):983.

81. Carroll DM, Cole A. Racial/ethnic group comparisons of quit ratios and prevalences of cessation-related factors among adults who smoke with a quit attempt. Am J Drug Alcohol Abuse 2022;48(1):58–68.

82. Grobe JE, Goggin K, Harris KJ, et al. Race moderates the effects of Motivational Interviewing on smoking cessation induction. Patient Educ Couns 2020;103(2):350–8.

83. Escobar-Chavez JJ, Dominguez-Delgado CL, Rodriguez-Cruz IM. Targeting nicotine addiction: the possibility of a therapeutic vaccine. Drug Des Devel Ther 2011;5:211–24.

84. Xu A, Kosten TR. Current status of immunotherapies for addiction. Ann N Y Acad Sci 2021;1489(1):3–16.

85. Hartmann-Boyce J, Cahill K, Hatsukami D, et al. Nicotine vaccines for smoking cessation. Cochrane Database Syst Rev 2012;(8):CD007072.

86. Cornuz J, Zwahlen S, Jungi WF, et al. A vaccine against nicotine for smoking cessation: a randomized controlled trial. PLoS One 2008;3(6):e2547.

87. Hatsukami DK, Jorenby DE, Gonzales D, et al. Immunogenicity and smoking-cessation outcomes for a novel nicotine immunotherapeutic. Clin Pharmacol Ther 2011;89(3):392–9.

88. Truong TT, Kosten TR. Current status of vaccines for substance use disorders: A brief review of human studies. J Neurol Sci 2022;434:120098.

89. Johnson MW, Griffiths RR. Potential Therapeutic Effects of Psilocybin. Neurotherapeutics 2017;14(3):734–40.

90. Johnson MW, Garcia-Romeu A, Griffiths RR. Long-term follow-up of psilocybin-facilitated smoking cessation. Am J Drug Alcohol Abuse 2017;43(1):55–60.

91. Johnson MW, Garcia-Romeu A, Johnson PS, et al. An online survey of tobacco smoking cessation associated with naturalistic psychedelic use. J Psychopharmacol 2017;31(7):841–50.

Electronic Cigarette Use, Misuse, and Harm

Hasmeena Kathuria, MD

KEYWORDS

- Electronic cigarettes • Vaping • E-cigarette respiratory health effects • EVALI
- Youth nicotine addiction • Harm reduction • Tobacco control policy

KEY POINTS

- Newer generations of e-cigarettes are capable of delivering high nicotine concentrations and lead to youth addiction and subsequent combustible cigarette use.
- Studies suggest that e-cigarettes can compromise respiratory health over time.
- Some studies suggest reduced harm when individuals switch from smoking cigarettes to vaping e-cigarettes, but further study is needed.
- The combination of e-cigarettes and cigarettes is more harmful than using e-cigarettes alone or to smoking cigarettes alone.
- Some studies suggest that e-cigarettes may be effective as smoking-cessation aids when used as a therapeutic intervention, but not when used as a consumer product.

INTRODUCTION

Vaping involves inhaling an aerosol that is created by heating an electronic liquid (e-liquid) containing a variety of substances that usually include nicotine and/or cannabinoids, flavorings, and additives (eg, glycerol or propylene glycol).[1] E-cigarettes are most commonly battery-operated devices used to generate this aerosol.[2] Understanding these devices, the components in the e-liquids, and vaping practices is critical in understanding the various health effects, including adolescent nicotine addition, attributable to the use of these products.

Epidemiology of Vaping

While e-cigarette use among adults had increased between 2014 and 2019, the National Health Interview Survey showed a decline in 2020 to 3.7%.[3,4] However, among young adults (18–24 years), e-cigarette use has increased in 2020 to 9.4%.[3] Most adults who use e-cigarettes have currently or previously smoked cigarettes.[5]

The Pulmonary Center, Boston University School of Medicine, 72 East Concord Street R304, Boston, MA 02118, USA
E-mail address: hasmeena@bu.edu

Med Clin N Am 106 (2022) 1081–1092
https://doi.org/10.1016/j.mcna.2022.07.009
0025-7125/22/© 2022 Elsevier Inc. All rights reserved.

In 2021, 2.06 million youths used e-cigarettes.[6] The 2020 and 2021 National Youth Tobacco Survey suggest a trend reversal of e-cigarette use in both middle and high school students after an upward trend between 2013 and 2019,[6–8] but caution is warranted in comparing results as survey methodology changed during the COVID-19 pandemic. In 2021, 11.3% of high school students and 2.8% of middle school students reported current use of e-cigarettes.[6]

E-Cigarette Devices

The essential components of an e-cigarette device include a mouthpiece, e-liquid, a battery, and an atomizer, which is the heating element (often heating-coils made of metals) that converts the e-liquid to aerosol.[2] E-cigarette design has evolved over time as described below and in **Fig. 1**.[2]

First-generation e-cigarettes, often referred to as cig-a-likes, were designed for one-time use and had fixed, low-voltage batteries in which inhalation triggered heating of the e-liquid. Later modifications to first-generation devices made them reusable.

Second-generation e-cigarettes have larger rechargeable batteries, removable atomizers, and higher volume refillable e-liquid reservoirs (tanks) that enables the user to regulate the power delivery and adjust the e-liquid components. They can be medium size (pen style) or large size (tank style).

Third-generation e-cigarettes are known as modifiable e-cigarettes (mods) and feature adjustable atomizers, cartridges, and high-capacity batteries that allow the user to control the concentration and speed of aerosol delivery. They can also contain sub-Ohm resistance heating coils allowing large aerosol production.

Fourth-generation e-cigarettes, known as pod-mods, have a replaceable prefilled e-liquid cartridge (pod) sold separately and a rechargeable mod system that consists of a battery, atomizer, and mouthpiece built into 1 device. These systems (eg, the

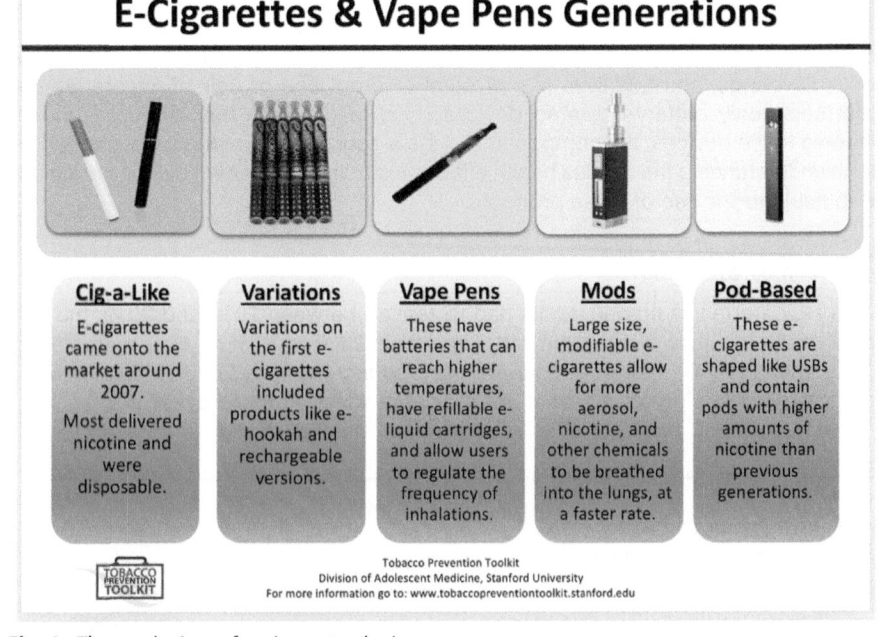

Fig. 1. The evolution of e-cigarette devices.

common brand JUUL) can deliver much higher concentrations of nicotine than earlier devices.[9]

E-Liquid Components

Nicotine

Most e-liquids contain nicotine; however, the amount inhaled depends on many factors including e-cigarette design (eg, devices that use high-capacity batteries deliver more nicotine), nicotine concentration in the e-liquid, the use of nicotine salts, other components in the e-liquid, vaping technique, and puffing intensity.[2,9] An acidic pH (pH 5.5–6) facilitates inhalation of nicotine, whereas an alkaline pH (pH 7) facilitates oral absorption. Earlier forms of e-liquids used freebase nicotine (higher pH) which resulted in throat irritation; newer products (eg, JUUL) use nicotine salts (lower pH) which reduces throat irritation and allows inhalation of higher doses of nicotine.[1,2,10]

Flavorings

Flavorings increase the attractiveness of e-cigarettes particularly to youth, resulting in initiation and persistence of e-cigarette use and reduced harm perception of tobacco products.[11] There are over 7000 available flavors. Of adolescents who have vaped, most start with flavored or menthol products; the first e-cigarette used by 81% of youth ever-users were flavored products.[12] Nearly 80% of current youth e-cigarette users vape flavored e-cigarettes.[6]

While little is known about the health effects of most flavorings, it is known that some flavorings such as diacetyl found in sweet flavorings is associated with bronchitis obliterans (also known as "popcorn lung").[13]

Additives

Most e-cigarettes contain propylene glycol or glycerol, used as humectants to aerosolize e-cigarettes. The safety of propylene glycol and vegetable glycerin at levels inhaled by e-cigarette users remains uncertain. During the heating process to create aerosol, thermal degradation of propylene glycol and glycerol can form reactive carbonyl compounds (formaldehyde, acetaldehyde, acrolein) that can reach sufficient concentration for potential damage to the respiratory tract[13]; increased battery voltage results in higher concentrations of these carbonyls. In addition to respiratory effects, acrolein and formaldehyde are listed as group I carcinogenic compounds by the International Agency for Research on Cancer, and acetaldehyde is a group 2B possibly carcinogenic compound.[14]

Tetrahydrocannabinol

Tetrahydrocannabinol (THC) can be inhaled through e-cigarette devices, and the amount inhaled can be high. Dry marijuana, oil concentrates, and waxes can be vaped through a variety of devices. As discussed below, vaping THC-containing products has been linked to e-cigarette, or vaping, product use-associated lung injury (EVALI).[15] The long-term pulmonary health effects of vaping marijuana are not known. Dabbing describes a form of vaping highly concentrated THC created by heating butane-extracted cannabis oil.[16] Case reports have shown an association between butane inhalation and acute respiratory distress syndrome.[17]

Synthetic nicotine and cannabinoids

Synthetic nicotine is made in the laboratory and not derived from tobacco. Some e-cigarette manufactures that used tobacco-derived nicotine switched to synthetic nicotine to avoid regulation by the Food and Drug Administration (FDA). In March 2022, this loophole was closed; the FDA's Center for Tobacco Products now has the authority to regulate synthetic nicotine products. It is unknown if the health effects of synthetic nicotine differ from those of tobacco-derived nicotine.

Vaping synthetic cannabinoids has increased in popularity and can be highly addictive.[18] Individuals can present with acute intoxication with presenting symptoms including delirium, respiratory depression, and even death. The long-term health effects are unknown.

Modifications and Individual Use Characteristics

User puff topography, such as the length of inhalation, puff volume, and the frequency of use, can also influence the health effects of e-cigarettes. Dripping is a common modification that involves directly adding e-liquid onto the atomizer, resulting in immediate aerosolization of the e-liquid. This method produces a thicker aerosol cloud.[19] One study showed that this method had greater emission of volatile aldehydes (eg, formaldehyde).[20] Hacking includes any postmarket modifications to the device not intended by the manufacturer.

HEALTH EFFECTS OF E-CIGARETTES
Effects of Nicotine Exposure

Nicotine toxicity
Nicotine exposure whether from vaping or smoking can increase heart rate and blood pressure.[21] Until 2009, nicotine poisoning was a rare occurrence since nicotine toxicity generally requires significantly higher concentrations than those derived from smoking a cigarette. In 2021, poison control centers reported over 4500 tobacco-related exposure cases with e-cigarette devices or liquid nicotine.[22]

Nicotine effects on brain development
The brain is developing until the mid-twenties; nicotine exposure during this timeframe can rewire the brain and cause deficits in working memory, attention, auditory processing, impulsivity, as well as learning difficulties, anxiety, and mood swings.[23]

Nicotine addiction
E-cigarette use, particularly with increased use of nicotine salts and devices capable of delivering high nicotine concentrations, can increase the risk to nicotine dependence and combustible tobacco use. This gateway effect is suggested by observational studies showing that e-cigarette use precedes cigarette smoking.[24,25] A meta-analyses of longitudinal studies in adolescents and young adults aged 14 to 30 years showed that e-cigarette ever users had a higher probability of initiating cigarette smoking than e-cigarette never users.[26] E-cigarette use has also been associated with increased odds of marijuana, stimulant, and polysubstance use.[27]

All adolescents who use e-cigarettes should be provided with options for behavioral cessation support.[28] Currently there are no FDA-approved medications for the treatment of nicotine or tobacco dependence in adolescents younger than 18 years. The American Academy of Pediatrics recommends considering off-label use of nicotine replacement therapy (NRT) in adolescents with moderate to severe nicotine dependence.[29]

E-Cigarette, or Vaping, Product Use-Associated Lung Injury

EVALI is an acute or subacute respiratory illness in individuals who used e-cigarettes in the prior 90 days.[30,31] The Centers for Disease Control and Prevention (CDC) initiated an investigation of EVALI in August 2019, and as of February 18, 2020, 2807 hospitalized cases were reported to the CDC; among the reported cases, there were 68 deaths.[31]

EVALI cases peaked in September 2019, followed by a gradual decline likely due to increased public awareness and the removal of vitamin E acetate, a diluent added to THC-containing e-cigarettes linked to the outbreak of EVALI. The CDC stopped collecting data in February 2020 although cases continue to be reported, suggesting that other compounds or unknown additives in THC- and non-THC-containing e-cigarettes may also be causative. The exact pathogenesis of EVALI is unknown but point to varying degrees of acute lung injury with pathologic findings that include diffuse alveolar damage, organizing pneumonia, or acute fibrinous pneumonitis.[32]

Patients most often present with respiratory symptoms (eg, dyspnea, cough, chest pain, and hemoptysis), and one-third may progress to acute respiratory failure. Gastrointestinal symptoms (nausea, vomiting, abdominal pain, and diarrhea) and subjective fevers are commonly reported.[30] The CDC provides case definition criteria for EVALI (below).[33] These criteria were formed before the COVID-19 pandemic; a negative nucleic acid test for severe acute respiratory syndrome coronavirus 2 should also be included.

- Use of an e-cigarette or related product in the previous 90 days
- Pulmonary infiltrates on chest radiograph or computed tomography
- Exclusion of lung infection based on negative results on all other clinically indicated respiratory infectious disease testing
- Absence of a likely alternative diagnosis (cardiac, rheumatologic, or neoplastic process).

Patients who have worsening symptoms and hypoxemia are usually initiated on systemic glucocorticoids.[34] The mainstay of treatment is close monitoring and supportive care focused on ensuring adequate oxygenation and vaping cessation.[33]

Effects of E-Cigarette Aerosol Inhalation on the Lungs

The health effects of vaping are difficult to study and largely unknown given that the levels of toxins and manifestations of lung disease vary depending on the e-cigarette liquid components, evolution of devices, and user characteristics (eg, dual use, topography).[35] A comprehensive review of the effects of e-cigarettes on respiratory health from human, animal, and in vivo laboratory studies has been recently reported.[21,36,37] Some of the epidemiologic and biomarker studies are outlined below.

Epidemiologic studies

Epidemiologic studies, including meta-analyses, cross-sectional studies, and longitudinal studies, have reported associations between e-cigarettes and respiratory disease.[37–39] The Population Assessment of Tobacco and Health (PATH) study is an ongoing longitudinal cohort study on tobacco use behavior, attitudes and beliefs, and tobacco-related health outcomes. Using data from the PATH study, Xie and colleagues found that in adults, e-cigarette use was associated with an increased risk of developing respiratory diseases (COPD, emphysema, chronic bronchitis, and asthma) independent of cigarette smoking.[40] Another study of young adults (18–24 years) with no prevalent respiratory disease or symptoms demonstrated that former and current e-cigarette use was associated with higher odds of developing wheezing-related respiratory symptoms, after accounting for cigarette smoking and other combustible tobacco product use.[41]

Lung function studies

Randomized clinical trials of acute and chronic e-cigarette use on lung function have shown variable results, with some showing reductions in lung function[21,36,42] and others showing no change.[21,36,43] A study that compared 30 healthy daily users of e-cigarettes to 30 controls with spirometry for a minimum of 1 hour after use found that e-cigarette users had lower forced expiratory volume in one second (FEV1) and a lower percentage of the forced vital capacity (FVC) expired in one second (FEV1/FVC ratio) than controls.[42]

Biomarkers of lung inflammation and injury

Increased mucin levels are a biomarker of chronic bronchitis[44]; increased MUC5AC levels have been found in bronchial epithelia and in airway secretion in e-cigarette users.[45] Proteomic studies of sputum from e-cigarette users showed an altered profile of innate defense proteins in airway secretions, including higher levels of neutrophil activation.[45] Smokers exposed to e-cigarette aerosol resulted in impaired gas exchange in association with an increase in the lung damage biomarker CC16, suggesting that e-cigarettes may cause acute injury to the small airways.[46] Another study found elevated neutrophil elastase, matrix metalloproteinase-2 (MMP-2), and matrix metalloproteinase-9 (MMP-9) activities and protein levels in e-cigarette users' and smokers' bronchoalveolar lavage fluid (BAL) relative to nonsmokers, suggesting that e-cigarette users and smokers are at risk of developing chronic lung disease.[47]

Respiratory Effects of Dual Use of Combustible Cigarettes and Cigarettes

Several studies provide epidemiologic evidence that the combination of e-cigarettes and combustible cigarettes is more harmful than using either one alone. In a population-based study, associations of e-cigarette use with respiratory symptoms (chronic cough, sputum, or wheeze) were strongest among dual users with combustible cigarettes.[48] A longitudinal analysis using PATH data showed that dual use of e-cigarettes and combustible cigarettes has higher risk of developing respiratory disease than using either product alone.[39] Goniewicz and colleagues found that dual users had higher amounts of almost all toxic substances (3 tobacco-specific nitrosamines, 5 polycyclic aromatic hydrocarbons, and 13 volatile organic compounds) than cigarette-only users.[49]

Effects of Switching from Combustible Cigarettes to E-Cigarettes on Lung Health

A systematic literature review of epidemiologic studies that compared respiratory outcomes among former smokers who transitioned to e-cigarettes versus current exclusive smokers showed that former smokers who transitioned to e-cigarettes had ~ 40% lower odds of respiratory outcomes than current exclusive smokers.[50]

Several studies have studied symptom scores and spirometry among chronic smokers who transition to e-cigarettes; smokers who have been studied after transitioning to e-cigarettes have had either no change or slight improvements in spirometry.[51] In patients with preexisting lung conditions, switching from smoking to vaping did not improve lung function.[52,53] Longer trials are needed to determine whether switching from smoking to vaping can improve lung function; changes in spirometry can reliably be detected only after years of cigarette smoking.[54]

IS THERE A ROLE FOR E-CIGARETTES TO PROMOTE SMOKING CESSATION?

Evidence from clinical trials suggest that e-cigarettes may be effective as smoking cessation aids when used as a therapeutic intervention with counseling.[55–57] In a Cochrane systematic review that included 16,000 individuals who smoked cigarettes, quit rates were higher with nicotine e-cigarettes than with NRT and with nicotine e-cigarettes than with non-nicotine e-cigarettes. The authors highlighted the need for more evidence on the newer e-cigarette devices. Although e-cigarettes may facilitate smoking cessation, they are not associated with a reduction in nicotine dependency[58] and may lead to dual use of e-cigarettes and cigarettes.

Observational trials provide evidence on how e-cigarette devices are used in actual practice rather than in clinical trials; in general, the effects of e-cigarettes in promoting smoking cessation are less favorable. In a recent meta-analysis of observational studies of adults who smoke cigarettes, e-cigarette consumer product use was not significantly associated with cigarette smoking cessation.[57]

The American Thoracic Society Clinical Practice Guideline recommends varenicline rather than e-cigarettes for smoking cessation.[59] The US Preventive Services Task Force concludes that the evidence is insufficient to fully evaluate the harms and benefits of e-cigarettes for smoking cessation.[60] There are 7 FDA-approved medications to treat tobacco use disorder; e-cigarette is not FDA-approved to treat tobacco use disorder. If individuals are using e-cigarettes to try to stop smoking, information should be provided on the uncertainties about the long-term health risks, and they should be counseled on tobacco cessation using guideline-recommended approaches; the goal should be to stop using all tobacco products, including e-cigarettes.

DISCUSSION

Opinions differ about whether possible harm-reduction benefits of switching from cigarettes to e-cigarettes could outweigh adverse effects of e-cigarette use among individuals who have never smoked, those who have switched and continue to use e-cigarettes, and dual users of e-cigarettes and cigarettes.[61] There is uncertainty of the long-term effects of e-cigarettes and differing interpretations on the effectiveness in promoting smoking cessation. Evidence from clinical trials suggest that e-cigarettes may be effective as smoking-cessation aids when used as a therapeutic intervention with counseling. However, meta-analysis of observational studies shows that e-cigarette consumer products—as used in real-world settings—are not associated with smoking abstinence. The high prevalence of e-cigarette use among youth and the concerning evidence that e-cigarette use is a strong risk factor for subsequent smoking cigarettes[13] support a more restrictive regulatory policy on e-cigarettes.

In the Unites States, the FDA regulates e-cigarettes through its Center for Tobacco Products and assesses population as well as individual impacts for the products as actually used by the general population. These regulations require that manufacturers demonstrate their e-cigarette products meet the FDA standard of providing a net public health benefit or face removal from the market. Since flavorings are a key driver of youth tobacco use,[11,62,63] and therefore cannot meet the public health standard that the law requires, it is of utmost importance that no flavored tobacco products be allowed to remain on the market.

SUMMARY

E-cigarette devices are rapidly evolving over time. The true health effects of e-cigarettes are difficult to study and remain largely unknown given that the levels of toxins and manifestations of lung disease vary depending on the e-cigarette liquid components, evolution of devices, and user practices. E-cigarette use, particularly with increased use of nicotine salts and devices that are capable of delivering high nicotine concentrations, can increase the risk to nicotine dependence and combustible tobacco use, a particular concern given the high rates of e-cigarette use among youth. Epidemiologic studies show an association between e-cigarette use and incidence pulmonary disease, and biomarker studies show tissue damage in both the airway and parenchyma after acute exposure, suggesting that e-cigarettes compromise respiratory health over time. Some studies suggest reduced harm from e-cigarette use compared with smoking, but this requires further study. Most adults who use e-cigarettes also smoke cigarettes; the combination of e-cigarettes and cigarettes is more harmful than using either product alone. Clinicians should strongly advise youth and nonsmokers against initiating e-cigarettes and should educate individuals on the health effects of dual use of e-cigarettes and cigarettes.

CLINICS CARE POINTS

- E-cigarette devices are rapidly evolving over time, and it is therefore difficult to assess the true health effects of e-cigarettes.
- Newer generations of e-cigarettes are capable of delivering high nicotine concentrations and lead to youth addiction and subsequent combustible cigarette use.
- Flavored tobacco products are a major driver for youth tobacco use.
- Studies suggest that e-cigarettes can compromise respiratory health over time.
- Some studies suggest reduced harm when individuals switch from smoking cigarettes to vaping e-cigarettes, but further study is needed.
- The combination of e-cigarettes and cigarettes is more harmful than using either alone.
- Some studies suggest that e-cigarettes may be effective as smoking cessation aids when used as a therapeutic intervention with counseling but less likely to be effective when used as a consumer product.
- There are 7 Food and Drug Administration-approved medications for promoting smoking cessation; e-cigarettes are not an FDA-approved tool for promoting smoking cessation.
- The evidence is clear that youth and individuals who never smoked should not start using e-cigarettes.

DISCLOSURE

H. Kathuria is a section editor for UpToDate (Tobacco Dependence Treatment).

REFERENCES

1. Boyer EW, Levy S, Smelson D, et al. The Clinical Assessment of Vaping Exposure. J Addict Med 2020;14(6):446–50.
2. DeVito EE, Krishnan-Sarin S. E-cigarettes: Impact of E-Liquid Components and Device Characteristics on Nicotine Exposure. Curr Neuropharmacol 2018;16(4): 438–59.
3. Cornelius ME, Loretan CG, Wang TW, et al. Tobacco Product Use Among Adults - United States, 2020. MMWR Morb Mortal Wkly Rep 2022;71(11):397–405.
4. Dai H, Leventhal AM. Prevalence of e-Cigarette Use Among Adults in the United States, 2014-2018. JAMA 2019;322(18):1824–7.
5. Mayer M, Reyes-Guzman C, Grana R, et al. Demographic Characteristics, Cigarette Smoking, and e-Cigarette Use Among US Adults. JAMA Netw Open 2020; 3(10):e2020694.
6. Gentzke AS, Wang TW, Cornelius M, et al. Tobacco Product Use and Associated Factors Among Middle and High School Students - National Youth Tobacco Survey, United States, 2021. MMWR Surveill Summ 2022;71(5):1–29.
7. Jamal A, Gentzke A, Hu SS, et al. Tobacco Use Among Middle and High School Students - United States, 2011-2016. MMWR Morb Mortal Wkly Rep 2017;66(23): 597–603.

8. Miech R, Johnston L, O'Malley PM, et al. Trends in Adolescent Vaping, 2017-2019. N Engl J Med 2019;381(15):1490–1.

9. Goniewicz ML, Boykan R, Messina CR, et al. High exposure to nicotine among adolescents who use Juul and other vape pod systems ('pods'). Tob Control 2019;28(6):676–7.

10. Cheng T. Chemical evaluation of electronic cigarettes. Tob Control 2014;23(Suppl 2):ii11–7.

11. Health NCfCDPaHPUOoSa. E-Cigarette Use Among Youth and Young Adults: A Report of the Surgeon General. 2016.

12. Ambrose BK, Day HR, Rostron B, et al. Flavored Tobacco Product Use Among US Youth Aged 12-17 Years, 2013-2014. JAMA 2015;314(17):1871–3.

13. National Academies of Sciences, Engineering, and Medicine. Public health consequences of E-cigarettes. Washington, DC: The National Academies Press; 2018. https://doi.org/10.17226/24952.

14. Canistro D, Vivarelli F, Cirillo S, et al. E-cigarettes induce toxicological effects that can raise the cancer risk. Sci Rep 2017;7(1):2028.

15. Blount BC, Karwowski MP, Shields PG, et al. Vitamin E Acetate in Bronchoalveolar-Lavage Fluid Associated with EVALI. N Engl J Med 2019. https://doi.org/10.1056/NEJMoa1916433.

16. Stogner JM, Miller BL. The Dabbing Dilemma: A Call for Research on Butane Hash Oil and Other Alternate Forms of Cannabis Use. Subst Abus 2015;36(4):393–5.

17. Ahmed A, Shapiro D, Su J, et al. Vaping Cannabis Butane Hash Oil Leads to Severe Acute Respiratory Distress Syndrome-A Case of EVALI in a Teenager With Hypertrophic Cardiomyopathy. J Intensive Care Med May 2021;36(5):617–21.

18. Blount BC, Karwowski MP, Morel-Espinosa M, et al. Evaluation of Bronchoalveolar Lavage Fluid from Patients in an Outbreak of E-cigarette, or Vaping, Product Use-Associated Lung Injury - 10 States, August-October 2019. MMWR Morb Mortal Wkly Rep 2019;68(45):1040–1.

19. Guy MC, Helt J, Palafox S, et al. Orthodox and Unorthodox Uses of Electronic Cigarettes: A Surveillance of YouTube Video Content. Nicotine Tob Res 2019; 21(10):1378–84.

20. Talih S, Balhas Z, Salman R, et al. Direct Dripping": A High-Temperature, High-Formaldehyde Emission Electronic Cigarette Use Method. Nicotine Tob Res 2016;18(4):453–9.

21. Neczypor EW, Mears MJ, Ghosh A, et al. E-Cigarettes and Cardiopulmonary Health: Review for Clinicians. Circulation 2022;145(3):219–32.

22. American Association of Poison Control Centers - E-Cigarettes and Liquid Nicotine [Internet]. [cited March 13 2022]. Available at: https://www.aapcc.org/track/ecigarettes-liquid-nicotine.

23. Yuan M, Cross SJ, Loughlin SE, et al. Nicotine and the adolescent brain. J Physiol 2015;593(16):3397–412.

24. Leventhal AM, Strong DR, Kirkpatrick MG, et al. Association of Electronic Cigarette Use With Initiation of Combustible Tobacco Product Smoking in Early Adolescence. JAMA 2015;314(7):700–7.

25. Primack BA, Soneji S, Stoolmiller M, et al. Progression to Traditional Cigarette Smoking After Electronic Cigarette Use Among US Adolescents and Young Adults. JAMA Pediatr 2015;169(11):1018–23.

26. Soneji S, Barrington-Trimis JL, Wills TA, et al. Association Between Initial Use of e-Cigarettes and Subsequent Cigarette Smoking Among Adolescents and Young

Adults: A Systematic Review and Meta-analysis. JAMA Pediatr 2017;171(8): 788–97.

27. Bentivegna K, Atuegwu NC, Oncken C, et al. E-cigarette Use Is Associated with Non-prescribed Medication Use in Adults: Results from the PATH Survey. J Gen Intern Med 2019;34(10):1995–7.

28. Graham AL, Amato MS, Cha S, et al. Effectiveness of a Vaping Cessation Text Message Program Among Young Adult e-Cigarette Users: A Randomized Clinical Trial. JAMA Intern Med 2021;181(7):923–30.

29. Farber HJ, Walley SC, Groner JA, et al. Clinical Practice Policy to Protect Children From Tobacco, Nicotine, and Tobacco Smoke. Pediatrics 2015;136(5):1008–17.

30. Layden JE, Ghinai I, Pray I, et al. Pulmonary Illness Related to E-Cigarette Use in Illinois and Wisconsin - Final Report. N Engl J Med 2020;382(10):903–16.

31. Centers for Disease Control and Prevention (CDC). Outbreak of lung injury associated with the use of e-cigarette, or vaping, products. Available at: https://www. cdc.gov/tobacco/basic_information/e-cigarettes/severe-lung-disease.html# latest-information. Accessed on May 06, 2022.

32. Butt YM, Smith ML, Tazelaar HD, et al. Pathology of Vaping-Associated Lung Injury. N Engl J Med 2019;381(18):1780–1.

33. Schier JG, Meiman JG, Layden J, et al. Severe Pulmonary Disease Associated with Electronic-Cigarette-Product Use - Interim Guidance. MMWR Morb Mortal Wkly Rep 2019;68(36):787–90.

34. Hayes D, Board A, Calfee C, et al. Pulmonary and Critical Care Considerations for E-Cigarette, or Vaping, Product Use-Associated Lung Injury. Chest 2022. https:// doi.org/10.1016/j.chest.2022.02.039.

35. Kosmider L, Sobczak A, Fik M, et al. Carbonyl compounds in electronic cigarette vapors: effects of nicotine solvent and battery output voltage. Nicotine Tob Res 2014;16(10):1319–26.

36. Gotts JE, Jordt SE, McConnell R, et al. What are the respiratory effects of e-cigarettes? BMJ 2019;366:l5275.

37. Wills TA, Soneji SS, Choi K, et al. E-cigarette use and respiratory disorders: an integrative review of converging evidence from epidemiological and laboratory studies. Eur Respir J 2021;57(1). https://doi.org/10.1183/13993003.01815-2019.

38. McConnell R, Barrington-Trimis JL, Wang K, et al. Electronic Cigarette Use and Respiratory Symptoms in Adolescents. Am J Respir Crit Care Med 2017; 195(8):1043–9.

39. Bhatta DN, Glantz SA. Association of E-Cigarette Use With Respiratory Disease Among Adults: A Longitudinal Analysis. Am J Prev Med 2020;58(2):182–90.

40. Xie W, Kathuria H, Galiatsatos P, et al. Association of Electronic Cigarette Use With Incident Respiratory Conditions Among US Adults From 2013 to 2018. JAMA Netw Open 2020;3(11):e2020816.

41. Xie W, Tackett AP, Berlowitz JB, et al. Association of Electronic Cigarette Use with Respiratory Symptom Development among US Young Adults. Am J Respir Crit Care Med 2022. https://doi.org/10.1164/rccm.202107-1718OC.

42. Meo SA, Ansary MA, Barayan FR, et al. Electronic Cigarettes: Impact on Lung Function and Fractional Exhaled Nitric Oxide Among Healthy Adults. Am J Mens Health 2019;13(1). 1557988318806073.

43. Polosa R, Cibella F, Caponnetto P, et al. Health impact of E-cigarettes: a prospective 3.5-year study of regular daily users who have never smoked. Sci Rep 2017; 7(1):13825.

44. Kesimer M, Ford AA, Ceppe A, et al. Airway Mucin Concentration as a Marker of Chronic Bronchitis. N Engl J Med 2017;377(10):911–22.

45. Reidel B, Radicioni G, Clapp PW, et al. E-Cigarette Use Causes a Unique Innate Immune Response in the Lung, Involving Increased Neutrophilic Activation and Altered Mucin Secretion. Am J Respir Crit Care Med 2018;197(4):492–501.

46. Chaumont M, van de Borne P, Bernard A, et al. Fourth generation e-cigarette vaping induces transient lung inflammation and gas exchange disturbances: results from two randomized clinical trials. Am J Physiol Lung Cell Mol Physiol 2019; 316(5):L705–19.

47. Ghosh A, Coakley RD, Ghio AJ, et al. Chronic E-Cigarette Use Increases Neutrophil Elastase and Matrix Metalloprotease Levels in the Lung. Am J Respir Crit Care Med 2019;200(11):1392–401.

48. Hedman L, Backman H, Stridsman C, et al. Association of Electronic Cigarette Use With Smoking Habits, Demographic Factors, and Respiratory Symptoms. JAMA Netw Open 2018;1(3):e180789.

49. Goniewicz ML, Smith DM, Edwards KC, et al. Comparison of Nicotine and Toxicant Exposure in Users of Electronic Cigarettes and Combustible Cigarettes. JAMA Netw Open 2018;1(8):e185937.

50. Goniewicz ML, Miller CR, Sutanto E, et al. How effective are electronic cigarettes for reducing respiratory and cardiovascular risk in smokers? A systematic review. Harm Reduct J 2020;17(1):91.

51. Cibella F, Campagna D, Caponnetto P, et al. Lung function and respiratory symptoms in a randomized smoking cessation trial of electronic cigarettes. Clin Sci (Lond) 2016;130(21):1929–37.

52. Polosa R, Morjaria JB, Caponnetto P, et al. Persisting long term benefits of smoking abstinence and reduction in asthmatic smokers who have switched to electronic cigarettes. Discov Med 2016;21(114):99–108.

53. Bowler RP, Hansel NN, Jacobson S, et al. Electronic Cigarette Use in US Adults at Risk for or with COPD: Analysis from Two Observational Cohorts. J Gen Intern Med 2017;32(12):1315–22.

54. Woodruff PG, Barr RG, Bleecker E, et al. Clinical Significance of Symptoms in Smokers with Preserved Pulmonary Function. N Engl J Med 2016;374(19): 1811–21.

55. Hajek P, Phillips-Waller A, Przulj D, et al. A Randomized Trial of E-Cigarettes versus Nicotine-Replacement Therapy. N Engl J Med 2019;380(7):629–37.

56. Hartmann-Boyce J, McRobbie H, Lindson N, et al. Electronic cigarettes for smoking cessation. Cochrane Database Syst Rev 2021;4:CD010216.

57. Wang RJ, Bhadriraju S, Glantz SA. E-Cigarette Use and Adult Cigarette Smoking Cessation: A Meta-Analysis. Am J Public Health 2021;111(2):230–46.

58. Hanewinkel R, Niederberger K, Pedersen A, et al. E-cigarettes and nicotine abstinence: a meta-analysis of randomised controlled trials. Eur Respir Rev 2022;(163):31. https://doi.org/10.1183/16000617.0215-2021.

59. Leone FT, Zhang Y, Evers-Casey S, et al. Initiating Pharmacologic Treatment in Tobacco-Dependent Adults. An Official American Thoracic Society Clinical Practice Guideline. Am J Respir Crit Care Med 2020;202(2):e5–31.

60. Krist AH, Davidson KW, Mangione CM, et al. Interventions for Tobacco Smoking Cessation in Adults, Including Pregnant Persons: US Preventive Services Task Force Recommendation Statement. JAMA 2021;325(3):265–79.

61. Kalkhoran S, Glantz SA. Modeling the Health Effects of Expanding e-Cigarette Sales in the United States and United Kingdom: A Monte Carlo Analysis. JAMA Intern Med 2015;175(10):1671–80.

62. Feirman SP, Lock D, Cohen JE, et al. Flavored Tobacco Products in the United States: A Systematic Review Assessing Use and Attitudes. Nicotine Tob Res 2016;18(5):739–49.

63. Zare S, Nemati M, Zheng Y. A systematic review of consumer preference for e-cigarette attributes: Flavor, nicotine strength, and type. PLoS One 2018;13(3): e0194145.

Marijuana and the Lung
Evolving Understandings

Manish Joshi, MD, FCCP[a,b,*], Anita Joshi, BDS, MPH[c],
Thaddeus Bartter, MD, FCCP[a,b]

KEYWORDS

- Marijuana • Cannabis smoking • Chronic obstructive pulmonary disease
- Lung cancer

KEY POINTS

- Marijuana can cause bronchitis and may have some impacts on pulmonary physiology, but, even when smoked, does not cause COPD.
- Data with respect to lung cancer and marijuana are suboptimal, but a summary of current collective data argues against causality.
- Marijuana use for recreational purposes should be discouraged in teens.

Very few drugs, if any, have such a tangled history as a medicine. In fact, prejudice, superstition, emotionalism, and even ideology have managed to lead cannabis to ups and downs concerning both its therapeutic properties and its toxicological and dependence-inducing effects.

—*E. A. Carlini*[1]

INTRODUCTION

Marijuana is the second most widely smoked substance after tobacco.[2] Globally, in 2019 an estimated 200 million persons aged 15 to 64 years (4% of the adult population) used cannabis products.[2,3] The usage is increasing. The overall number of people who used cannabis in the past year is estimated to have increased by nearly 18% over the past decade (2010–2019), greater than the 10% increase in the global population over the same period.[2,3] In the United States, the past-year and past-month prevalences of cannabis use among the adult population have increased by 60% and

[a] Pulmonary and Critical Care Division, University of Arkansas for Medical Sciences, 4301 West Markham, Little Rock, AR 72205, USA; [b] Central Arkansas Veterans Healthcare System, Little Rock, Arkansas, USA; [c] Department of Epidemiology, Fay W. Boozman College Public Health, University of Arkansas for Medical Sciences, 4300 West Markham, Little Rock, AR 72205, USA
* Corresponding author. University of Arkansas for Medical Sciences, 4301 West Markham, Mail Slot #555, Little Rock, AR 72205.
E-mail address: mjoshi@uams.edu

Med Clin N Am 106 (2022) 1093–1107
https://doi.org/10.1016/j.mcna.2022.07.010
0025-7125/22/© 2022 Elsevier Inc. All rights reserved.
medical.theclinics.com

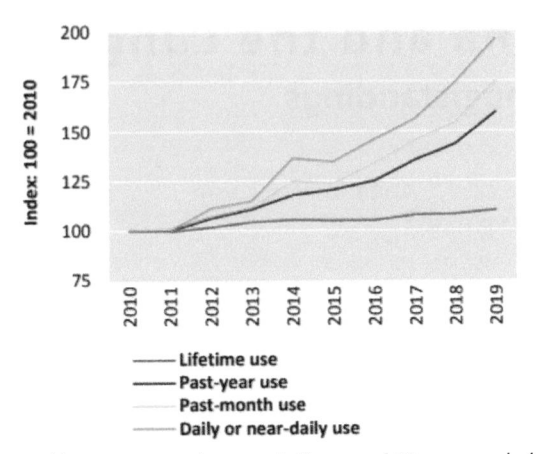

Fig. 1. Trends in cannabis use among the population aged 18 years and older, United States, 2010 to 2019 (*Data from* United States, substance abuse and mental health services administration (no permission required).)

75%, respectively; the prevalence of daily or near-daily use has doubled over the period 2010 to 2019[3] (**Fig. 1**).

Marijuana has been subjected to fascinating cross-currents of medicine, politics, prejudice, and economics. Marijuana has been and is being used medicinally while at the same time being labeled by some as highly dangerous. We know of no other drug/product that is simultaneously legal (some state laws) and illegal (federal law). Categorization of marijuana by some societies as "illicit" has limited both transparency and research, and bias pervades existing literature, with flagrant contradictions not supported by data. The goal of this review is to cover current understanding about physiologic impact, applications, and potential injury related to the use of marijuana with the hope of minimizing bias by relying on the limited but growing body of available data. This review concentrates on pulmonary implications but includes important contextual information.

Biology of Cannabis

The taxonomy of marijuana is confusing and somewhat vague. There are 2 prevalent subspecies of the Cannabaceae (sativa and indica) and 4 varieties.[4] These 2 are often hybridized and vary with respect to characteristics.[4] Usage ranges from utilitarian (rope, with the plant commonly named *hemp*) to medicinal/psychoactive. The medicinal applications are produced from the dried and crumbled leaves and flowering tops of the cannabis plant and are produced and consumed in almost every country. By contrast, cannabis resin, the concentrated extract of cannabis flowers and plants, is produced mainly in a few countries in North Africa, the Middle East, and Southwest Asia.[2,4] Hash oil is a cannabis product that can be extracted from any part of the plant. An increasing number of *cannabis* extracts is being produced from the dried flowering tops and leaves of the female plant, expanding the options for ingestion and inhalation of the active components.[2,4]

The main psychoactive ingredient in marijuana is delta-9-tetrahydrocannabinol (Δ9-THC); however, more than 120 compounds (cannabinoids) have been identified within the cannabis plant with cannabidiol (CBD) being the principal cannabinoid.[4–6] Δ9-THC is used for both recreational and medical purposes, whereas the applications of other CBDs are primarily medical.[4–6] CB1 and CB2 receptors, which bind both Δ9-THC and cannabinoids, were discovered in 1990 and 1993, respectively, followed by the discovery of endogenous ligands that attach to those receptors.[5,6] This endocannabinoid system (our understanding of which is still in its infancy) is widely distributed throughout the body, with cannabinoid receptors suspected to be the most numerous single receptor type in the human brain.[5,6]

Marijuana History

Members of the Cannabaceae family have been used by humans for millennia[5–8]; they have been used by multiple civilizations. Uses have ranged from utilitarian to medicinal to religious. In India, medical and religious usage of cannabis probably began around 1000 years BC.[5,7,8] Medicinal applications have ranged from analgesic to anti-inflammatory to tranquilizer to anticonvulsant. Cannabis was introduced into Western medicine during the nineteenth century when W. B. O'Shaughnessy, an Irish physician working in Calcutta in the 1830s, wrote a paper extolling cannabis titled, "Indian Hemp. Traditional Eastern Medicine met Western."[7,8] By the mid-nineteenth century, the medical use of cannabis had received official legitimacy—it was listed in the United States and British Pharmacopeia, and cannabis extracts or tinctures were used extensively by physicians in the Western world. The availability and usage of medical marijuana reached a climax in the last decade of that century.[7,8]

In the United States, marijuana was used medicinally as a bronchodilator and analgesic until 1941, when it was dropped from the US Pharmacopeia.[1,7,8] The Controlled Substances Act, passed in 1970, classified marijuana as a schedule I drug, defined by the Drug Enforcement Administration as follows: "Schedule I drugs, substances, or chemicals are defined as drugs with no currently accepted medical use and a high potential for abuse. Schedule I drugs are the most dangerous of all drugs of all the drug schedules with potentially severe psychological or physical dependence" (http://www.justice.gov/dea/druginfo/ds.shtml). This definition is inaccurate, although it persists to this day.[1,7,8] The labeling was political, not medical. In fact, in the 1930s the American Medical Association lobbied Congress against rendering marijuana federally illegal.[8]

Marijuana and the Lung

The most common route of acquisition of marijuana compounds is via smoke inhalation. Smoke is usually inhaled from combusted compacted and rolled leaves (a "joint"), analogous to a cigarette, or from a water pipe ("bong").[4,7] Most studies quantify exposure to cannabis smoke in "joint-years"; 1 joint-year is equivalent to 1 joint smoked daily for a year. When marijuana is smoked, THC is absorbed into the bloodstream via the lungs.[5,9] Marijuana smoke contains a complex mixture of chemicals that has significant overlap with tobacco smoke.[10,11] In addition, the authors' colleagues have demonstrated that cigarette smoke particles and marijuana smoke particles are similar in both size and distribution when studied with an electrical aerosol analyzer.[12] Given these commonalities, the widespread and increasing use of marijuana has raised concerns that it may cause short- and long-term respiratory complications including bronchitis, pneumothorax/pneumomediastinum, and chronic lung diseases such as chronic obstructive pulmonary disease (COPD), interstitial lung disease, and lung cancers. For this review of respiratory implications of marijuana use, inhalation will be the route of absorption in the cited studies unless specifically stated otherwise.

EFFECTS OF SHORT-TERM AND LONG-TERM MARIJUANA SMOKING ON LUNG FUNCTION
Acute Physiologic Impact

Acutely, cannabis is a bronchodilator; it was listed as such in early pharmacopeias from the mid-1800s until its reclassification as a schedule I product in 1941.[1,5,7,8]

Formal studies postdated this usage, with publications in the 1970s by Tashkin and colleagues[13] and Vachon and colleagues.[14] Tashkin and colleagues[13] demonstrated that after smoking marijuana, there was an immediate increase in specific airway conductance, which peaked at 15 minutes after smoking and remained elevated at 60 minutes; this finding was also demonstrated for ingestion; after ingestion of 10, 15, and 20 mg Δ^9-THC subjects' specific airway conductance increased significantly when compared with placebo. Bronchodilation reached peak levels 3 hours after ingestion, and airway conductance remained elevated for 4 to 6 hours.[13] Tashkin and colleagues[15,16] subsequently reported a similar bronchodilator effect of cannabis in patients with mild asthma and in patients with methacholine- and exercise-induced bronchospasm.

Long-Term Usage and Lung Function

Given that cigarette smoke and marijuana smoke share many components,[10–12] one would have expected long-term marijuana to cause spirometric impairment. Multiple cross-sectional and longitudinal studies have evaluated the long-term effects of marijuana on lung function and compared lung function in marijuana smokers with that of nonsmokers, tobacco smokers, and smokers of marijuana and tobacco[17–30] (**Table 1**). Most of the studies have several limitations such as difficulty in obtaining accurate information for an illicit drug, quantifying its use, and small proportions of marijuana-only smokers (and even smaller numbers of very heavy users). Another possible source of error is a large variation in volume of marijuana smoked; inclusion criteria for the data that are available vary widely, from 50 joints over a lifetime to more than 40 joint-years (>10,000 joints in lifetime). One can, nevertheless, reach some conclusions that seem to be supported by the literature. Key studies are listed in **Table 1**, and key findings are summarized in the following sections.

Long-Term Usage: Marijuana Alone

Results have been conflicting (see **Table 1**). After an early study suggested that marijuana caused a decrease in forced vital capacity (FVC), 2 meta-analyses (with far greater numbers of subjects) came to the opposite conclusion—that marijuana does not cause spirometric impairment.[31,32] One large study found statistically significant nonlinearity for marijuana smokers, with increases of both forced expiratory volume in the first second of expiration (FEV_1) and FVC at low levels of exposure (up to 7 joint-years of lifetime exposure) followed by decreases in FEV_1 at higher levels of exposure.[27] However, the more recent larger cohort studies have shown that the FEV_1 is not impacted.[28,29] Some studies, including the largest cohort study by Kempker and colleagues[28] have demonstrated a decrease in the FEV_1/FVC ratio.[26,27,29,30] This decrease was caused not by a decrease in FEV_1, but by a significant ($P = .0001$) increase in FVC_1 (of note, there is no known disease process that increases the FVC; tobacco reduces the FEV_1/FVC ratio, but by causing a decrease in FEV_1). Every study that looked at diffusing capacity has found no significant impact from marijuana (in never-tobacco-smokers). These collective data suggest that marijuana may have some impact on lung function, but that if it does the nature of those changes differs distinctly from those caused by tobacco.

Long-Term Marijuana Usage Coupled with Cigarette Use

The results of a comparative study by Aldington and colleagues[24] suggest that persons who consume both cannabis and tobacco have a pattern of response similar to tobacco-only users, although, surprisingly, it may be mildly attenuated. Tan and colleagues[25] reported that concomitant usage was associated with increased risk

Table 1

Effects of the use of marijuana on lung function measures in comparison with nonsmoking subjects with adjustment for tobacco use in those who have smoked both marijuana and tobacco

Study/Year/Design	Cohort Size	Age, years	Marijuana Use Average	FEV$_1$	FVC	FEV$_1$/FVC	TLC	D$_{LCO}$
Tashkin et al,[17] USA 1980 Cross-sectional	148	24.1	3 d per week (several times per d) for more than 2–5 y	↕	↑	NR	↑	↕
Tashkin et al,[18] USA 1987 Cross-sectional	446	25–49	54.4 MJ joint years	↓	↑	↓	↑	↓
Bloom et al,[19] USA 1987 Cross-sectional	990	15–40	58.2 MJ joint years	↓	NR	↓	NR	NR
Sherrill et al,[20] USA 1991 Longitudinal	1802	15–60	5–5.5 MJ cigarettes per week	←	NR	←	NR	NR
Tashkin et al,[21] USA 1997 Longitudinal	394	25–49	>3.5 MJ joints per day	↕	NR	↓	NR	NR
Taylor et al,[22] 2000 NZ Longitudinal	900	Birth–26	230 times in the past year	↕	NR	←	NR	NR
Moore et al,[23] 2005 USA Cross-sectional	6728	20–59	10.2 d in last month	NR	NR	↑	NR	NR
Aldington et al,[24] 2007 NZ Cross-sectional	339	18–75	Mean 54.2 MJ joint years	↕	↑	↓	↕	↕
Tan et al,[25] 2009 USA Longitudinal	856	56.3	Lifetime median number of MJ joints: 80.5–208	→	→	↓	NR	NR

(continued on next page)

Table 1
(continued)

Study/Year/Design	Cohort Size	Age, years	Marijuana Use Average	FEV₁	FVC	FEV₁/FVC	TLC	DLCO
Hancox et al,[26] 2010 NZ Longitudinal	967	Birth–32	≤1 MJ joint-year 461/967 >1 MJ joint-year 222/967	↕	→	↕	→	↕
Pletcher et al,[27] 2012 USA Longitudinal	5115	18–30	2–3 times of use in past 30 d	↑	→	↑	NR	NR
Kempker et al,[28] 2015 USA Cross-sectional	7716	18–59	15.8 MJ joint-years 12 d of use/month	↕	→	←	NR	NR
Morris et al,[29] 2018 USA Cross-sectional	2304	40–80	30.15 MJ joint years	→	→	↕	NR	NR
Hancox et al,[30] 2022 NZ Longitudinal	881	Birth–45	≤5 MJ joint-year 433/881 >5 MJ joint-year 107/881	↕	→	←	→	←

Abbreviations: ↑, Increase; ↓, decrease; ↔, no association; DLCO, diffusing capacity for carbon monoxide; FEV₁, forced expiratory volume; FVC, forced vital capacity; FEV₁/FVC, ratio; ; MJ, marijuana; NR, not reported; NZ, New Zealand; TLC, total lung capacity; RV, residual volume.

(compared with tobacco use alone) of COPD (odds ratio [OR], 2.90; 95% confidence interval [CI], 1.53–5.51) when the lifetime dose of marijuana exceeded 50 marijuana cigarettes, suggesting synergy between marijuana and tobacco. The findings of Morris and colleagues[29] are consistent with mild attenuation of injury when marijuana is added to tobacco. When these data are combined, it is reasonable to conclude that tobacco is the dominant cause of injury in those who use both products, with an unclear contribution from marijuana.

Clearly there are some contradictory data, some of which suggest that marijuana may cause some lung injury and some of which suggests that marijuana has a protective effect on lung function even in smokers. When changes have been documented, they are not consistent with the pathophysiology of COPD. Given the collected data, it is now reasonable to make 2 conclusions: (1) marijuana in the short term is a bronchodilator and (2) the cumulative effects of long-term marijuana use are minor, and smoking marijuana does not cause COPD. That marijuana smoke contains somewhat counterbalancing injurious and beneficial components is a plausible construct. In contrast to the sometimes contradictory results for marijuana, all cited studies (see **Table 1**) that followed cohorts of tobacco-only smokers consistently showed the expected pattern of lung injury.

RESPIRATORY SYMPTOMS IN MARIJUANA SMOKERS

Associations between marijuana smoking (alone or in combination with tobacco) and respiratory symptoms have been systematically examined in 11 cross-sectional observational studies[18–20,22–25,29,33–35] **(Table 2)**. Despite its documented bronchodilation, marijuana smoking is consistently associated with wheeze, cough, and increased sputum production. This apparent contradiction may be related to anatomic considerations. Respiratory symptoms in marijuana smokers are likely due to inflammatory changes in large airway mucosa. Fligiel and colleagues[36] demonstrated large airway inflammation on endobronchial biopsy specimens of habitual marijuana smokers. The histopathologic abnormalities reported were goblet cell hyperplasia, loss of ciliated epithelial cells, and intraepithelial and subepithelial inflammation; the investigators concluded that smoking of marijuana alone caused at least as extensive histopathologic abnormalities in the tracheobronchial mucosa as tobacco alone, including metaplastic changes and nuclear alterations that could be premalignant. Another study of healthy (relatively asymptomatic) habitual marijuana smokers correlated visual changes from bronchoscopy with biopsies.[37] Marijuana smokers (compared with nonsmokers) had significantly higher bronchitis index scores (based on central airway erythema, edema, and airway secretions). These visual changes were confirmed on bronchial biopsies.[37] Cessation does lead to symptom resolution implying normalization of histopathology, but there are no studies involving biopsies in prior users.[33]

The collective data suggest that chronic marijuana smoking is often associated with large airway inflammation, which can be symptomatic. There is no good evidence for the distal airway/alveolar injury that leads to COPD. The dichotomous areas of involvement may explain the contradictions noted earlier.

MARIJUANA AND LUNG CANCER

Moir and colleagues[11] extensively examined the compositions of both mainstream and side-stream smoke from marijuana and tobacco cigarettes and showed many qualitative similarities and some quantitative differences. In addition, the histopathologic and immunohistologic evidence in marijuana users, including bronchial squamous metaplasia and overexpression of molecular markers of pretumor

Table 2

Effects of the use of marijuana on respiratory symptoms when compared with nonsmoking subjects or with adjustment for tobacco use

Study/Design	Cohort Size	Age, Years	Marijuana Use Average	Dyspnea	Wheeze	Cough	Sputum
Tashkin et al,[18] 1987 USA Cross-sectional	446	25–49	54.4 MJ joint-years	↕	→	→	→
Bloom et al,[19] 1987 USA Cross-sectional	990	15–40	58.2 MJ joint-years	↕	→	↕	→
Sherrill et al,[20] 1991 USA Longitudinal	1802	15–60	5–5.5 MJ cigarettes per week	↕	→	→	→
Taylor et al,[22] 2000 NZ Longitudinal	900	Birth–26	230 times in the past year	→	→	→	→
Moore et al,[23] 2005 USA Cross-sectional	6728	20–59	10.2 d in last month	↕	→	→	→
Aldington et al,[24] 2007 NZ Cross-sectional	339	18–75	Mean 54.2 MJ joint years	NR	→	→	→
Tan et al,[25] 2009 USA Longitudinal	856	56.3	Lifetime median number of MJ joints: 80.5–208	→	→	↕	NR

Study	N	Age	MJ exposure				
Tashkin et al,[21] 2012 USA Longitudinal	299	33.4	30 MJ joint-years	↕	→	→	→
Macleod et al,[34] 2015 UK Cross-sectional	500	37	Men: 104.5 MJ joint-years Women: 53.2 MJ joint-years	↕	→	→	→
Hancox et al,[30] 2015 NZ Longitudinal	943	Birth–38	≤1 MJ joint-year 99 >1 MJ joint-year 146	→	→	→	→
Morris et al,[29] 2018 USA Cross-sectional	2304	40–80	30.15 MJ joint-years	↕	→	↕	↕

Abbreviations: ↑, Increase; ↓, decrease; ↔, no association; MJ, marijuana; NR: Not reported; NZ, New Zealand.

progression, are consistent with a lung cancer risk from marijuana.[36,38] Taking this evidence a step further, Maertens and colleagues[39] used a toxicogenomics approach and used murine lung epithelial cells to compare and contrast the toxicologic molecular pathways affected by marijuana smoke condensate (MSC) and tobacco smoke condensate (TSC). Both TSC and MSC exposure were associated with the expression of genes involved in xenobiotic metabolism, oxidative stress, inflammation, and DNA damage response. It is interesting that the MSC was more potent than TSC in dose-response analyses for most common pathways. The data clearly demonstrate pathways affected by MSC that are similar to those for TSC. This study strengthens the link supporting the biological plausibility of marijuana smoking as a risk factor for the development of lung cancer.

Given the aforementioned data, it is surprising that the collective clinical data do not prove an association between marijuana and lung cancer. The current epidemiologic evidence with respect to marijuana smoking and lung cancer is conflicting and sparse with the net balance to date against causation. A pooled analysis of few older case-control studies from Tunisia, Morocco, and Algeria did find that the OR for lung cancer was increased for cannabis smoker after adjusting for lifetime tobacco pack-years (OR, 2.4; 95% CI, 1.6–3.8), raising concerns of oncogenicity.[40] Another population-based Swedish cohort study with 40-year follow-up found a 2-fold risk of lung cancer (CI, 1.08–4.14) in the 831 subjects who reported heavy cannabis use (defined by lifetime use of more than 50 times for their study).[41] A more recent study by Zhang and colleagues[42] contradicts the aforementioned studies. The investigators pooled data on 2159 lung cancer cases and 2985 controls from 6 case-control studies in the United States, Canada, United Kingdom, and New Zealand within the International Lung Cancer Consortium. The overall pooled OR for habitual marijuana smokers versus nonhabitual or never users was 0.96 (95% CI, 0.66–1.38) after adjusting for sociodemographic factors, tobacco smoking status, and pack-years.[42] Another case-control study including 611 lung cancers found no association between use of marijuana and lung cancers (with ORs <1 regardless of intensity of marijuana usage).[43] A recent meta-analysis by Ghasemiesfe and colleagues[44] concluded that evidence of any association between marijuana use and incident lung cancer was insufficient due to confounders.

To summarize, one would expect marijuana to be associated with an increased risk for lung cancer. Older studies corroborated that impression, with more recent studies negating it. Once again, there is a suggestion that marijuana smoke may contain both injurious and beneficial substances. None of these conclusions should be considered to be final; studies have been subject to confounding by concomitant use of tobacco, small sample sizes, young age of participants, and, most important, underreporting.[40–44] It has been proved that marijuana has far less toxicity than does tobacco, but it is reasonable to suggest caution against regular heavy marijuana use.

EMPHYSEMATOUS BULLAE, BAROTRAUMA (PNEUMOTHORAX), AND INTERSTITIAL LUNG DISEASE IN MARIJUANA SMOKERS?

In 2007, Beshay and colleagues[45] reported an unusual increase in the number of young patients at their surgical emergency unit in Switzerland who presented with pneumothorax and history of marijuana smoking. The investigators analyzed and reported their observations as the first and largest case series of spontaneous pneumothorax in heavy marijuana smokers. The radiographic findings on chest computed tomography showed large apical bullae, up to 12 cm in size, which were not present in controls (patients with pneumothorax and no history of marijuana smoking) over the same interval (2002–2004). In another review, 36 case reports of apical bullous lung disease attributable to heavy cannabis smoking have been reported in young adults.[46] It is evident that marijuana smokers tend to have deeper inhalations and hold their breath for up to 4 times longer than cigarette smokers, sometimes accompanied by Valsalva maneuvers, which may predispose them to barotrauma.[47] It had been postulated that this smoking technique (rather than cannabis itself) is responsible for cases of spontaneous pneumothorax and bullous lung disease reported in young marijuana smokers.[46,47] Contradicting the aforementioned reports, the recent study by Morris and colleagues[29] showed that marijuana smokers had a decrease in emphysema and no evidence for bullous disease, bringing into doubt any association of marijuana with bullae and pneumothorax.

Fligiel and colleagues[48] reported interstitial fibrosis in 24 rhesus monkeys inhaling marijuana on autopsy. No studies have been found showing such effects in humans. Interestingly, in a case report of interstitial disease in a marijuana smoker, biopsies demonstrated particulate matter consistent with talc pneumoconiosis, implicating talcum adulteration and not the marijuana itself.[49]

MEDICINAL USE AND NONPULMONARY ADVERSE EFFECTS OF MARIJUANA

A detailed discussion of nonpulmonary adverse effects and of medicinal use of marijuana is beyond the scope of this review. However, the authors briefly touch on some of them because they are all germane to the issue of marijuana use. There have been substantial changes to the cannabis policy landscape in the twenty-first century; in the last 2 decades almost all states and the District of Columbia have legalized cannabis in some form for the treatment of medical conditions. Marijuana and other cannabinoids (including synthetic cannabinoids) are modestly effective in symptom palliation in patients with cancer; one of the earliest recognized indications for cannabinoids was chemotherapy-induced nausea and vomiting.[50] However, the first milestone was reached in 2018 when the US Food and Drug Administration approved a cannabinoid derived from marijuana to treat severe forms of childhood epilepsy.[51] The available literature suggests that it is also effective in alleviating pain related to cancer, especially neuropathic pain.[50,52] In fact, the comprehensive 2017 consensus report on cannabis compiled by the National Academies of Sciences states that there is conclusive or substantial evidence that cannabis is effective for treating chronic pain in adults, as an antiemetic in chemotherapy-induced nausea/vomiting, and in improving patient-reported spasticity in multiple sclerosis.[53]

No evidence that recreational cannabis use improves general health has been found. The main acute adverse effects for some marijuana users include tachycardia, anxiety, and panic, especially in occasional or naive users.[53,54] Marijuana can be considered to be addictive, and is especially so when individuals start using it in their teens.[48] Marijuana smoking can lead to impairment of cognition, coordination, and judgment and can result in automobile accidents.[55,56] A systematic review of high-quality studies by Asbridge and colleagues[57] concluded that acute cannabis consumption nearly doubles the risk of a collision resulting in serious injury or death. (Ironically, marijuana is less toxic than alcohol, the dominant legal cause of impaired cognition and automobile accidents.) Data suggesting long-term harmful effects of cannabis on neuropsychological function in the developing brain of adolescents are emerging and caution strongly against recreational use in teens.[54,55]

SUMMARY

Marijuana has been used throughout the world for thousands of years. The vilification of marijuana was a relatively recent political—not medical—intervention, which has negatively impacted our capacity to use and study its components. Although confounded by several factors, knowledge does continue to evolve. The delineation of the prevalence of endocannabinoid receptors has led to a better mechanistic understanding of its capacity to affect us. It is known that different components help (or may help) in the treatment of epilepsy, nausea, anorexia, chronic pain, depression, and possibly cancer.

There are 2 caveats with respect to the use of marijuana. First, it contains mind-altering substances. Any use of marijuana needs to be tempered by knowledge of contexts in which this can cause harm. Second, apart perhaps from focused medicinal uses, marijuana presents a danger to the developing brain, with increased risk of addiction and possibly of cognitive impairment.

The literature on inhaled marijuana and the lung, the primary topic of this review, is somewhat contradictory, but some principles have emerged. That marijuana smoke contains both injurious and protective substances is a reasonable conclusion given what is known today. Marijuana can cause large airway inflammation, but it is also a bronchodilator and does not seem to cause small airway injury. Marijuana does not cause COPD. The collective literature suggests that marijuana does not cause lung cancer. (The authors would argue that any conclusions with respect to the heavy habitual marijuana user should be tentative, because the data are too sparse for this subpopulation.) The data support continued evaluation of the potential benefits of marijuana and its components and of alternative means of acquisition that bypass airway inflammation. Finally, the data on marijuana contrast starkly with the consistent demonstration of injury from tobacco, the greatest legalized killer in the world today. Any possible toxicity of marijuana pales in comparison.

CLINICS CARE POINTS

- Marijuana smoking can cause respiratory symptoms but does not cause COPD.
- Marijuana and tobacco smoke share many components, but a summary of current collective data argues against marijuana and lung cancer causality
- Marijuana use for recreational purposes should be strongly discouraged in teens.

DISCLOSURE

There are no financial conflicts to disclose for all the authors.

REFERENCES

1. Carlini EA. The good and the bad effects of (-) trans-delta-9-tetrahydrocannabinol (delta 9-THC) on humans. Toxicon 2004;44(4):461–7.
2. World Drug Report 2021 (United Nations publication, Sales No. E.21.XI.8). Available at: WDR 2021_Booklet 3 (unodc.org) (Accessed March 10, 2022).
3. 2019 National survey of Drug use and health. Rockville, MD: Substance Abuse and Mental Health Services Administration. Available at: https://www.samhsa.gov/data/release/2019-national-survey-drug-use-and-health-nsduh-releases. Accessed March 10, 2022.
4. WHO Expert Committee on Drug Dependence: Fortieth report. Available at: https://apps.who.int/iris/bitstream/handle/10665/279948/9789241210225-eng.pdf. Accessed March 10, 2022.

5. Pertwee RG. Cannabinoid pharmacology: the first 66 years. Br J Pharmacol 2006;147(Suppl 1):S163–71.

6. Mechoulam R, Parker LA. The endocannabinoid system and the brain. Annu Rev Psychol 2013;64:21–47.

7. Zuardi AW. History of cannabis as a medicine: a review. Rev Bras Psiquiatr 2006; 28(2):153–7.

8. Aggarwal SK, Carter GT, Sullivan MD, et al. Medicinal use of cannabis in the United States, 2009 States: historical perspectives, current trends, and future directions. J Opioid Manag 2009;5(3):153–68.

9. Grotenhermen F. Pharmacokinetics and pharmacodynamics of cannabinoids. Clin Pharmacokinet 2003;42:327–60.

10. Lee ML, Novotny M, Bartle KD. Gas chromatography/mass spectrometric and nuclear magnetic resonance spectrometric studies of carcinogenic polynuclear aromatic hydrocarbons in tobacco and marijuana smoke condensates. Anal Chem 1976;48(2):405–16.

11. Moir D, Rickert WS, Levasseur G, Larose Y, Maertens R, White P, et al. A comparison of mainstream and sidestream marijuana and tobacco cigarette smoke produced under two machine smoking conditions. Chem Res Toxicol 2008;21:494–502.

12. Anderson PJ, Wilson JD, Hiller FC. Particle size distribution of mainstream tobacco and marijuana smoke. Am Rev Respir Dis 1989;140:202–5.

13. Tashkin DP, Shapiro BJ, Frank IM. Acute pulmonary physiologic effects of smoked marijuana and oral Δ9-tetrahydrocannabinol in healthy young men. N Engl J Med 1973;289:336–41.

14. Vachon L, Fitzgerald, Solliday NH, Gould IA, Gaensler EA. Single-dose effect of marijuana smoke: bronchial dynamics and respiratorycenter sensitivity in normal subjects. N Engl J Med 1973;288:985–9.

15. Tashkin DP, Shapiro BJ, Frank IM. Acute effects of smoked marijuana and oral Δ9-tetrahydrocannabinol on specific airway conductance in asthmatic subjects. Am Rev Respir Dis 1974;109:420–8.

16. Tashkin DP, Shapiro BJ, Frank IM. Acute effects of marihuana on airway dynamics in spontaneous and experimentally induced bronchial asthma. In: Braude M, Szara S, editors. Pharmacology of marihuana. New York: Raven Press; 1976. p. 785–801.

17. Tashkin DP, Calvarese BM, Simmons MS, Shapiro BJ. Respiratory status of seventy-four habitual marijuana smokers. Chest 1980;78:699–706.

18. Tashkin DP, Coulson AH, Clark VA, Simmons M, Bourque LB, Duann S, et al. Respiratory symptoms and lung function in habitual heavy smokers of marijuana alone, smokers of marijuana and tobacco, smokers of tobacco alone, and nonsmokers. Am Rev Respir Dis 1987;135:209–16.

19. Bloom JW, Kaltenborn WT, Paoletti P, Camilli A, Lebowitz MD. Respiratory effects of non-tobacco cigarettes. Br Med J (Clin Res Ed) 1987;295:1516–8.

20. Sherrill DL, Krzyzanowski M, Bloom JW, Lebowitz MD. Respiratory effects of non-tobacco cigarettes: a longitudinal study in general population. Int J Epidemiol 1991;20:132–7.

21. Tashkin DP, Simmons MS, Sherrill DL, Coulson AH. Heavy habitual marijuana smoking does not cause an accelerated decline in FEV1 with age. Am J Respir Crit Care Med 1997;155:141–8.

22. Taylor DR, Poulton R, Moffitt TE, Ramankutty P, Sears MR. The respiratory effects of cannabis dependence in young adults. Addiction 2000;95:1669–77.

23. Moore BA, Augustson EM, Moser RP, Budney AJ. Respiratory effects of marijuana and tobacco use in a US sample. J Gen Intern Med 2004;20:33–7.
24. Aldington S, Williams M, Nowitz M, et al. Effects of cannabis on pulmonary structure, function and symptoms. Thorax 2007;62:1058–63.
25. Tan WC, Lo C, Jong A, Xing L, et al. Vancouver Burden of Obstructive Lung Disease (BOLD) Research Group. Marijuana and chronic obstructive lung disease— a population-based study. CMAJ 2009;180:814–20.
26. Hancox RJ, Poulton R, Ely M, et al. Effects of cannabis on lung function: a population-based cohort study. Eur Respir J 2010;35:42–7.
27. Pletcher MJ, Vittinghoff E, Kalhan R, et al. Association between marijuana exposure and pulmonary function over 20 years. JAMA 2012;307:173–81.
28. Kempker JA, Honig EG, Martin GS. The effects of marijuana exposure on expiratory airflow. A study of adults who participated in the U.S. National Health and Nutrition Examination Study. Ann Am Thorac Soc 2015;12:135–41.
29. Morris MA, Jacobson SR, Kinney GL, Tashkin DP, Woodruff PG, Hoffman EA, et al. Marijuana use associations with pulmonary symptoms and function in tobacco smokers enrolled in the Subpopulations and Intermediate Outcome Measures in COPD Study (SPIROMICS). Chronic Obstr Pulm Dis 2018;5:46–56.
30. Hancox RJ, Gray AR, Zhang X, Poulton R, Moffitt TE, Caspi A, et al. Differential effects of cannabis and tobacco on lung function in mid–adult life. Am J Respir Crit Care Med 2022;205:1179–85.
31. Tetrault JM, Crothers K, Moore BA, et al. Effects of marijuana smoking on pulmonary function and respiratory complications: a systematic review. Arch Intern Med 2007;167:221–8.
32. Ghasemiesfe M, Ravi D, Vali M, Korenstein D, et al. Marijuana Use, Respiratory Symptoms, and Pulmonary Function: A Systematic Review and Meta-analysis. Ann Intern Med 2018;169(2):106–15.
33. Tashkin DP, Simmons M, Tseng C-H. Impact of changes in regular use of marijuana and/or tobacco on chronic bronchitis. COPD 2012;9:367–74.
34. Macleod J, Robertson R, Copeland L, McKenzie J, Elton R, Cannabis Reid P. tobacco smoking, and lung function: a cross-sectional observational study in a general practice population. Br J Gen Pract 2015;65:e89–95.
35. Hancox RJ, Shin HH, Gray AR, Poulton R, Sears MR. Effects of quitting cannabis on respiratory symptoms. Eur Respir J 2015;46:80–7.
36. Fligiel SEG, Roth MD, Kleerup EC, Barsky SH, Simmons MS, Tashkin DP. Tracheobronchial histopathology in habitual smokers of cocaine, marijuana, and/or tobacco. Chest 1997;112:319–26.
37. Roth MD, Arora A, Barsky SH, Kleerup EC, Simmons M, Tashkin DP. Airway inflammation in young marijuana and tobacco smokers. Am J Respir Crit Care Med 1998;157:928–37.
38. Barsky SH, Roth MD, Kleerup EC, Simmons M, Tashkin DP. Histopathologic and molecular alterations in bronchial epithelium in habitual smokers of marijuana, cocaine and/or tobacco. J Natl Cancer Inst 1998;90:1198–205.
39. Maertens RM, White PA, Williams A, Yauk CL. A global toxicogenomic analysis investigating the mechanistic differences between tobacco and marijuana smoke condensates in vitro. Toxicology 2013;308:60–73.
40. Berthiller J, Straif K, Boniol M, et al. Cannabis smoking and risk of lung cancer in men: a pooled analysis of three studies in Maghreb. J Thorac Oncol 2008;3: 1398–403.
41. Callaghan RC, Allebeck P, Sdorchuk A. Marijuana use and risk of lung cancer: a 40-year cohort study. Cancer Causes Control 2013;24:1811–20.

42. Zhang LR, Morgenstern H, Greenland S, et al. Cannabis and Respiratory Disease Research Group of New Zealand. Cannabis smoking and lung cancer risk: pooled analysis in the International Lung Cancer Consortium. Int J Cancer 2015;136(4):894–903.
43. Hashibe M, Morgenstern H, Cui Y, et al. Marijuana use and the risk of lung and upper aerodigestive tract cancers: results of a population-based case-control study. Cancer Epidemiol Biomarkers Prev 2006;15(10):1829–34.
44. Ghasemiesfe M, Barrow B, Leonard S, et al. Association Between Marijuana Use and Risk of Cancer: A Systematic Review and Meta-analysis. JAMA Netw Open 2019;2(11):e1916318.
45. Beshay M, Kaiser H, Niedhart D, et al. Emphysema and secondary pneumothorax in young adults smoking marijuana. Eur J Cardiothorac Surg 2007;32(6): 834–8.
46. Lee MH, Hancox RJ. Effects of smoking cannabis on lung function. Expert Rev Respir Med 2011;5:537–46.
47. Wu TC, Tashkin DP, Djahed B, et al. Pulmonary hazards of smoking marijuana as compared with tobacco. N Engl J Med 1988;318(6):347–51.
48. Fligiel SE, Beals TF, Tashkin DP, et al. Marijuana exposure and pulmonary alterations in primates. Pharmacol Biochem Behav 1991;40:637–42.
49. Scheel AH, Krause D, Haars H, Schmitz I, Junker K. Talcum induced pneumoconiosis following inhalation of adulterated marijuana, a case report. Diagn Pathol 2012;7:1746–96.
50. Bowles DW, O'Bryant CL, Camidge DR, Jimeno A. The intersection between cannabis and cancer in the United States. Crit Rev Oncol Hematol 2012;83:1–10.
51. FDA Approves First Drug Comprised of an Active Ingredient Derived from Marijuana to Treat Rare, Severe Forms of Epilepsy. Available at: https://www.fda.gov/news-events/press-announcements/fda-approves-first-drug-comprised-active-ingredient-derived-marijuana-treat-rare-severe-forms. Accessed April 20, 2022.
52. Joshi M, Bartter T, Joshi A. The Role of Science in the Opioid Crisis. N Engl J Med 2017;377(18):1797.
53. The Health Effects of Cannabis and Cannabinoids. The Current State of Evidence and Recommendations for Research. Available at: https://www.ncbi.nlm.nih.gov/books/NBK425741. Accessed April 20, 2022.
54. Volkow ND, Baler RD, Compton WM, Weiss SRB. Adverse health effects of marijuana use. N Engl J Med 2014;370:2219–27.
55. Hall W, Degenhardt L. Adverse health effects of non-medical cannabis use. Lancet 2009;374:1383–91.
56. Blows S, Ivers RQ, Connor J, Ameratunga S, Woodward M, Norton R. Marijuana use and car crash injury. Addiction 2005;100:605–11.
57. Asbridge M, Hayden JA, Cartwright JL. Acute cannabis consumption and motor vehicle collision risk: systematic review of observational studies and meta-analysis. BMJ 2012;344:e536.

The Survival of the Surviving Sepsis Campaign

Rory Spiegel, MD[a,b,*], Max Hockstein, MD[a,b], Jessica Waters, MD[a],
Munish Goyal, MD[a]

KEYWORDS

- Sepsis • Treatment bundles • Surviving sepsis campaign

KEY POINTS

- Care of the patient with sepsis should be individualized to the patient's needs and guided by the treating clinician.
- Volume resuscitation in patients with sepsis should be undertaken with caution.
- Lactic acid provides minimal insight into resuscitation progress.

INTRODUCTION

Even well-intentioned policies have great potential to cause harm. This statement is vividly illustrated by the influential, yet controversial, Surviving Sepsis Campaign (SSC) guidelines and subsequent CMS benchmarks. Despite low-quality evidence, tendentious industry ties, and rebuke from the Infectious Disease Society of America (IDSA), these benchmarks continue to eschew therapy driven by clinician expertise and individual patient needs in favor of mandating an arbitrary, one-size-fits-all approach that suspends clinical judgment and promotes indiscriminate use of treatments that have the potential to cause great harm.[1]

HISTORICAL PERSPECTIVE OF THE SURVIVING SEPSIS CAMPAIGN

The creation of current SSC guidelines and treatment bundles has been surrounded by controversy regarding both industry influence and the validity of their now-mandated recommendations. The campaign published its first guidelines in 2004 in *Critical Care Medicine*.[2] The original sepsis guidelines were underpinned by the principles of Early Goal-Directed Therapy (EGDT). EDGT was supported by a then-landmark, though subsequently nonreproducible, study by Rivers and colleagues, a small, single-center study that found mortality benefit in patients who received a

---

[a] Department of Emergency Medicine, Medstar Washington Hospital Center, 110 Irving St, Washington, DC 20010, USA; [b] Department of Critical Care Medicine, Medstar Washington Hospital Center, Washington, DC 20010, USA
* Corresponding author. Department of Emergency Medicine, Medstar Washington Hospital Center, Washington, DC 20010.
E-mail address: rory.j.spiegel@medstar.net

Med Clin N Am 106 (2022) 1109–1117
https://doi.org/10.1016/j.mcna.2022.08.006
0025-7125/22/© 2022 Elsevier Inc. All rights reserved.

medical.theclinics.com

protocol of therapies targeting measured goals for central venous pressure (CVP), mean arterial pressure, and ScvO$_2$.[3–6]

Beyond its shaky evidential foundation, controversy regarding industry funding influencing committee recommendations plagued the SSC from its inception. The SSC guidelines were initially developed by Eli Lilly as part of a commercial marketing strategy for its product, Xigris (recombinant human activated protein C).[7] Although the touted benefits of Xigris were later disproved and subsequently removed from the SCC's recommendations, early ties to pharmaceutical companies continue to tarnish the guidelines' legitimacy.[8]

The first SSC care bundles were released as guidelines for clinicians in 2005 and have been repeatedly updated when evidence supporting individual interventions were refuted.[5,8,9] The Severe Sepsis and Septic Shock Performance Measure Bundle, known as SEP-1, is a performance measure (PM) initially developed by a number of SCCM members, modeled closely after the SSC guidelines and was similarly muddied by industry ties.[10] In 2008, Henry Ford Hospital initially submitted its PM to the National Quality Forum (NQF), which evaluates performance metrics for CMS. It was not endorsed in its entirety until 2012, when it was approved despite both Henry Ford Hospital and one of the PM investigators holding the patent to a CVP and ScvO$_2$ catheter that would allow for implementation of a measure requiring CVP and ScvO$_2$-guided hemodynamic support, an intervention later found to have no benefit over usual care and that was subsequently dropped.[4,10,11]

After endorsement by the NQF, SEP-1 was formally adopted by CMS in 2015, tying hospital reimbursement to implementation of 3-hour and 6-hour target bundles. By 2017, this required reporting of up to 7 unproven hemodynamic interventions and potential completion of up to 141 tasks within 3 hours for one patient.[12] An examination of the evidence supporting the hemodynamic interventions mandated by SEP-1 found that the CMS guidelines relied on low-quality studies without proven mortality benefit.[11] In 2018, the SCC updated their recommendations, dissolving the 3- and 6-hour bundles that many hospitals have struggled to implement in favor of a 1-hour bundle.[13,14] The evolution of the SCC bundles can be seen in **Table 1**.

THE SURVIVING SEPSIS CAMPAIGN: A PROBLEMATIC PROTOCOL

The first unproven assumption is whether treatment bundles similar to those promoted by the SSC are beneficial. It is important to note that protocolized care has never been definitively demonstrated to be superior to individualized treatment guided by the bedside clinician. Arguments for the use of protocolized care have their roots in early goal-directed therapy, citing its overwhelming superiority compared with standard care. But the benefits seen in this small, single-center study were not replicated in any of the 3 subsequent large, high-quality, multicenter randomized controlled trials (RCTs). All of those studies demonstrated no benefit to protocolized hemodynamic resuscitation when compared with the unstructured judgment of the treating physician.[3–6]

Second, the SCC guidelines and similar bundles assume that earlier treatment is universally better. Support of such beliefs can be attributed to a number of datasets reporting a temporal benefit associated with earlier completion of the sepsis bundle.[15–19] The common finding of these studies is a statistically significant increase in mortality for every hour delay. Unfortunately, due to the methodological shortcomings and concomitant bias inherent to these studies, we are incapable of reaching the conclusion that early care is universally better care. To illustrate these flaws, the authors examine the largest and most well-done study used to support bundled care,

Table 1
The historical evolution of the Surviving Sepsis Campaign treatment bundles

2004[2] 2008[34]	2012[35]	2018[14]
6 hours	**3 hours**	**1 hour**
• CVP 8–12 mm Hg • MAP 65 mm Hg • UO 0.5 mL/kg1/h • ScvO2 ≥ 70% If aforementioned goals are not achieved, transfuse packed red blood cells to achieve a hematocrit of 30% and/or administer a dobutamine infusion to achieve this goal.	• Measure lactate level • Obtain blood cultures before administration of antibiotics • Administer broad spectrum antibiotics • Administer 30 mL/kg crystalloid for hypotension or lactate ≥ 4 mmol/L *2018*: apply vasopressors if patient is hypotensive during or after fluid resuscitation to MAP ≥ 65 mm Hg	

24 hours
• Low-dose steroids
• Human activated protein C
• Glucose 70–150 mg/dL
• Median plateau pressure < 30 cm H₂O
	6 hours
	• Vasopressors (for hypotension that does not respond to initial fluid resuscitation) to maintain MAP ≥ 65 mm Hg
	• In the event of persistent arterial hypotension despite volume resuscitation or initial lactate ≥ 4 mmol/L:
	  ○ Measure CVP
	  ○ Measure ScvO2
	  ○ Remeasure lactate if initial lactate was elevated	

Time to Treatment and Mortality during Mandated Emergency Care for Sepsis, published in the NEJM in 2017 by Seymour and colleagues.[17]

The investigators performed a retrospective analysis of 185 hospitals involved in the New York State Department of Health sepsis registry database. Patients were included in this analysis if they were treated according to a prespecified 3-hour treatment bundle within 6 hours of presentation to the Emergency Department. Although the bundles varied from hospital to hospital, all participating centers were required to obtain blood cultures before administering antibiotics, measure serum lactate level, and administer broad-spectrum antibiotics. The investigators included patients older than 17 years who had either severe sepsis or septic shock as defined by the 2001 International Sepsis Definitions.[20]

Seymour and colleagues examined 49,331 patients seen at 149 Emergency Departments from April 2014 to June 2016. The median time to complete the 3-hour bundle was 1.30 hours, to administer broad-spectrum antibiotics was 0.95 hours, and to complete the initial fluid bolus (30 mL/kg) was 2.56 hours. Using an internally derived and validated risk model using 10% of the cohort, the investigators performed a multivariable regression on the remaining 90% of the cohort and determined that each hour required to complete the 3-hour bundle was associated with a statistically significant increase in mortality (odds ratio of 1.04/h; 95% confidence interval [CI], 1.02–1.05; P < 0.001). This same association was seen with the time to administration of broad-spectrum antibiotics (odds ratio 1.04/h; 95% CI, 1.03–1.06; P < 0.001), time to completion of blood cultures (odds ratio 1.04/h; 95% CI, 1.02–1.06; P < 0.001), and time to obtaining serum lactate (odds ratio 1.04/h; 95% CI, 1.02–1.06; P < 0.001), the latter two presumably serving as surrogates for the prior. Notably, this association was not demonstrated when the time to completion of fluid bolus was examined in isolation (odds ratio for mortality 1.01/h; 95% CI, 0.99–1.02; P = 0.21).

Despite rigorous design, such retrospective analyses have inherent methodological issues, limiting the conclusions one can draw from such data. All of these studies including the one highlighted earlier by Seymour and colleagues are observational cohorts that separate patients by time to intervention. As patients were not randomized to receive treatment at a certain time threshold, causative statements cannot be made. Hershey and colleagues[21] illustrate a progressive decrease in sepsis-related mortality, describing that sepsis-related mortality has been falling over time nationwide, with or without mandatory bundled care.

Further, even if one is to disregard their methodology, the effect sizes reported in these trials are minimal and driven by those patients with septic shock. The analysis by Seymour and colleagues[17] published in the NEJM reports a 1.04 (95% CI, 1.03–1.06) increase in the odds of death for every hour delay to completion of the 3-hour sepsis bundle. Essentially, for every 148 patients in whom the completion of the sepsis bundle is delayed by 1 hour, one additional person will die. These temporal benefits for early treatment were only present in the sickest subset of patients, suggesting that when applied to a general ED population, any benefit that may exist in this selected cohort will be diluted out.

In fact, the only prospective RCT evaluating early antibiotic administration in an undifferentiated cohort of patients with suspected infection found no benefit. The PHANTASi trial, published by Alam and colleagues[22] in the Lancet, examined the effects of prehospital antibiotics in a cohort of patients with suspected infection. The investigators randomized patients with a diagnosed or suspected infection, to either usual care (typically intravenous (IV) fluid resuscitation and supplemental O_2) or traditional care plus open-label IV ceftriaxone.

Between June 2014 and June 2016, the investigators enrolled 2698 patients, of whom 1548 were assigned to the intervention and 1150 to the usual care group. The prehospital administration of antibiotics reduced the time to antibiotic administration by 96 minutes. Despite this temporal benefit, the investigators reported no difference in their primary outcome, 28-day mortality, between the prehospital antibiotic group and standard care (8% in both groups). Nor did they observe a difference in 90-day mortality (12% in both groups), the rate of intensive care unit (ICU) admissions (10% vs 9%), and hospital or ICU length of stay. Notably, less than 4% of study participants had septic shock limiting extrapolation of this finding to the sickest subset of septic patients.

A third flawed assumption is that all components of the bundle are equally efficacious and Should be applied with uniform zeal. Although early appropriate antibiotic administration is paramount to the management of septic shock, the remainder of the current bundle has very little evidence supporting its use. When Seymour and colleagues examined the individual components of the sepsis bundle, they noted that time to antibiotic administration showed similar temporal benefits to completion of the entire sepsis bundle, whereas the time to fluid bolus administration did not. Andrews and colleagues further question the benefit of early protocolized care in their

RCT of a 6-hour hemodynamic resuscitation protocol versus usual, clinician-directed care performed in a resource-limited setting in adults with sepsis and hypotension. Although participants randomized to protocolized care received more fluid and were more likely to receive vasopressors in the first 6 hours of their care, in-hospital mortality was 15% higher than those randomized to usual care.[23] The investigators observed that the rates of resolution of shock were equal between groups. In contrast, signs of harm from fluid overload were far more prevalent in the protocolized care group; this calls into question the hemodynamic utility of a fluid bolus and whether timely source control is enough.

The use of serum lactate to guide ongoing resuscitation as recommended by the SSC is not only not supported by evidence, given our current understanding of the cause of hyperlactatemia in sepsis, but also it is nonsensical. Since William Huckabee's publications in 1958, lactate has been an understood byproduct of anaerobic metabolism.[24] For patients in states of hypoperfusion, delivery of oxygen to tissues decreases, lowering its availability to act as the final electron acceptor in oxidative phosphorylation. As such, cellular metabolism shifts to anaerobic from aerobic metabolism resulting in type A lactic acidosis. The logical pathway that follows is that elevated serum lactate levels in sepsis are due to shock, leading to end-organ hypoperfusion. IV fluid administration will increase venous return and cardiac output, thus improving end-organ perfusion and subsequently clearing elevated lactate levels. Unfortunately, this physiological rationale falls apart at every step when examined closely.

First, the mechanisms for elevated lactate values in sepsis are multifactorial. They are primarily driven by circulating endogenous catecholamines and metabolic disturbances caused by sepsis-induced inflammatory mediators.[25] As end-organ hypoperfusion is not the principal driver of lactate values in sepsis, the assumption that using lactate as a therapeutic end point of fluid-resuscitation is misguided. Second, an elevated lactate value neither defines shock type nor guides its management if shock is present. Serum lactate levels can be elevated in all forms of shock, which have varied responses to IV fluid administration. Third, even in patients with shock due to sepsis, serum lactate levels do not differentiate patients who will augment their cardiac output from patients who will not. Finally, among patients who improve their cardiac output following IV fluid administration, these improvements are often transient, a return to baseline levels shortly following the fluid administration.

These flaws in a lactate-guided resuscitation strategy were illustrated by the findings of the ANDROMEDA-SHOCK investigation.[26] The investigators found that patients randomized to the lactate-driven protocol did notably worse than their counterparts randomized to a protocol driven by capillary refill. Lactate reduction at fixed time points (eg, 6 h) is associated with improved mortality; however, a number of confounders, for example, the initiation of concomitant vasoactive infusions, prevent what may seem to be a straightforward interpretation.[27] As such, although lactate should be viewed as a prognostic marker of ongoing resuscitative efforts, it should be detached from the ongoing decisions of IV fluid administration.

Finally, most of the studies examining the temporal benefit of various treatments in sepsis approach this question from a very finite vantage. By examining only the patients retrospectively determined to have sepsis, investigators excluded patients without sepsis who are exposed to all the risks associated with broad spectrum antibiotics, large volume fluid resuscitation, and having blood cultures obtained without any potential for benefit. As such, the harm they are exposed to from overtreatment is purged from the subsequent analysis and unquantifiable. It is these unintended and unmeasured consequences that are most concerning. Each of us has been witness to the victims of overzealous sepsis care: in a patient presenting with suspected pneumonia only after the CMS-mandated 30 mL/kg fluid challenge does it become apparent their symptoms were not infectious but due to underlying cardiac infirmity. How many patients receive broad-spectrum antibiotics and large volume fluid resuscitation needlessly? And what about blood cultures? How many patients experience the pain from multiple needle sticks let alone the added expense, antimicrobial exposure, and hospital length of stay associated with false positives? How many patients do we screen in order to identify the few that may benefit from aggressive care?

No one would argue against an aggressive and timely resuscitation in the face of a patient presenting with septic shock, but this is not the mandate the SSC guideline promotes. Achieving the 3-hour treatment bundle is challenging enough for most hospitals; most centers increase sepsis-bundle compliance not by improving the quality of care but by entering anyone with even the smallest sign of physiological derangement into the sepsis pathway.[28,29] Compressing the time required to complete these quality measures will only heighten these "beat the clock strategies." Filbin and colleagues[30] report that despite implementation of a robust sepsis screening and treatment protocol, 71% of the patients were unable to reach the 1-hour treatment mandate outlined by the 2018 SSC. This resource-heavy protocolized metric of care is based on an overreaching interpretation of evidence, which when reviewed in totality, suggests the futility of such bluntly applied endeavors.

WHAT LIES BEYOND THE SURVIVING SEPSIS CAMPAIGN TREATMENT BUNDLES?

Although the SSC experienced wide-spread support for many years, recently there has been a growing dissent due to the guidelines' lack of high-quality evidence supporting most of their claims and the logistical burdens these guidelines have placed on health care systems. The Infectious Disease Society of America (IDSA) and the American College of Emergency Physicians (ACEP) have published their own position articles on the management of patients with sepsis and septic shock.

Compared with the SSC, these guidelines limit their recommendations to what is supported by the current evidence. For example, the SSC continues to recommend an empiric 30 mL/kg initial fluid bolus and to guide ongoing resuscitative efforts using serum lactate levels. The ACEP clinical policy does not endorse an empirical fluid bolus but rather recommends individualized fluid resuscitation needs for each patient. Nor do they recommend the use of serum lactate levels to guide ongoing IV fluid resuscitation, as it has not been found to be an accurate marker of ongoing fluid needs. The SSC continues to recommend the SIRS criteria as a tool to screen patients with sepsis and septic shock despite evidence demonstrating its poor diagnostic accuracy. In the IDSA's position article, the investigators recommend against using the SIRS criteria due to its poor specificity, recommending instead using the simple criteria of suspected infection and signs of shock.

In the end, guidance documents published on the management of sepsis and septic shock should discuss how best to identify patients who will truly benefit from timely aggressive care and what interventions are supported by the current evidence. Policy makers need to understand the interplay between sensitivity and specificity when recommending a screening tool. We will never be able to identify every patient who goes on to develop sepsis at time zero, without broadening our catchment population so large as to render the screening tool functionally useless. Rather, when selecting a tool to aid clinicians in identifying patients with sepsis, it should focus on identifying the subset of patients who truly do benefit from timely care.

Moreover, future policies should embrace the concept that sepsis is not a monolith. Rather it is a syndrome that originates from a multitude of sources, and the physiological derangements observed in any one patient are a result of the interplay of the host's specific physiology, environmental factors, and infectious source. It is naive to think such complexities can be addressed by blunt tools such as treatment bundles. Policy makers should encourage early evaluation by a clinician experienced in the management of sepsis and treatment individualized to each specific patient's underlying physiologic perturbations. Most importantly, they should avoid policies mandating care bundles that do not have compelling evidence to support their implementation. They must consider the inevitable burdens and opportunity costs mandates create on clinicians and hospital systems alike.

SUMMARY

Although well intentioned, the Surviving Sepsis guidelines in all their iterations have laid a heavy weight on already overstressed health care systems,[31] all without any evidence of benefit, nor knowledge of the logistical consequences such recommendations will cost.[32,33] Consider the consequences of blindly adhering to these broad-reaching, resource-laden protocols, not only for the patients with sepsis, but for those without, needlessly exposed to these aggressive treatment bundles. Consider the consequences for the hospitals charged with the task of differentiating the sick from the well and applying radial traction to their already scarce resources. If we fail to do so, there may come a time in the not-so-distant future when we look back upon our marginal gains in sepsis care, only to discover we have quite literally drowned an entire populace in our endeavors.

CLINICS CARE POINTS

- In the care of patients with sepsis, protocolized care has never been definitively demonstrated to be superior to individualized treatment guided by the bedside clinician.

- Although it is assumed, earlier treatment is universally better in the care of patients with sepsis; this too is not supported by the evidence.

- Because end-organ hypoperfusion is not the principal driver of lactate values in sepsis, the assumption that using lactate as a therapeutic end point of fluid-resuscitation is misguided.

DISCLOSURE

The authors have nothing to disclose.

REFERENCES

1. IDSA Sepsis Task Force. Infectious diseases society of america (IDSA) POSITION STATEMENT: why IDSA did not endorse the surviving sepsis campaign guidelines. Clin Infect Dis 2018;66(10):1631–5.
2. Dellinger RP, Carlet JM, Masur H, et al. Surviving Sepsis Campaign Management Guidelines Committee. Surviving Sepsis Campaign guidelines for management of severe sepsis and septic shock. Crit Care Med 2004;32(3):858–73.
3. Rivers E, Nguyen B, Havstad S, et al, Early Goal-Directed Therapy Collaborative Group. Early goal-directed therapy in the treatment of severe sepsis and septic shock. N Engl J Med 2001;345(19):1368–77.

4. ProCESS Investigators, Yealy DM, Kellum JA, et al. A randomized trial of protocol-based care for early septic shock. N Engl J Med 2014;370(18):1683–93.
5. ARISE Investigators, ANZICS Clinical Trials Group, Peake SL, Delaney A, Bailey M, et al. Goal-directed resuscitation for patients with early septic shock. N Engl J Med 2014;371(16):1496–506.
6. Mouncey PR, Osborn TM, Power GS, et al. ProMISe Trial Investigators. Trial of early, goal-directed resuscitation for septic shock. N Engl J Med 2015;372(14): 1301–11.
7. Eichacker PQ, Natanson C, Danner RL. Surviving sepsis–practice guidelines, marketing campaigns, and Eli Lilly. N Engl J Med 2006;355(16):1640–2.
8. Ranieri VM, Thompson BT, Barie PS, et al, PROWESS-SHOCK Study Group. Drotrecogin alfa (activated) in adults with septic shock. N Engl J Med 2012;366(22): 2055–64.
9. Sprung CL, Annane D, Keh D, et al, CORTICUS Study Group. Hydrocortisone therapy for patients with septic shock. N Engl J Med 2008;358(2):111–24.
10. Jaswal DS, Natanson C, Eichacker PQ. Endorsing performance measures is a matter of trust. BMJ 2018;360:k703.
11. Wang J, Strich JR, Applefeld WN, et al. Driving blind: instituting SEP-1 without high quality outcomes data. J Thorac Dis 2020;12(Suppl 1):S22–36.
12. Pepper DJ, Jaswal D, Sun J, et al. Evidence underpinning the centers for medicare & medicaid services' severe sepsis and septic shock management bundle (SEP-1): a systematic review. Ann Intern Med 2018;168(8):558–68.
13. Baghdadi JD, Wong MD, Uslan DZ, et al. Adherence to the SEP-1 Sepsis Bundle in Hospital-Onset v. Community-Onset Sepsis: a Multicenter Retrospective Cohort Study. J Gen Intern Med 2020;35(4):1153–60.
14. Levy MM, Evans LE, Rhodes A. The Surviving Sepsis Campaign Bundle: 2018 update. Intensive Care Med 2018;44(6):925–8.
15. Damiani E, Donati A, Serafini G, et al. Effect of performance improvement programs on compliance with sepsis bundles and mortality: a systematic review and meta-analysis of observational studies. PLoS One 2015;10(5):e0125827.
16. Rhodes A, Phillips G, Beale R, et al. The Surviving Sepsis Campaign bundles and outcome: results from the International Multicentre Prevalence Study on Sepsis (the IMPreSS study). Intensive Care Med 2015;41(9):1620–8.
17. Seymour CW, Gesten F, Prescott HC, et al. Time to Treatment and Mortality during Mandated Emergency Care for Sepsis. N Engl J Med 2017;376(23):2235–44.
18. Liu VX, Morehouse JW, Marelich GP, et al. Multicenter Implementation of a Treatment Bundle for Patients with Sepsis and Intermediate Lactate Values. Am J Respir Crit Care Med 2016;193(11):1264–70.
19. Leisman DE, Doerfler ME, Ward MF, et al. From Compliance With a Simplified 3-Hour Sepsis Bundle in a Series of Prospective, Multisite, Observational Cohorts. Crit Care Med 2017;45(3):395–406.
20. Levy MM, Fink MP, Marshall JC, et al. SCCM/ESICM/ACCP/ATS/SIS. 2001 SCCM/ESICM/ACCP/ATS/SIS International Sepsis Definitions Conference. Crit Care Med 2003;31(4):1250–6.
21. Hershey TB, Kahn JM. State sepsis mandates - a new era for regulation of hospital quality. N Engl J Med 2017;376(24):2311–3.
22. Alam N, Oskam E, Stassen PM, et al. PHANTASi Trial Investigators and the ORCA (Onderzoeks Consortium Acute Geneeskunde) Research Consortium the Netherlands. Prehospital antibiotics in the ambulance for sepsis: a multicentre, open label, randomised trial. Lancet Respir Med 2018;6(1):40–50.

23. Andrews B, Semler MW, Muchemwa L, et al. Effect of an early resuscitation protocol on in-hospital mortality among adults with sepsis and hypotension: a randomized clinical trial. JAMA 2017;318(13):1233–40.
24. Huckabee WE. Relationships of pyruvate and lactate during anaerobic metabolism. I. Effects of infusion of pyruvate or glucose and of hyperventilation. J Clin Invest 1958;37(2):244–54.
25. Vincent JL, Bakker J. Blood lactate levels in sepsis: in 8 questions. Curr Opin Crit Care 2021;27(3):298–302.
26. Hernández G, Ospina-Tascón GA, Damiani LP, et al, The ANDROMEDA SHOCK Investigators and the Latin America Intensive Care Network (LIVEN). Effect of a resuscitation strategy targeting peripheral perfusion status vs serum lactate levels on 28-day mortality among patients with septic shock: the ANDROMEDA-SHOCK randomized clinical trial. JAMA 2019;321(7):654–64.
27. Ryoo SM, Lee J, Lee YS, et al. Lactate level versus lactate clearance for predicting mortality in patients with septic shock defined by sepsis-3. Crit Care Med 2018;46(6):e489–95.
28. Venkatesh AK, Slesinger T, Whittle J, et al. Preliminary performance on the new CMS sepsis-1 national quality measure: early insights from the emergency quality network (E-QUAL). Ann Emerg Med 2018;71(1):10–5.e1.
29. Deis AS, Whiles BB, Brown AR, et al. Three-Hour Bundle Compliance and Outcomes in Patients With Undiagnosed Severe Sepsis. Chest 2018;153(1):39–45.
30. Filbin MR, Thorsen JE, Zachary TM, et al. Antibiotic delays and feasibility of a 1-hour-from-triage antibiotic requirement: analysis of an emergency department sepsis quality improvement database. Ann Emerg Med 2020;75(1):93–9.
31. Matthias T, Ranasinghe T, Mallawaarachchi C, et al. A study on adherence to surviving sepsis campaign bundle at a tertiary care hospital in Sri Lanka. Int J Infect Dis 2020;101:217.
32. Ko BS, Choi SH, Shin TG, et al. Impact of 1-hour bundle achievement in septic shock. J Clin Med Res 2021;10(3). https://doi.org/10.3390/jcm10030527.
33. Kalantari A, Rezaie SR. Challenging the one-hour sepsis bundle. West J Emerg Med 2019;20(2):185–90.
34. Dellinger RP, Levy MM, Carlet JM, et al. Surviving Sepsis Campaign: international guidelines for management of severe sepsis and septic shock: 2008. Intensive Care Med 2008;34(1):17–60.
35. Dellinger RP, Levy MM, Rhodes A, et al. Surviving Sepsis Campaign Guidelines Committee including the Pediatric Subgroup. Surviving sepsis campaign: international guidelines for management of severe sepsis and septic shock: 2012. Crit Care Med 2013;41(2):580–637.

UNITED STATES POSTAL SERVICE®

Statement of Ownership, Management, and Circulation
(All Periodicals Publications Except Requester Publications)

1. Publication Title	2. Publication Number	3. Filing Date
MEDICAL CLINICS IN NORTH AMERICA	337 – 340	9/18/2022

4. Issue Frequency	5. Number of Issues Published Annually	6. Annual Subscription Price
JAN, MAR, MAY, JUL, SEP, NOV	6	$316.00

7. Complete Mailing Address of Known Office of Publication (Not printer) (Street, city, county, state, and ZIP+4®)

ELSEVIER INC.
230 Park Avenue, Suite 800
New York, NY 10169

Contact Person
Malathi Samayan
Telephone (Include area code)
+44 42994507

8. Complete Mailing Address of Headquarters or General Business Office of Publisher (Not printer)

ELSEVIER INC.
230 Park Avenue, Suite 800
New York, NY 10169

9. Full Names and Complete Mailing Addresses of Publisher, Editor, and Managing Editor (Do not leave blank)

Publisher (Name and complete mailing address)

DOLORES MELONI, ELSEVIER INC.
1600 JOHN F KENNEDY BLVD. SUITE 1800
PHILADELPHIA, PA 19103-2899

Editor (Name and complete mailing address)

TAYLOR HAYES, ELSEVIER INC.
1600 JOHN F KENNEDY BLVD. SUITE 1800
PHILADELPHIA, PA 19103-2899

Managing Editor (Name and complete mailing address)

PATRICK MANLEY, ELSEVIER INC.
1600 JOHN F KENNEDY BLVD. SUITE 1800
PHILADELPHIA, PA 19103-2899

10. Owner (Do not leave blank. If the publication is owned by a corporation, give the name and address of the corporation immediately followed by the names and addresses of all stockholders owning or holding 1 percent or more of the total amount of stock. If not owned by a corporation, give the names and addresses of the individual owners. If owned by a partnership or other unincorporated firm, give its name and address as well as those of each individual owner. If the publication is published by a nonprofit organization, give its name and address.)

Full Name	Complete Mailing Address
WHOLLY OWNED SUBSIDIARY OF REED/ELSEVIER, US HOLDINGS	1600 JOHN F KENNEDY BLVD. SUITE 1800 PHILADELPHIA, PA 19103-2899

11. Known Bondholders, Mortgagees, and Other Security Holders Owning or Holding 1 Percent or More of Total Amount of Bonds, Mortgages, or Other Securities. If none, check box ▶ ☐ None

Full Name	Complete Mailing Address
N/A	

12. Tax Status (For completion by nonprofit organizations authorized to mail at nonprofit rates) (Check one)
The purpose, function, and nonprofit status of this organization and the exempt status for federal income tax purposes:
☒ Has Not Changed During Preceding 12 Months
☐ Has Changed During Preceding 12 Months (Publisher must submit explanation of change with this statement)

PS Form 3526, July 2014 [Page 1 of 4 (see instructions page 4)] PSN: 7530-01-000-9931 PRIVACY NOTICE: See our privacy policy on www.usps.com.

---

13. Publication Title	14. Issue Date for Circulation Data Below
MEDICAL CLINICS IN NORTH AMERICA	JULY 2022

15. Extent and Nature of Circulation		Average No. Copies Each Issue During Preceding 12 Months	No. Copies of Single Issue Published Nearest to Filing Date
a. Total Number of Copies (Net press run)		452	392
b. Paid Circulation (By Mail and Outside the Mail)	(1) Mailed Outside-County Paid Subscriptions Stated on PS Form 3541 (Include paid distribution above nominal rate, advertiser's proof copies, and exchange copies)	265	234
	(2) Mailed In-County Paid Subscriptions Stated on PS Form 3541 (Include paid distribution above nominal rate, advertiser's proof copies, and exchange copies)	0	0
	(3) Paid Distribution Outside the Mails Including Sales Through Dealers and Carriers, Street Vendors, Counter Sales, and Other Paid Distribution Outside USPS®	129	116
	(4) Paid Distribution by Other Classes of Mail Through the USPS (e.g. First-Class Mail®)	0	0
c. Total Paid Distribution (Sum of 15b (1), (2), (3), and (4))	▶	394	350
d. Free or Nominal Rate Distribution (By Mail and Outside the Mail)	(1) Free or Nominal Rate Outside-County Copies Included on PS Form 3541	39	27
	(2) Free or Nominal Rate In-County Copies Included on PS Form 3541	0	0
	(3) Free or Nominal Rate Copies Mailed at Other Classes Through the USPS (e.g. First-Class Mail)	0	0
	(4) Free or Nominal Rate Distribution Outside the Mail (Carriers or other means)	0	0
e. Total Free or Nominal Rate Distribution (Sum of 15d (1), (2), (3) and (4))	▶	39	27
f. Total Distribution (Sum of 15c and 15e)	▶	433	377
g. Copies not Distributed (See Instructions to Publishers #4 (page 83))	▶	19	15
h. Total (Sum of 15f and g)	▶	452	392
i. Percent Paid (15c divided by 15f times 100)	▶	90.99%	92.83%

* If you are claiming electronic copies, go to line 16 on page 3. If you are not claiming electronic copies, skip to line 17 on page 3.

PS Form 3526, July 2014 (Page 2 of 4)

16. Electronic Copy Circulation		Average No. Copies Each Issue During Preceding 12 Months	No. Copies of Single Issue Published Nearest to Filing Date
a. Paid Electronic Copies	▶		
b. Total Paid Print Copies (Line 15c) + Paid Electronic Copies (Line 16a)	▶		
c. Total Print Distribution (Line 15f) + Paid Electronic Copies (Line 16a)	▶		
d. Percent Paid (Both Print & Electronic Copies) (16b divided by 16c × 100)	▶		

☒ I certify that 50% of all my distributed copies (electronic and print) are paid above a nominal price.

17. Publication of Statement of Ownership

☒ If the publication is a general publication, publication of this statement is required. Will be printed in the NOVEMBER 2022 issue of this publication. ☐ Publication not required.

18. Signature and Title of Editor, Publisher, Business Manager, or Owner

Malathi Samayan - Distribution Controller

Malathi Samayan

Date 9/18/2022

I certify that all information furnished on this form is true and complete. I understand that anyone who furnishes false or misleading information on this form or who omits material or information requested on the form may be subject to criminal sanctions (including fines and imprisonment) and/or civil sanctions (including civil penalties).

PS Form 3526, July 2014 (Page 3 of 4) PRIVACY NOTICE: See our privacy policy on www.usps.com

Moving?

Make sure your subscription moves with you!

To notify us of your new address, find your **Clinics Account Number** (located on your mailing label above your name), and contact customer service at:

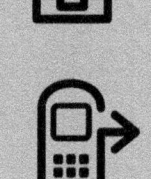

Email: journalscustomerservice-usa@elsevier.com

800-654-2452 (subscribers in the U.S. & Canada)
314-447-8871 (subscribers outside of the U.S. & Canada)

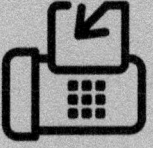

Fax number: 314-447-8029

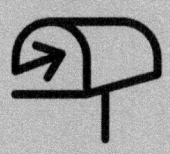

Elsevier Health Sciences Division
Subscription Customer Service
3251 Riverport Lane
Maryland Heights, MO 63043

*To ensure uninterrupted delivery of your subscription, please notify us at least 4 weeks in advance of move.

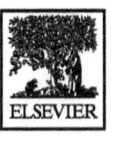

Printed and bound by CPI Group (UK) Ltd, Croydon, CR0 4YY

03/10/2024

01040474-0001